DRUG TARGETING AND DELIVERY
Concepts in Dosage Form Design

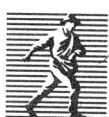

ELLIS HORWOOD SERIES IN PHARMACEUTICAL TECHNOLOGY
incorporating Pharmacological Sciences
Series Editor: Professor Michael H Rubinstein, Professor of Pharmaceutical Technology, Liverpool John Moores University, School of Pharmacy

Author(s)	Title
Armstrong & James	UNDERSTANDING EXPERIMENTAL DESIGN AND INTERPRETATION IN PHARMACEUTICS (Available in Cloth and Paperback)
Bloomfield et al	MICROBIAL QUALITY ASSURANCE IN PHARMACEUTICALS, COSMETICS, TOILETRIES
Broadley	AUTONOMIC PHARMACOLOGY
Cartwright & Matthews	PHARMACEUTICAL PRODUCT LICENSING: Requirements for Europe
Cartwright & Matthews	INTERNATIONAL PHARMACEUTICAL PRODUCT REGISTRATION: Quality, Safety, Efficacy
Clark & Moos	DRUG DISCOVERY TECHNOLOGIES
Cole	PHARMACEUTICAL PRODUCTION FACILITIES: Design and Application
Cole, Hogan, Aulton	PHARMACEUTICAL TABLET COATING TECHNOLOGY
Cook	POTASSIUM CHANNELS: Structure, Classification, Function and Therapeutic Potential
Craig & Newton	DIELECTRIC ANALYSIS OF PHARMACEUTICAL SYSTEMS
D'Arcy & McElnay	PHARMACY AND PHARMACOTHERAPY OF ASTHMA
Denyer & Baird	GUIDE TO MICROBIOLOGICAL CONTROL IN PHARMACEUTICS
Doods & Van Meel	RECEPTOR DATA FOR BIOLOGICAL EXPERIMENTS: A Guide to Drug Selectivity
Evans et al	POTASSIUM CHANNEL MODULATOR DRUGS: From Synthesis to Clinical Experience
Field & Goldthorpe	DRUG RESISTANCE IN VIRUSES: Principles, Mechanisms and Clinical Perspectives
Ford & Timmins	PHARMACEUTICAL THERMAL ANALYSIS: Techniques and Applications
Glasby	DICTIONARY OF ANTIBIOTIC-PRODUCING ORGANISMS
Gould	PHYSICOCHEMICAL PROPERTIES OF DRUGS: A Handbook for Pharmaceutical Scientists
Hardy et al	DRUG DELIVERY TO THE GASTROINTESTINAL TRACT
Harvey	DRUGS FROM NATURAL PRODUCTS: Pharmaceuticals and Agrochemicals
Hider & Barlow	POLYPEPTIDE AND PROTEIN DRUGS: Production, Characterization, Formulation
Ioannides & Lewis	DRUGS, DIET AND DISEASE VOLUME 1 Mechanistic Approaches to Cancer
Izquierdo	NATURALLY OCCURING BENZODIAZEPINES: Structure, Distribution and Function
Junginger	DRUG TARGETING AND DELIVERY: Concepts in Dosage Form Design
Krogsgaard-Larsen & Hansen	EXCITATORY AMINO ACID RECEPTORS: Design of Agonists and Antagonists
Kourounakis & Rekka	STEROIDS, DRUG RESPONSE AND METABOLISM: Pharmacochemical Approach to Defensive Steroids
Labaune	HANDBOOK OF PHARMACOKINETICS: The Toxicity Asssessment of Chemicals
Law	IMMUNOASSAY PROCEDURES: A Practical Guide
Martinez	PEPTIDE HORMONES AS PROHORMONES
Rainsford	ANTI-RHEUMATIC DRUGS: Actions and Side Effects
Ramabhadran	PHARMACEUTICAL DESIGN AND DEVELOPMENT: A Molecular Biological Approach
Ridgway Watt	TABLET MACHINE INSTRUMENTATION IN PHARMACEUTICS: Principles and Practice
Roth et al	PHARMACEUTICAL CHEMISTRY Volume 1 Drug Synthesis
Roth et al	PHARMACEUTICAL CHEMISTRY Volume 2 Drug Analysis
Rubinstein	PHARMACEUTICAL TECHNOLOGY Controlled Drug Release Volume 1
Rubinstein	PHARMACEUTICAL TECHNOLOGY Tableting Technology Volume 1
Rubinstein	PHARMACEUTICAL TECHNOLOGY Drug Stability
Russell & Chopra	UNDERSTANDING ANTIBACTERIAL ACTION AND RESISTANCE (Cloth & Paper)
Rutherford	PHARMACEUTICAL SPECIFICATIONS: Standards for Drugs
Taylor & Kennewell	MODERN MEDICINAL CHEMISTRY (Available in Cloth and Paperback)
Theobald	RADIOPHARMACEUTICALS: Using Radioactive Compounds in Pharmaceutics and Medicine
Thomas & Thurston	CHEMISTRY FOR PHARMACY, PHARMACOLOGY AND THE HEALTH SCIENCES (Available in Cloth and Paperback)
Tweed	CLINICAL TRIALS FOR THE PHARMACEUTICAL INDUSTRY
Van Meel, Hauel, Shelley	CARDIOTONIC AGENTS FOR THE TREATMENT OF HEART FAILURE
Vergnaud	CONTROLLED DRUG RELEASE OF ORAL DOSAGE FORMS
Washington	PARTICLE SIZE ANALYSIS IN PHARMACEUTICS AND OTHER INDUSTRIES
Washington et al	PHARMACOKINETIC MODELLING USING STELLA ON THE APPLE MACINTOSH (TM)
Wells	PHARMACEUTICAL PREFORMULATION
Wells & Rubinstein	PHARMACEUTICAL TECHNOLOGY Controlled Drug Release Volume 2
Wells & Rubinstein	PHARMACEUTICAL TECHNOLOGY Tableting Technology Volume 2
Wells & Rubinstein	PHARMACEUTICAL TECHNOLOGY Tableting Technology Volume 3
Wilson & Washington	PHYSIOLOGICAL PHARMACEUTICS: Biological Barriers to Drug Absorption

The above is a complete list of all Ellis Horwood titles in the pharmaceutical and pharmacological sciences, both published and in preparation. Further details can be obtained from Simon and Schuster International Group 0442 – 881900.

DRUG TARGETING AND DELIVERY
Concepts in Dosage Form Design

Editor:
H.E. JUNGINGER, Ph.D., M.D.
Professor of Pharmaceutical Technology,
Center for Bio-Pharmaceutical Sciences,
Leiden University, The Netherlands

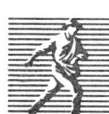

ELLIS HORWOOD
NEW YORK   LONDON   TORONTO   SYDNEY   TOKYO   SINGAPORE

FIRST INDIAN REPRINT, 2010
First published in 1992 by
ELLIS HORWOOD LIMITED
Market Cross House, Cooper Street,
Chichester, West Sussex, PO19 1EB, England

 A division of
Simon & Schuster International Group
A Paramount Communications Company

© Ellis Horwood Limited, 1992

All rights reserved. No part of this publication may be reproduced, stored in a retrieval system, or transmitted, in any form, or by any means, electronic, mechanical, photocopying, recording or otherwise, without the prior permission, in writing, of the publisher

Printed and bound in India by Nutech Photolithographers, New Delhi

British Library Cataloguing in Publication Data
A catalogue record for this book is available from the British Library

ISBN 0–13–220468–1

Library of Congress Cataloging-in-Publication Data
Available from the publishers
FOR SALE IN SOUTH ASIA ONLY

Table of contents

Preface vii

List of contributors ix

PART I PARENTERAL ROUTE

1 Transport of macromolecules across the microvascular endothelium 1
   V. W. M. van Hinsbergh

2 Receptor-dependent uptake of macromolecules by specific hepatic cells ... 13
   Th. J. C. van Berkel

3 Novel immunoliposome targeting system avoiding reticuloendothelial cell
   interactions 26
   A. Mori, Dexi Liu and Leaf Huang

PART II GASTROINTESTINAL AND BUCCAL ROUTES

4 Structure and barrier function of the epithelium of gastrointestinal and
   oral mucosa 45
   C. A. Squier

5 Buccal drug delivery: mucoadhesion requirements and transmucosal
   transport barriers 57
   H. E. Boddé, M. E. de Vries, C.-M. Lehr, J. A. Bouwstra, J. C. Verhoef, M. Ponec,
   W. H. M. Craane-van Hinsberg and H. E. Junginger

6 Colloidal drug delivery systems for gastrointestinal application 71
   J.-P. Devissaguet, H. Fessi, N. Ammoury and G. Barratt

7 Intestinal bioadhesive drug delivery systems 92
   C.-M. Lehr, J. A. Bouwstra, A. G. de Boer, J. C. Verhoef, D. D. Breimer and H. E. Junginger

8 Pellets and multi-unit dosage forms: state of the art 101
   J. G. Fokkens

9 Oral uptake of microparticles across the gastrointestinal mucosa 113
A. T. Florence and P. U. Jani

PART III PULMONAL ROUTE

10 Pulmonary surfactant: basic physiology and its use for replacement therapy 129
B. Lachmann and E. P. Eijking

11 Molecular aspects of lung surfactant proteins and their use as pulmonal carriers 155
K. P. Schäfer

PART IV DERMAL AND TRANSDERMAL ROUTES

12 Skin penetration enhancers 169
J. Hadgraft and K. A. Walters

13 Skin cell cultures: reconstructed skin as a tool in the development of dermatological drugs and formulations 178
P. J. J. Wauben-Penris

14 Trends in transdermal drug delivery systems 190
W. Fischer

15 Interactions between liposomes and human stratum corneum *in vitro* ... 203
J. A. Bouwstra, H. E. J. Hofland, F. Spies, G. S. Gooris and H. E. Junginger

PART V NASAL ROUTE

16 Nasal membranes — structure and permeability 223
W. A. Lee and P. A. Baldwin

17 Present and future trends in pharmaceutical dosage forms for nasal application 237
F. W. H. M. Merkus, W. A. J. J. Hermens, N. G. M. Schipper, S. G. Romeijn and J. C. Verhoef

Index 247

Preface

New discoveries regarding structure and function of biological membranes and other cellular barriers to drug transport promise to yield new, innovative methods for establishing drug delivery and targeting. This may lead to new concepts for drug delivery systems enabling the (targeted) delivery of drugs for which to date no suitable dosage forms are available. An important issue is, however, whether implementation of such new methods will be feasible in the near future, or that they should rather be looked upon as interesting but 'futuristic'.

This book originates from the manuscripts of the invited speakers of a symposium entitled 'Overcoming cellular barriers to drug targeting and delivery', held at the Center for Bio-Pharmaceutical Sciences, Leiden University, in May 1991. The speakers have been asked to address this issue and a special set-up has been chosen: the various routes of drug application (parenteral route, gastrointestinal and buccal routes, pulmonal route, dermal and transdermal route and nasal route) have been treated firstly with respect to their biological characteristics as function, structure, uptake mechanisms, etc. Secondly, from the viewpoint of pharmaceutics mainly, the 'translation' of biological concepts into novel and sophisticated dosage forms was aimed at. In principle the same set-up is chosen for the book, too, in order to try bridging the gap between biological sciences and the rational design of novel dosage forms and creating a new interface between different sciences.

Leiden, 1992   H. E. Junginger

List of contributors

Dr N. Ammoury URA 1218 CNRS, Faculty of Pharmacy, University of Paris-Sud, 92296 Chatenay-Malabry Cdex, France.
Dr P. A. Baldwin Drug Delivery Department, California Biotechnology Inc., 2450 Bayshore Parkway, Mountain View, CA 94043, USA.
Dr G. Barratt URA 1218 CNRS, Faculty of Pharmacy, University of Paris-Sud, 92296 Chatenay-Malabry Cdex, France.
Professor Dr Th. J. C. van Berkel Center for Bio-Pharmaceutical Sciences, Department of Biopharmaceutics, P.O. Box 9503, 2300 RA Leiden, The Netherlands.
Dr H. E. Bodd Center for Bio-Pharmaceutical Sciences, Department of Pharmaceutical Technology, P.O. Box 9502, 2300 RA Leiden, The Netherlands.
Dr A. G. de Boer Center for Bio-Pharmaceutical Sciences, Depatment of Pharmacology Leiden University, P.O. Box 9503, 2300 RA Leiden, The Netherlands.
Dr J. A Bouwstra Center for Bio-Pharmaceutical Sciences, Department of Pharmaceutical Technology, P.O. Box 9502, 2300 RA Leiden, The Netherlands.
Professor Dr D. D. Breimer Center for Bio-Pharmaceutical Sciences, Department of Pharmacology Leiden University, P.O. Box 9502, 2300 RA Leiden, The Netherlands.
W. H. M. Craane-van Hinsberg Center for Bio-Pharmaceutical Sciences, Departmet of Pharmaceutical Technology Leiden University, P.O. Box 9502, 2300 RA Leiden, The Netherlands.
Professor Dr J. Ph. Devissaguet URA 1218 CNRS, Faculty of Pharmacy, University of Paris-Sud, 92296 Chatenay-Malabry, France.
E. P. Eijking Department of Anaesthesiology. Erasmus University, P.O. Box 1738, 3000 DR Rotterdam, The Netherlands.
Dr H. Fessi URA 1218 CNRS, Faculty of Pharmacy, University of Paris-Sud, 92296 Chatenay-Malabry Cdex, France.
Dr W. Fischer Hexal Pharma, Industriestr. 25, 8150 Holzkirchen, Germany.
Professor Dr A. T. Florence Centre for Drug Delivery Research, University of London, School of Pharmacy, 29/39 Brunswick Square London WC1N 1AX, UK.
Dr J. G. Fokkens Solvay Duphar B. V., P.O. Box 900, 1300 DA Weesp, The Netherlands.

List of contributors

G. S. Gooris Center for Bio-Pharmaceutical Sciences, Department of Pharmaceutical Technology Leiden University, P.O. Box 9502, 2300 RA Leiden, The Netherlands.

Professor Dr J. Hadgraft University of Wales, The Welsh School of Pharmacy, Division of Pharmaceutical Chemistry, P.O. Box 13, Cardiff CF1 3XF, UK.

Dr W. A. J. J. Hermens Center for Bio-Pharmaceutical Sciences, Subdivision of Pharmaceutical Technology and Biopharmaceutics Leiden University, P.O. Box 9502, 2300 RA Leiden, The Netherlands.

Dr V. van Hinsbergh Gaubius Laboratorium IVVO/TNO, P.O. Box 430, 2300 AK Leiden, The Netherlands.

Dr H. E. Hofland Center for Bio-Pharmaceutical Sciences, Department of Pharmaceutical Technology Leiden University, P.O. Box 9502, 2300 RA Leiden, The Netherlands.

Professor Dr. L. Huang Department of Pharmacology, University of Pittsburgh School of Medicine, Pittsburgh, PA 15261, USA.

Dr Praful U. Jani Center for Drug Delivery Research, The School of Pharmacy, University of London, 29/39 Brunswick Square, London WC1N 1AX, UK.

H. E. Junginger Center for Bio-pharmaceutical Sciences, Department of Pharmaceutical Technology Leiden University, P.O. Box 9502, 2300 RA Leiden, The Netherlands.

Professor Dr B. Lachmann Erasmus University, Department of Anaesthesiology, P.O. Box 1738, 3000 DR Rotterdam, The Netherlands.

Dr William A. Lee Drug Delivery Department, California Biotechnology Inc., Mountain View, CA 94043, USA.

Dr C.-M. Lehr Center for Bio-Pharmaceutical Sciences, Department of Pharmaceutical Technology, P.O. Box 9502, 2300 RA Leiden, The Netherlands.

Dexi Liu Department of Molecular and Cell Biology, Division of Biochemistry and Molecular Biology, University of California Berkeley, CA 94720, USA.

Professor Dr F. W. H. M. Merkus Center for Bio-Pharmaceutical Sciences, Subdivision of Pharmaceutical Technology and Biopharmaceutics, P.O. Box 9502, 2300 RA Leiden, The Netherlands.

Atsuhide Mori Department of Pharmacology, University of Pittsburgh School of Medicine, Pittsburgh, PA 15261, USA.

Dr M. Ponec Department of Dermatology, University Hospital, Leiden University, Rijnsburgerweg 10, 2333 AA Leiden, The Netherlands.

S. G. Romeijn Center for Bio-Pharmaceutical Sciences, Subdivision of Pharmaceutical Technology and Biopharmaceutics Leiden University, P.O. Box 9502, 2300 RA Leiden, The Netherlands.

Professor Dr K. P. Schäfer Byk Gulden Pharmazeutika, Byk-Gulden-Strasse 2, P.O. Box 10 03 10, D-7750 Konstanz, Germany.

N. G. M. Schipper Centre for Bio-Pharmaceutical Sciences, Subdivision of Pharmaceutical Technology and Biopharmaceutics Leiden University, P.O. Box 9502, 2300 RA Leiden, The Netherlands.

Dr F. Spies Laboratory for Electron Microscopy, Leiden University, Rdnsburger Weg 10, 2333 AA Leiden, The Netherlands.

Professor Dr Chr.A. Squier The University of Iowa, College of Dentistry, Dows Institute for Dental Research, Department of Oral Pathology, Iowa City, IA 52242, USA.

Dr J. C. Verhoef Center for Bio-Pharmaceutical Sciences, Leiden University, Subdivision of Pharmaceutical Technology and Biopharmaceutics P.O. Box 9502, 2300 RA Leiden, The Netherlands.

Dr M. E. de Vries Faculty of Medicine, University of Amsterdam, Meibeydreef 15, Amsterdam, The Netherlands.

Dr Kenneth A. Walters AN-eX Analytic Services Ltd., Redwood Building, Cardiff CFI 3XF, UK.

Dr P. J. J. Wauben-Penris Brocades Pharma, P.O. Box 5009, 2600 GA Delft, The Netherlands.

Part I
Parenteral route

1

Transport of macromolecules across the microvascular endothelium

Victor W. M. van Hinsbergh

INTRODUCTION

The vascular system provides the mechanism by which oxygen, nutrients and hormones are supplied to the tissues. The exchange between blood and tissues occurs in capillaries and postcapillary venules of the microvasculature. The endothelium is the main component of the wall of capillaries and postcapillary venules and represents an active and selective barrier for fluid, solutes, macromolecules and white blood cells between the blood and the tissue. The overall mass of the endothelium in the adult human body is estimated to be about 720 g, of which the capillaries and postcapillary venules represent more than 600 g (Wolinsky, 1980). All together the endothelial cells represent an organ with maximal exposure to the blood and with many different functions, including the regulation of vascular permeability (Table 1). Extravasation of molecules is actively and selectively controlled by the endothelium and varies in different parts of the body. Orally and intravenously administered drugs will encounter the active and selective endothelial barrier on their way to target tissues. This endothelial barrier may interfere with the efficiency of a drug, but, on the other hand, the differences in the various endothelia of the body may be used to address a drug to a specific target organ. In this chapter present knowledge about microvascular permeability is briefly surveyed. First, the barrier aspects of various types of capillaries are summarized, followed by the structures that may be involved in exchange of solutes and macromolecules over the endothelium. Subsequently, the permeability pathways for solutes and macromolecules over the microvascular endothelium are discussed. Finally, the mechanism of vascular leakage during endothelial activation is described and possible improvements to the barrier function of the endothelium are discussed.

Table 1. Functions of the vascular endothelium	
(1)	Regulation of vascular permeability.
(2)	Prevention of coagulation and platelet deposition.
(3)	Contribution to the regulation of the vascular tone in muscular blood vessels by the production of factors and the conversion of vasoactive substances.
(4)	Synthesis and secretion of many specific proteins, including basal membrane proteins.
(5)	Expression of many, often specifically localized receptors and binding sites, e.g. insulin and transferrin receptors and binding sites for lipoprotein lipase.
(6)	Homing, margination and extravasation of various types of white blood cells.
(7)	Contribution to local and systemic response to inflammatory stimuli.
(8)	Angiogenesis.

THE ENDOTHELIUM OF CAPILLARIES AND POSTCAPILLARY VENULES

Essentially, the endothelium can be considered as a highly attenuated epitheloid monolayer, which during its development has acquired many mechanisms to cope with the regional needs of nutrition, hormone exchange and removal of waste products. Four major types of capillary endothelia are distinguished based on the presence or absence of fenestrae and gaps and the complexity of their barrier function.

Continuous capillaries

A common form of capillary is the continuous capillary found in muscle and connective tissues. The cells are extremely thin at their periphery (to less than 0.3 µm) and only thickened in the region of the nucleus. Their surface is covered with a thin glycocalyx which is negatively charged by anionic sites. Vesicular invaginations are frequently observed on both the luminal and basolateral plasma membranes of the cells. They have a diameter of 70–80 nm and their neck (about 60 nm diameter) is often covered with a thin neutral lining. In cross-sections many vesicle structures of identical diameter are found, which are in direct or indirect contact with the vesicular invaginations. Fine striped structures have been observed on the cytoplasmic surface of individual plasmalemmal vesicles, which were not found on the plasma membrane (Peters et al., 1985; Izumi et al., 1988). At their basal side the capillaries are enwrapped by a basal membrane, which is synthesized by the endothelium and in which pericytes can be encountered. In cross-section, capillaries contain one to five endothelial cells which are connected by an interdigitated junctional complex. In addition to folding of the plasma membrane these complexes contain tight junctions and sometimes gap junctions.

Fenestrated endothelia

Additional structures are encountered in specific capillaries. In visceral tissues, the capillaries contain fenestrae, small circular openings that are present in the extremely attenuated parts of the cells. These fenestrae are covered by a unique structure. Using scanning electron microscopy, a central knob and six to eight radiating spokes and wedge-like pores have been observed (Maul, 1971; Bearer *et al.*, 1985). Perfusion studies with electron-dense proteins and subsequent transmission electron microscopy have revealed that the luminal side of the diaphragms binds avidly cationic ferritin, while the basolateral side does not (Simionescu *et al.*, 1982). The polarly expressed anionic sites are contributed mostly by heparan sulphate proteoglycans (Simionescu *et al.*, 1981). To what extent the pores are patent or closed is not yet known. The expression of fenestrae can probably be regulated. *In vitro* studies have shown that diaphragms in bovine adrenal capillary endothelial cells easily disappear in culture, but can be partly restored by growing the cells on a basal lamina produced by Madin–Darby canine kidney (MDCK) cells for a prolonged period in the postconfluent state (Milici *et al.*, 1985). On the basis of the currently available fragmentaric electron microscopical data of fenestrated endothelia in various tissues it is likely that considerable variation exists. The endothelium of glomerular capillaries contains relatively large fenestrae without diaphragms.

Sinusoidal endothelial cells

In liver and bone marrow sinusoids, the endothelium has only a poorly developed basal membrane or none at all and is perforated by large and irregularly shaped gaps. Relative large molecules and particles, such as low density lipoproteins, can exchange easily between the blood and the space of Disse underneath the endothelium. Only very large particles such as chylomicrons are excluded and have to be partly catabolized in peripheral tissues before their remnants gain access to the hepatocytes. On the other hand, liver sinusoidal endothelial cells are very rich in receptors and in coated pits and vesicles, which are involved in the removal of specific and modified molecules from the circulation.

Brain capillaries

In several specialized regions of the body, in particular in the microvessels of the brain and the spinal cord, a very tight continuous endothelium is present. The barrier is two-fold. On one hand the tight junctions form complicated belts around the endothelial cells, comparable with tight junctions in epithelial cells. Solutes and macromolecules have to pass via specific receptors. On the other hand, the specialized metabolic activities of brain microvascular endothelial cells convert or degrade many molecules during their passage through the cell. Direct interaction between the endothelium and astrocytes is thought to be necessary for the maintenance of these specialized characteristics.

Postcapillary venules

The structure of the wall of the postcapillary venules is similar to that of continuous and fenestrated capillaries, although the diameter of the vessel is larger. As described below, the contractile response of the postcapillary venules to inflammatory or vasoactive substances results in intercellular gaps, suggesting an at least more complicated contractile structure around the cellular junctions than in true capillaries.

EXCHANGE ACROSS THE MICROVASCULAR ENDOTHELIUM
Passage pathways
The endothelium is a complex structure. On the basis of morphological observations, mainly by electron microscopy, a number of structures have been identified that may be involved in the permeation of gasses, fluid, solutes and macromolecules. Fig. 1 depicts an artificial combination of these structures. They comprise the following.

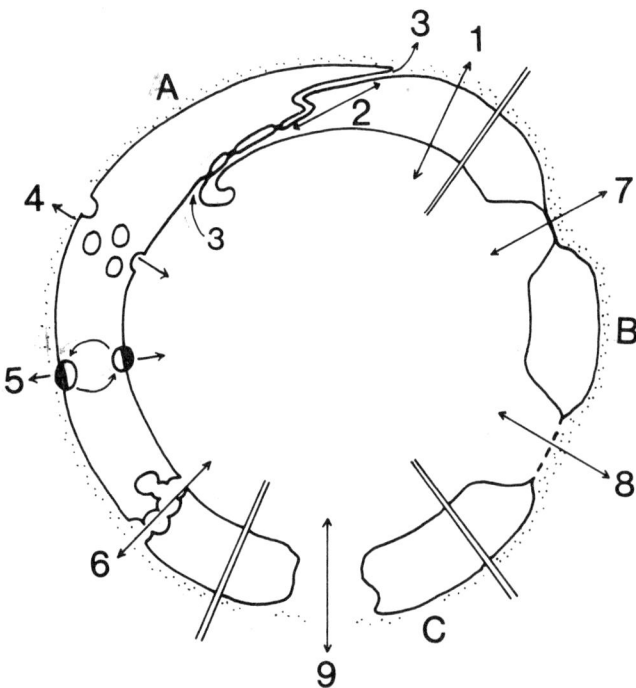

Fig. 1. Schematic representation of various exchange pathways which may be involved in the permeation of various nutrients, fluid and macromolecules across the endothelium: 1, diffusion through the cell membranes and the cytoplasm; 2, lateral diffusion of small lipophilic molecules through the lipid bilayers of the cellular junctions; 3, extracellular passage through the narrow slits of endothelial junctions; 4, vesicular exchange; 5, carrier-mediated exchange and receptor-mediated transport; 6, transendothelial channels which consist of fused vesicles; 7, closed diaphragms; 8, open diaphragms, in which the basal membrane and its surface charge act as main barrier; 9, extracellular exchange via intercellular gaps. The figure depicts an endothelial cell that encloses a capillary and combines exchange properties of continuous, fenestrated and sinusoidal endothelia. In part A the exchange pathways of continuous endothelia are depicted; the top part shows a junctional complex with three tight junctions. The fenestrae are specific for fenestrated endothelia (B). Gaps are only observed in sinusoidal endothelia and between endothelial cells in activated postcapillary venules (C).

(1) Direct diffusion through the two plasma membranes and the cytoplasm. Oxygen can be exchanged in this way.
(2) Lateral diffusion of small lipid molecules through the lipid bilayers of the intercellular junctions (Blanchette-Mackie and Scow, 1981).
(3) Exchange of fluid and solutes through the narrow slits of intercellular junctions. The permeability is regulated at the tight junctions and probably by a fibre matrix that fills the junctional areas.
(4) Bulk exchange of solutes and macromolecules via vesicles.
(5) Exchange of solutes and macromolecules via transendothelial channels, which are formed by several fused vesicles.
(6) Receptor-mediated transcytosis (active transport and facilitated diffusion) of macromolecules and essential nutrients via specific carrier proteins.
(7) Exchange of fluid, solutes and possibly macromolecules via fenestrae with closed diaphragms.
(8) Exchange of fluid, solutes and possible macromolecules via open diaphragms. The basal membrane underneath these openings can prevent the escape of many macromolecules by sieving and electrostatic repulsion.
(9) Bulk exchange of solutes and large macromolecules via gaps in sinusoidal endothelial cells of liver, bone marrow and spleen, and via intercellular gaps in postcapillary venules upon inflammatory activation.

Role of various pathways in the exchange of fluid, solutes and macromolecules
Curry *et al.* (1976) and Renkin (1985) have calculated that the bulk flow of water through capillary walls (90–92%) occurs through the cell membrane pathway, while only 8–10% passes through the intercellular (pore) pathway. Small lipophilic molecules can exchange by lateral diffusion via the intercellular junctions (Blanchette-Mackie and Scow, 1981), but may also partly be carried by albumin molecules across certain endothelial barriers (Galis *et al.*, 1988).

Hydrophilic molecules and proteins cannot permeate through cell membranes but have to pass through gaps between the cells, fenestrae or vesicular structures. The permeability of these molecules decreases with increasing molecular size, suggesting that the pathway available to them acts as a molecular sieve. From physiological studies on lymph flow, physiologists have developed a model that approximates the flux of small and large water soluble molecules. In this model the permeation of water-soluble molecules proceeds via two types of pores 'small pores' with an approximate radius of 4–6 nm and 'large pores' which have a diameter of 20–100 nm. Evidence is now accumulating that the passage of small water-soluble molecules proceeds via intercellular junctions in continuous endothelia (except at the blood–brain barrier and similar very tight endothelia where glucose and amino acids are transported via specific receptors). Hence the intercellular junctions are expected to represent the small pores. Such channels will allow convective flow of water and solutes as well as diffusion exchange of solutes. Under normal conditions the passage of larger water-soluble molecules is hindered not only by the slit width but probably also by complex interaction of macromolecules, the so-called fibre matrix. Albumin plays an important role in this fibre matrix and interacts by its positively charged amino acids with other components, probably glycosaminoglycans (Curry, 1986). It is likely that the large pores represent distended intercellular junctions (still filled with fibre matrix as they display molecular sieving characteristics). However, it remains difficult to confirm this using morphological techniques, as their frequency is two to four orders of magnitude less than that of small pores. Studies by Renkin indicate that the passage of macromolecules under non-stimulated conditions cannot be completely explained by small and large pore pathways. Whether the additional route is provided by vesicular exchange (Renkin, 1988) has still to be established.

Morphological studies on the extravasation of macromolecules
The use of electron dense tracers (ferritin, peroxidase, gold-labelled proteins) has provided new insights in the complexity of endothelial permeability. Whereas physiological measurements relate to complete microvascular beds (including capillaries and postcapillary venules) or single but selected and relatively large capillaries, electron microscopic studies can give information on local variation in capillary permeability. One of the sites of local variation may be the fenestrae, which are covered by a diaphragm with a highly anionic charge, and which may represent unique exchange structures. Also, the large lacunae in sinusoidal endothelial cells can be considered as a specific adaptation to allow maximal exchange of macromolecules. Whereas little confusion exists about the relatively easy extravasation of macromolecules through sinusoidal endothelia, the permeation pathways of macromolecules through continuous and fenestrated endothelium are still a matter of debate. Two conflicting opinions exist regarding the involvement of vesicles and intercellular clefts in macromolecular transport through continuous capillaries. In one view, substantiated by extensive evidence with electron-dense protein markers, the vesicles are the predominant site of transcytosis of proteins (see Palade, 1988, for review). In the other view, which is based on carefully conducted serial sectioning of frog mesenteric and cardiac muscle capillaries, nearly all vesicles are connected to the upper leaflet of the plasma membrane or to the basolateral part of the plasma membrane and hence provide extreme extensions of the surface of the plasma membrane (Frøkjær-Jensen, 1980; Bundgaard *et al.*, 1983). At most, 2% of the structures that are observed in cross-sections as vesicles appear to be true vesicles upon serial sectioning. However, these observations need not be as conflicting as it seems. First, the number of apparent vesicles is two orders of magnitude larger than is necessary to explain the exchange of albumin by vesicles. A small subpopulation of specific vesicle structures may explain the apparent difference. Secondly, receptor-mediated transcytosis, as is known for insulin and transferrin in blood-brain barrier capillaries, may be a more general phenomenon existing also in other capillaries. Evidence for high affinity binding and transcytosis of albumin to or via vesicular structures has been presented for various types of capillary endothelia (Milici *et al.*, 1987; Predescu *et al.*, 1988). Specific binding of insulin and transferrin has recently been demonstrated for various types of endothelial cells *in vitro*, but it is not yet clear whether these receptors are involved in protein transcytosis, in signal transduction or in receptor-mediated endocytosis via coated vesicles and subsequent lysosomal degradation. If receptor/carrier-mediated transcytosis is a general phenome-

non, there may exist a gradual transition between capillaries and postcapillary venules. In the proximal part receptor/carrier-mediated (vesicular) exchange may dominate, whereas in the distal part macromolecular exchange proceeds predominantly via intercellular junctions, which are regulated by cellular contraction. It is generally accepted that activation of the endothelium can open these junctions, resulting in a marked increase in the flow of fluid, solutes and macromolecules.

ENDOTHELIAL ACTIVATION AND VASCULAR LEAKAGE

Endothelial activation

Distension of the intercellular gaps in postcapillary venules is one of the features of endothelial activation. The vascular endothelium is a versatile tissue that adapts its properties in response to inflammatory, hormonal and local stimuli. These responses vary from very rapid responses which occur within minutes to responses that occur after hours or days (Fig. 2). The latter responses usually involve protein synthesis, e.g. the induction of leukocyte adhesion molecules, interleukin-6 and plasminogen activator inhibitor-1. In the early responses, receptor-mediated activation of cellular enzymes, often via second messengers, results in an immediate response of the cell. Among them are the rapid release of prostacyclin and nitric oxide, which are involved in vasorelaxation and in the prevention of platelet adhesion, the release of von Willebrand factor from Weibel-Palade bodies, the rapid release of tissue-type plasminogen activator, the main regulator of fibrinolysis in the blood compartment, and, in postcapillary venules, an increase in permeability via the formation of intercellular gaps.

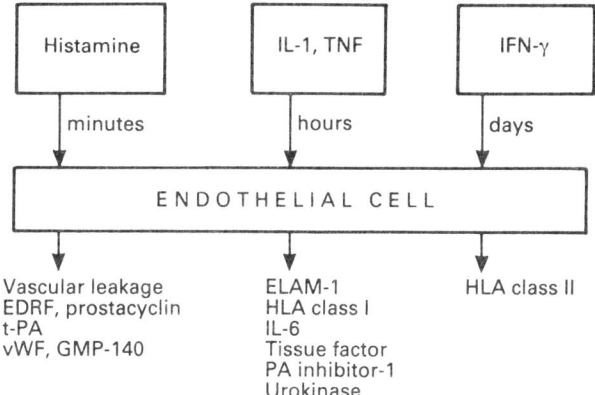

Fig. 2. Schematic and simplified scheme of events occuring during endothelial activation. Activation of endothelial cells occurs in successive stages by various mediators. After an initial rapid event, which can be evoked by many vasoactive agents including histamine and involves an increase of cytoplasmatic calcium ions or an activation of protein kinase C, slower responses include the synthesis of new proteins. Interleukin-1 (IL-1), tumour necrosis factor-α (TNF) and γ-interferon (IFN-γ) are given as examples; they do not exclusively act on the given time scale, but can also evoke other responses at shorter time intervals.

Vascular leakage

Three lines of evidence have contributed to the understanding of the mechanism of vascular leakage. By light and electron microscopic studies it has been shown by Majno and Palade (1961) and Majno et al. (1969) that histamine-type inflammatory mediators induce the formation of intercellular gaps in postcapillary venules large enough to trap carbon particles and even platelets. Majno concluded that this was due to contraction of endothelial cells, as the cells became thicker and the shape of the nucleus became more wrinkled. The increase in permeability proceeds via an H1 receptor and can also be demonstrated in monolayers of endothelial cells in culture (Langeler et al., 1989). Activation of the H1 receptor causes via a G protein the activation of phospholipase C, which results in the generation of diacyl-glycerol and inositol-triphosphate, with a subsequent rise in the intracellular concentration of calcium ions. Studies on cultured endothelial cells have demonstrated that cellular contraction indeed occurs and that calcium and magnesium ions, ATP, myosin light chain and myosin light chain kinase are involved (Wysolmerski and Lagunoff, 1990; Schnittler et al., 1990). Furthermore, the involvement of actin–myosin interaction in endothelial contraction has been effectively demonstrated by the use of myosin heads (S1 fragments) in permeabilized endothelial cells (Schnittler et al., 1990). Addition of S1 fragments prevented the interaction of actin and non-muscle myosin and endothelial contraction. S1 fragments that had been inactivated by N-ethylmaleimide did not interfere with these processes. Recent studies on single capillaries of the frog give further evidence for the involvement of calcium ions and cellular contraction in the increase in capillary permeability (He et al., 1990; Rutledge et al., 1990). Whether these observations can be generalized for other capillaries or are specific to relatively large capillaries has still to be established, but it further stresses the importance of the intercellular pathway in the extravasation of macromolecules.

Recent studies of Cuénoud, Joris and Majno have demonstrated that upon activation of the microvascular bed it is not only the postcapillary venules which can become permeable to macromolecules. Whereas postcapillary venules react directly upon histamine administration, arterioles can become leaky for macromolecules 6 h after the challenge of the vascular bed with histamine (Cuénoud et al., 1987). It has been suggested that this process, named focal arteriolar insudation, may be the result of a continued arterolar relaxation. As the endothelium is no longer capable of following the vascular distention, gaps may occur (Cuénoud et al., 1987). At present no information about the reversibility of this process is available. Furthermore, Joris et al. (1990) demonstrated that capillaries can also become permeable for macromolecules. They observed that, after a venular leakage phase in aseptic inflammation, a capillary leakage phase is induced by the inflammation reaction itself. This is possibly the result of diffuse angiogenesis. In this context it is challenging that vascular permeability factor is both an endothelial mitogen and an inducer of vascular leakage (Connolly et al., 1989).

Improving the barrier function of the endothelium

An understanding of the molecular interactions that underlie endothelial contraction and increased endothelial permeability also presents the opportunity to counteract these interactions and to prevent vascular leakage or to limit it to certain desired regions of the vascular bed. It has been known for many years that thrombocytopenia results in an increased microvascular permeability and that this increase can be counteracted by administration of platelets or platelet releasates (Roy and Djerrassi, 1972). The vascular leakage that occurs during preservation of graft organs can also be decreased by using a perfusion fluid with platelet factors instead of a platelet-free perfusate (Gimbrone et al., 1969). Serotonin and norepinephrine have been seen to improve the microvascular barrier function (Sweetman et al., 1981). Other agents, isoproterenol, terbutaline and xanthines, have also been demonstrated to be effective agents for counteracting microvascular leakage in experimental animals (Grega et al., 1988). These factors have in common that they can increase the cellular cAMP concentration. Recent studies *in vitro*, in which animal and human endothelial cells have been cultured on porous filters, have confirmed that an elevation of cyclic AMP results in a decreased endothelial permeability (Stelzner et al., 1989; Langeler et al., 1989; Langeler and van Hinsbergh, 1991). Interestingly, norepinephrine decreased endothelial permeability to a much larger extent than was expected on the basis of its cAMP increasing capacity (see Fig. 3). This suggests that additional mechanism(s) exist by which the barrier function of the endothelium can be improved (Langeler and van Hinsbergh, 1991).

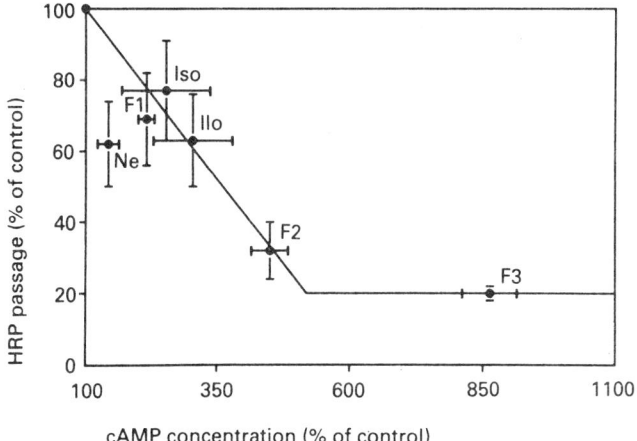

Fig. 3. Relative changes in endothelial permeability for horse radish peroxidase (HRP) vs relative changes in cyclic AMP concentration are given for monolayers of human umbilical artery endothelial cells cultured on porous filters that had been incubated with norepinephrine (Ne), isoproterenol (Iso), iloprost (Ilo) and various concentrations of forskolin (F1, F2 and F3). A correlation between these parameters has been found for isoproterenol, iloprost and 0.25 ad 2.5 µM forskolin (F1, F2). The effect of norepinephrine on permeability is stronger than expected on the basis of its cAMP enhancing effect. (From Langeler and van Hinsbergh (1991) with permission).

Interaction with pericytes and astrocytes

Cellular interactions may also contribute to a change in the barrier characteristic of the endothelium. An extreme example is the blood–brain barrier. The specific properties of the blood–brain barrier microvessels can be retained in endothelial cells in culture provided that the cells remain in contact with astrocytes. Both the complexity of the interendothelial junctions and several metabolic properties of the blood–brain microvascular endothelial cells, such as the expression of γ-glutamyl-transpeptidase and mono-amine oxidase, are only expressed when both types of cells are kept together (DeBault and Canncilla, 1980; Janzer and Raff, 1987). It is quite conceivable that future studies will reveal the extent to which pericytes affect the regulation of microvascular permeability and whether this can be influenced by pharmacological means.

CONCLUSION

How macromolecules pass through the microvascular endothelium is still a matter of debate. Several lines of evidence indicate that the increased extravasation of solutes and macromolecules occurs via intercellular gaps, which are widened by endothelial contraction. This process can be enhanced or counteracted by pharmacological means. On the other hand, under non-stimulated conditions, part of the extravasation of macromolecules appears to follow a different pathway, possibly vesicular exchange. In the near future, it will become clear whether receptor/carrier-mediated vesicular exchange is limited to brain capillaries or whether it is also a general phenomenon in other continuous capillaries. If this holds true — evidence for vesicular albumin binding and transcytosis has already been provided — there may exist a gradual transition between capillaries and postcapillary venules. In the proximal part receptor–carrier-mediated exchange may dominate, whereas in the distal part macromolecular exchange proceeds mainly via intercellular junctions. Insight into these mechanisms and the specialized structures involved will contribute to a rational approach to circumvent the endothelial barrier in targeting drugs to specific areas of the body.

REFERENCES

Bearer, E. L., Orci, L. and Sors, P. (1985) Endothelial fenestral diaphragms: a quick-freeze, deep-etch study. *J. Cell Biol.* **100** 418–428.

Blanchette-Mackie, E. J. and Scow, R. O. (1981) Lipolysis and lamellar structures in white adipose tissue of young rats: lipid movement in membranes. *J. Ultrastruct. Res.* **77** 295–318.

Bundgaard, M., Hageman, P. and Crone, C. (1983) The three-dimensional organization of plasmalemmal vesicular profiles in the endothelium of rat heart capillaries. *Microvasc. Res.* **25** 358–368.

Connolly, D. T., Heuvelman, D. M., Nelson, R., Olander, J. V., Eppley, B. L., Delfino, J. J., Siegel, N. R., Leimgruber, R. M. and Feder, J. (1989) Tumor vascular permeability factor stimulates endothelial cell growth and angiogenesis. *J. Clin. Invest.* **84** 1470–1478.

Cuénoud, H. F., Joris, I., Langer, R. S. and Majno, G. (1987) Focal arteriolar insudation. A response of arterioles to chronic nonspecific irritation. *Am. J. Pathol.* **127** 592–604.

Curry, F. E. (1986) Determinants of capillary permeability: a review of mechanisms based on single capillary studies in the frog. *Circ. Res.* **59** 367–380.

Curry, F. E., Mason, J. C. and Michel, C. C. (1976) Osmotic reflection coefficients of capillary walls to low molecular weight hydrophilic solutes measured in single capillaries of the frog mesentery. *J. Physiol. (London)* **261** 319–336.

DeBault, L. E. and Cancilla, P. A. (1980) γ-Glutamyl transpeptidase in isolated brain endothelial cells: induction by glial cells *in vitro*. *Science* **207** 653–655.

Frøkjær-Jensen, J. (1980) Three-dimensional organization of plasmalemmal vesicles in endothelial cells. An analysis by serial sectioning of frog mesenteric capillaries. *J. Ultrastruct. Res.* **73** 9–20.

Galis, Z., Ghitescu, L. and Simionescu, M. (1988) Fatty acids binding to albumin increases its uptake and transcytosis by the lung capillary endothelium. *Eur. J. Cell Biol.* **47** 358–365.

Gimbrone, M. A., Jr., Aster, R. H., Cotran, R. S., Corkery, J., Jandl, J. H. and Folkman, J. (1969) Preservation of vascular integrity in organs perfused *in vitro* with a platelet-rich medium. *Nature (London)* **222** 33–36.

Grega, G. J., Persson, C. G. A. and Svensjö, E. (1988) Endothelial cell reactions to inflammatory mediators assessed *in vivo* by fluid and solute flux analysis. In: Ryan, U. S. (ed.) *Endothelial Cells*, Vol. III. CRC Press Inc., Boca Raton, FL, pp. 103–119.

He, P., Pagakis, S. N. and Curry, F. E. (1990) Measurement of cytoplasmic calcium in single microvessels with increased permeability. *Am. J. Physiol.* **258** H1366–H1374.

Izumi, T., Shibata, Y. and Yamamoto, T. (1988) Striped structures on the cytoplasmic surface membranes of the endothelial vesicles of the rat aorta revealed by quick-freeze, deep-etching replicas. *Anat. Rec.* **220** 225–232.

Janzer, R. C. and Raff, M. C. (1987) Astrocytes induce blood–brain barrier properties in endothelial cells. *Nature (London)* **325** 253–257.

Joris, I., Cuénoud, H. F., Doern, G. V., Underwood, J. M. and Majno, G. (1990) Capillary leakage in inflammation. A study by vascular labeling. *Am. J. Pathol.* **137** 1353–1363.

Langeler, E. G. and van Hinsbergh, V. W. M. (1991) Norepinephrine and iloprost improve barrier function of human endothelial cell monolayers: role of cAMP. *Am. J. Physiol.* **260** C1052–C1059.

Langeler, E. G., Snelting-Havinga, I. and van Hinsbergh, V. W. M. (1989) Passage of low density lipoproteins through monolayers of human arterial endothelial cells. Effects of vasoactive substances in an *in vitro* model. *Arteriosclerosis* **9** 550–559.

Majno, G. and Palade, G. E. (1961) Studies on inflammation: I. The effect of histamine and serotonin on vascular permeability: an electron microscopic study. *J. Biophys. Biochem. Cytol.* **11** 571–605.

Majno, G., Shea, S. M. and Leventhal, M. (1969) Endothelial contraction induced by histamine-type mediators. An electron microscopic study. *J. Cell Biol.* **42** 647–672.

Maul, G. G. Y. (1971) Structure and formation of pores in fenestrated capillaries. *J. Ultrastruct. Res.* **36** 768–782.

Milici, A. J., Furie, M. B. and Carley, W. W. (1985) The formation of fenestrations and channels by capillary endothelium *in vitro*. *Proc. Natl. Acad. Sci. USA* **82** 6181–6185.

Milici, A. J., Watrous, N. E., Stukenbrok, H. and Palade, G. E. (1987) Transcytosis of albumin in capillary endothelium. *J. Cell Biol.* **105** 2603–2612.

Palade, G. E. (1988) The microvascular endothelium revisited. In Simionescu, N. and Simionescu, M. (eds) *Endothelial Cell Biology in Health and Disease*. Plenum, New York, pp. 3–21.

Peters, K.-R., Carley, W. W. and Palade, G. E. (1985) Endothelial plasmalemmal vesicles have a characteristic striped bipolar surface structure. *J. Cell Biol.* **101** 2233–2238.

Predescu, D., Simionescu, M., Simionescu, N. and Palade, G. E. (1988) Binding and transcytosis of glycoalbumin by the microvascular endothelium of the murine myocardium: evidence that glycoalbumin behaves as a bifunctional ligand. *J. Cell Biol.* **107** 1729–1738.

Renkin, E. M. (1985) Capillary transport of macromolecules: pores and other endothelial pathways. *J. Appl. Physiol.* **58** 315–325.

Renkin, E. M. (1988) Transport pathways and processes. In Simionescu, N. and Simionescu, M. (eds) *Endothelial Cell Biology in Health and Disease*. Plenum, New York, pp. 51–68.

Roy, A. J. and Djerassi, I. (1972) Effects of platelet transfusions: plug formation and maintenance of vascular integrity. *Proc. Soc. Exp. Biol. Med.* **139** 137–142.

Rutledge, J. C., Curry, F. E., Lenz, J. F. and Davis, P. A. (1990) Low density lipoprotein transport across a microvascular endothelial barrier after permeability is increased. *Circ. Res.* **66** 486–495.

Schnittler, H.-J., Wilke, A., Gress, T., Suttorp, N. and Drenckhahn, D. (1990) Role of actin and myosin in the control of paracellular permeability in pit, rat and human vascular endothelium. *J. Physiol.* **431** 379–401.

Simionescu, M., Simionescu, N., Silbert, J. E. and Palade, G. E. (1981) Differentiated microdomains on the luminal surface of the capillary endothelium. II. Partial characterization of their anionic sites. *J. Cell Biol.* **90** 614–621.

Simionescu, M., Simionescu, N. and Palade, G. E. (1982) Preferential distribution of anionic sites on the basement membrane and the abluminal aspect of the endothelium in fenestrated capillaries. *J. Cell Biol.* **95** 425–434.

Stelzner, T. J., Weil, J. V. and O'Brien, R. F. (1989) Role of cyclic adenosine monophosphate in the induction of endothelial barrier properties. *J. Cell Physiol.* **139** 157–166.

Sweetman, H. E., Shepro, D. and Hechtman, H. B. (1981) Inhibition of thrombocytopenic petechiae by exogeneous serotonin administration. *Haemostasis* **10** 65–78.

Wolinsky, H. (1980) A proposal linking clearance of circulating lipoproteins to tissue metabolic activity as a basis for understanding atherogenesis. *Circ. Res.* **47** 301–311.

Wysolmerski, R. B. and Lagunoff, D. (1990) Involvement of myosin light-chain kinase in endothelial cell retraction. *Proc. Natl. Acad. Sci. USA* **87** 16–20.

2

Receptor-dependent uptake of macromolecules by specific hepatic cells

Th. J. C. van Berkel

INTRODUCTION

Specific targeting of drugs can be achieved by utilizing the specific properties of the target cell. Because cell membranes are decisive for the primary interaction, it is obvious to relate the recognition marker of a drug or drug transport vehicle to the presence of specific receptors. In the present contribution the strategy is outlined to achieve targeting to specific cell types whereby the principle is illustrated for the liver. It is expected that the principles can be applied in a general sense in order to achieve delivery of drugs at various desired sites of action.

Currently utilized transport vehicles for drugs are (1) nanoparticles, (2) liposomes, (3) microemulsions, (4) proteins including monoclonal antibodies, (5) reconstituted viruses, erythrocytes, (6) steroids and (7) lipoproteins. In principle, all carriers give rise to a similar problem which is untimely capture by the reticuloendothelial system. This problem is more explicit with structures which are foreign to the body such as items (1)–(4), while for items (5)–(7) endogeneous transport routes are available. Because the experience within the Division of Biopharmaceutics is mostly related to item (7), I will use lipoproteins as a further example of the possibilities and limitations of the concept of drug targeting whereby the liver forms the desired targeting unit.

The liver is a heterogeneous tissue which contains, in addition to parenchymal cells (92.5% of liver protein), endothelial cells (3.3% of liver protein), Kupffer cells (2.5% of liver protein) and fat-storing cells (1.7% of liver protein). In order to determine uptake of substances in a certain cell type, a cell isolation method is needed which allows a quantitative recovery of the ligand in the purified cells.

The procedure as outlined in Scheme 1 prevents destruction of targeted ligands, because liver perfusion, cell separation and cell purification are performed at a low temperature (8°C). In addition, one is able to assess the recovery by comparing the radioactivity in the purified parenchymal, endothelial and Kupffer cells (all obtained from one liver) with the radioactivity originally present in the whole rat liver.

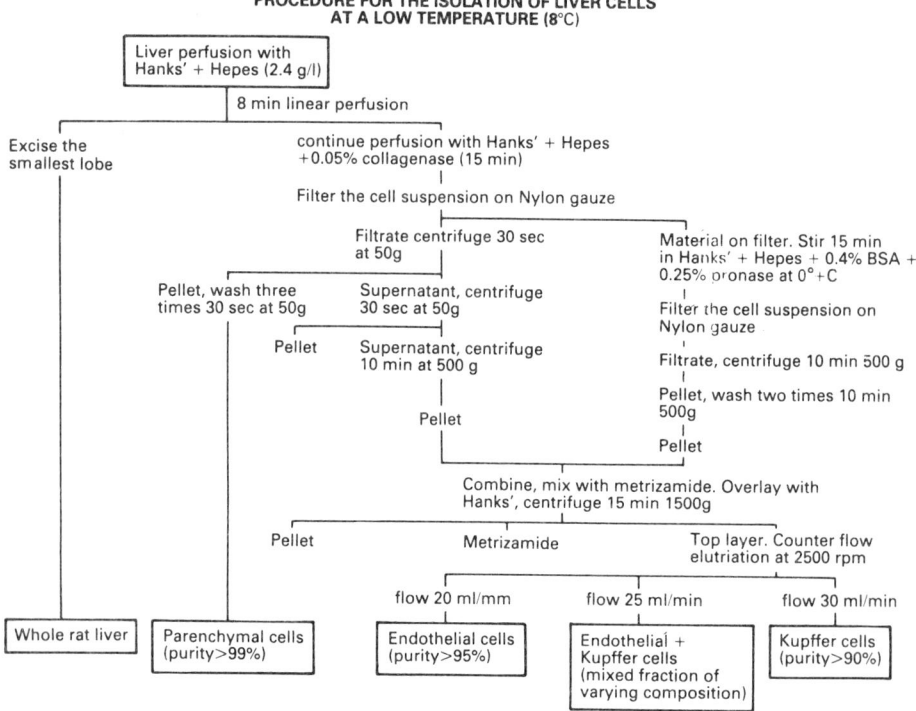

PROCEDURE FOR THE ISOLATION OF LIVER CELLS AT A LOW TEMPERATURE (8°C)

RESULTS

Chylomicrons

Chylomicrons are triglyceride-rich lipoproteins, synthesized by the small intestinal epithelium as vehicles to transport absorbed lipids to the plasma compartment. Electron micrographs have shown that chylomicrons are composed of a homogeneous core surrounded by a surface film. Although the protein moiety of chylomicrons is small (0.5-4% by weight), their role in the interaction with the liver is obvious. In particular, the relative amounts of apolipoproteins C and E are decisive for an interaction with the liver. A determinaton of the *in vivo* hepatic uptake of chylomicrons indicate that 65% of theinjected chylomicrons are recovered in the parenchymal cells (30 min after injection (Groot *et al.*, 1981)). This indicates that chylomicrons form a potential vehicle to transport drugs rapidly to the liver parenchymal cells. Furthermore incorporation of pure apolipoproteins might be utilized to modulate this function.

Very low density lipoproteins (VLDL)

Very low density lipoproteins are synthesized by the liver and transport lipids from the liver to extrahepatic sites. Their size is between 30 and 80 nm (Fig. 1) and they contain as apolipoproteins apo E, B and C. After injection of VLDL into the blood, uptake in the liver is induced, after conversion to so-called VLDL remnants of β-VLDL probably modulated by the apolipoproteins E and C (Fig. 2, (Harkes and van Berkel, 1984)). When at 10 min after injection the various liver cell types are isolated, it is clear that parenchymal liver cells form the major site of uptake (Fig. 3). So it can be concluded that in principle this particle might be utilized for rapid delivery of drugs to liver parenchymal cells (De Water *et al.*, 1990).

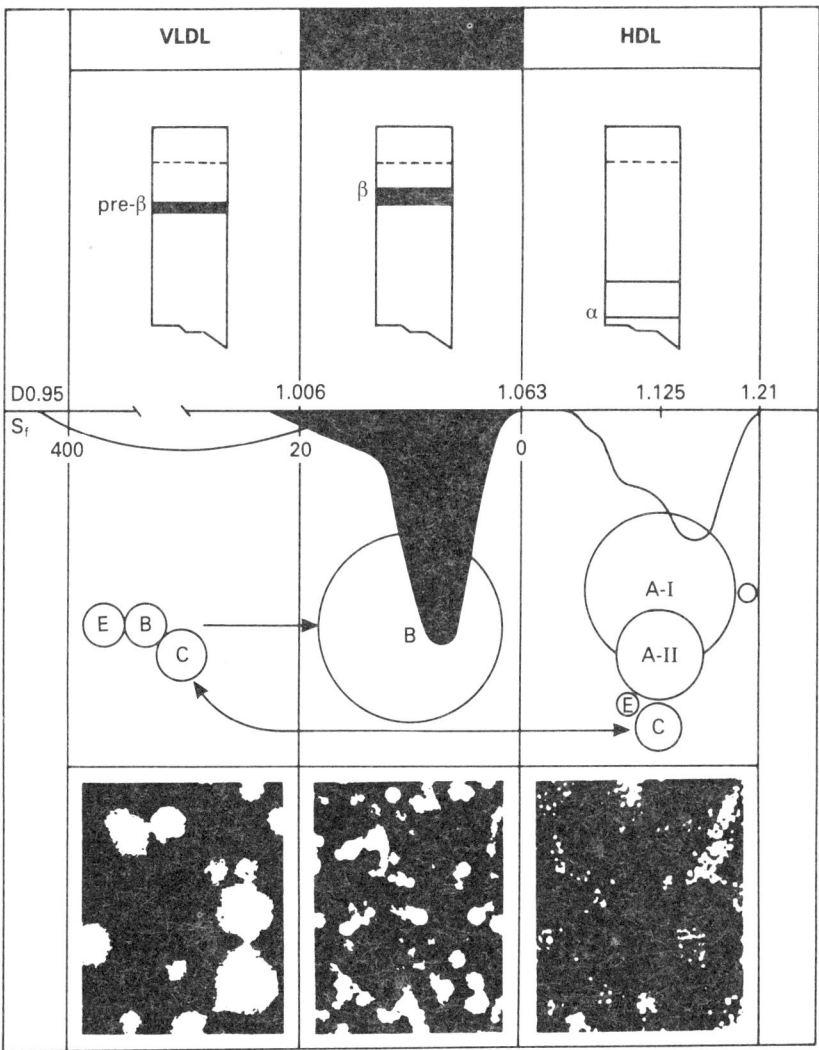

Fig. 1. Human serum lipoproteins. Electrophoretic mobility (top) ultracentrifugal distribution and apolipoprotein composition (middle), and electron micrographs (bottom).

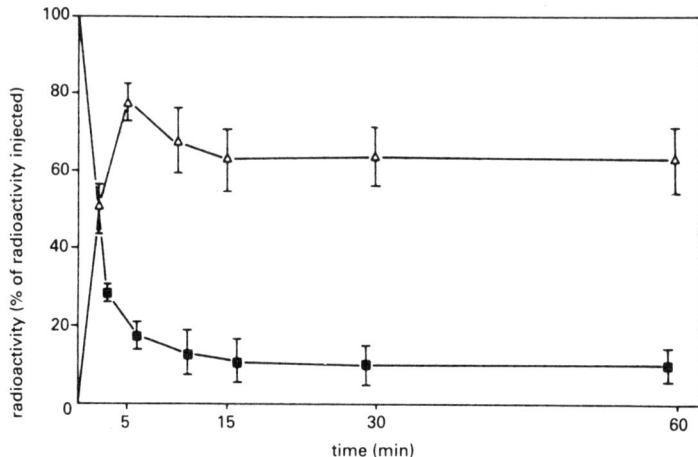

Fig. 2. Liver association and serum decay of [³H]cholesteryl-oleate-labelled β-VLDL. [³H]cholesteryl-oleate-labelled β-VLDL (50 μg apolipoprotein) was injected into anaesthetized rats. At the indicated time points, liver-associated radioactivity (■) and serum radioactivity (Δ) were determined. Data represent te mean of four experiments (±SD).

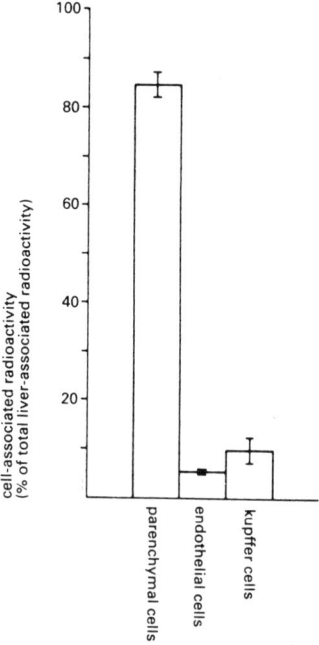

Fig. 3. Association of [³H]cholesteryl-oleate-labelled β-VLDL with parenchymal, endothelial and Kupffer cells *in vivo*. [³H]cholesterol-oleated-labelled β-VLDL (50 μg apolipoprotein) was injected into anaesthetized rats, and 10 min after injection liver perfusion was started. Multiplication of the percentage injected dose/mg cell protein by the amount of protein that each liver cell type contributes to total liver protein results in the [³H]cholesteryl-oleate-labelled β-VLDL uptake by each cell type. Data represent the mean of three experiments (±SD).

Low density (LDL) and high density lipoproteins (HDL)

Low density lipoproteins are a class of lipoproteins with a mean diameter of 23 nm while the high density lipoproteins are smaller (about 10 nm) (Fig. 1).

In order to determine the fate of LDL we labelled the apolipoprotein with ^{14}C-sucrose and determined the serum decay and liver uptake (Harkes and van Berkel, 1984). LDL is slowly removed for serum ($t_{1/2}$ of about 4.5 h) and for the major part (70–80%) recovered in the liver. A determinaton of the uptake in the various liver cells at 4.5 h after injection (Fig. 4) indicates that 71% of the total liver uptake of LDL is exerted by the Kupffer cells. When LDL is methylated, it loses its ability to interact with its specific receptor (van Berkel et al., 1985a). With parenchymal cells no significant difference in uptake between native LDL and methylated LDL was found, whereas it appears that only Kupffer cells internalize LDL in a receptor-dependent way. The data indicated that LDL can be used for drug transport to Kupffer cells with a relatively slow delivery rate.

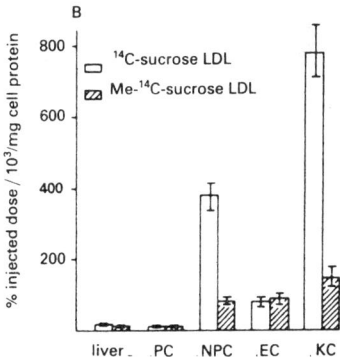

Fig. 4. Distribution of [^{14}C]sucrose-labelled LDL or [^{14}C]sucrose-labelled Me-LDL between parenchymal, endothelial and Kupffer cells.

Recently we synthesized the compound **I** (Kempen et al., 1984):

I. The structure of tris–gal–chol.

This compound was synthesized in order to utilize the active receptor for asialofetuin which is concentrated on liver parenchymal cells as a trigger for the uptake of various types of vesicles. The triantennary galactose-terminated cholesterol derivative (tris-gal–chol) dissolves easily in water and, upon mixing with liposomes, it is immediately incorporated into these particles. Tris-gal–chol addition to LDL leads to an immediate incorporation (Kempen et al., 1984).

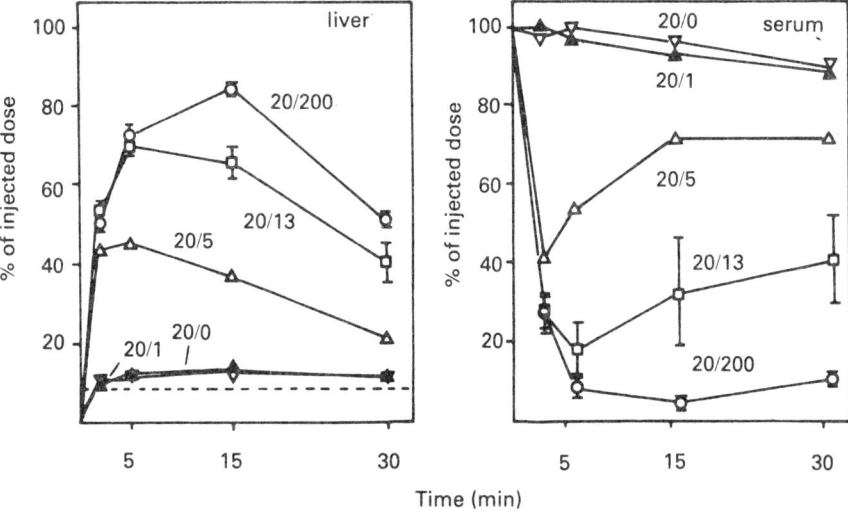

Fig. 5. Effect of tris–gal–chol on the liver association and serum decay of LDL. ^{125}I-LDL (20 µg of apolipoproteins) was mixed with 0 (∇), 1 (▲), 5 (Δ), 13 (□) or 200 (O) µg of tris–gal–chol. The mixture was injected into anaesthetized rats, and the liver association and serum decay were determined.

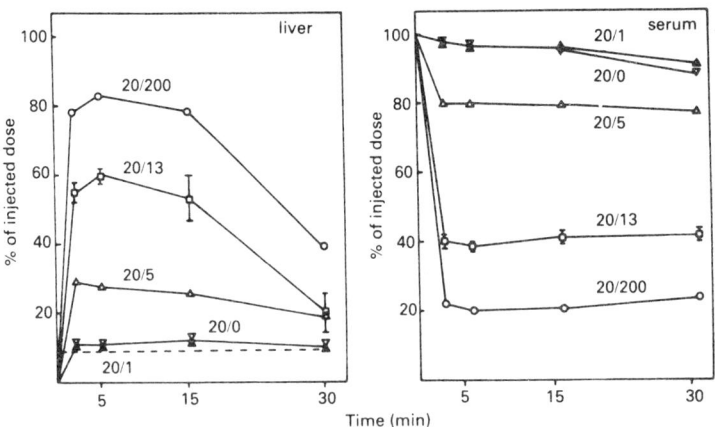

Fig. 6. Effect of tris–gal–chol on the liver association and serum decay of HDL. ^{125}I-HDL (20 µg of apolipoproteins) was mixed with 0 (∇), 1 (▲), 5 (Δ), 13 (□) or 200 (O) µg of tris–gal–chol. The mixture was injected into anaesthetized rats, and the liver association and serum decay were determined.

In Fig. 5 the decay of LDL in serum and uptake in liver is plotted after loading the particles with varying amounts of tris-gal–chol. Incorporation of tris-gal–chol into LDL leads to a markedly increased removal from serum paralleled with a quantitative recovery of the label in liver. Similar experiments performed with HDL show a similar induction of liver uptake by tris-gal–chol (Fig. 6).

The increased decay of tris-gal–chol LDL or tris-gal–chol in serum is nearly completely blocked by preinjection (1 min before the tris-gal–chol LDL) of 0.5 mmol/rat of N-acetylgalactosamine (GalNAc), while preinjection of the same dose of N-acetylglucosamine (GlcNAc) has no effect at all. This indicates that galactose residues mediate the increased liver interaction. When the various liver cell types are isolated at 10 min after injection (Fig. 7) it is clear that tris-gal–chol induces primarily uptake of LDL in Kupffer cells while with HDL uptake by parenchymal cells is highly stimulated. It thus appears that one compound may trigger different types of galactose receptors present on different cell types when incorporated in particles of different sizes (van Berkel et al., 1985a,b).

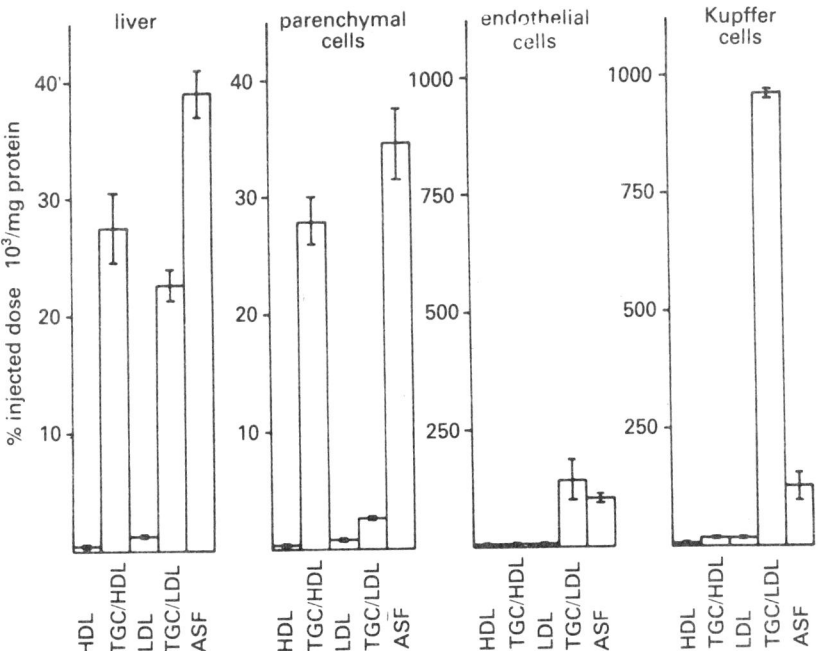

Fig. 7. The effect of tris–gal–chol on the association of HDL and LDL to parenchymal, endothelial and Kupffer cells in comparison with the association of asialofetuin (ASF). ^{125}I-HDL or ^{125}I-LDL (20 μg of apolipoprotein) were mixed with 13 μg of tris{gal–chol (TGC/HDL or TGC/LDL) or the equivalent amount of phosphate-buffered saline (HDL or LDL). 10 mins after injection of the apolipoprotein or ^{125}I-asialofetuin (9 μg), a liver perfusion was started, and the total liver association (after an 8 min perfusion at 8°C) and the association with the subsequently isolated (at 8°C) parenchymal, endothelial and Kupffer cells was determined.

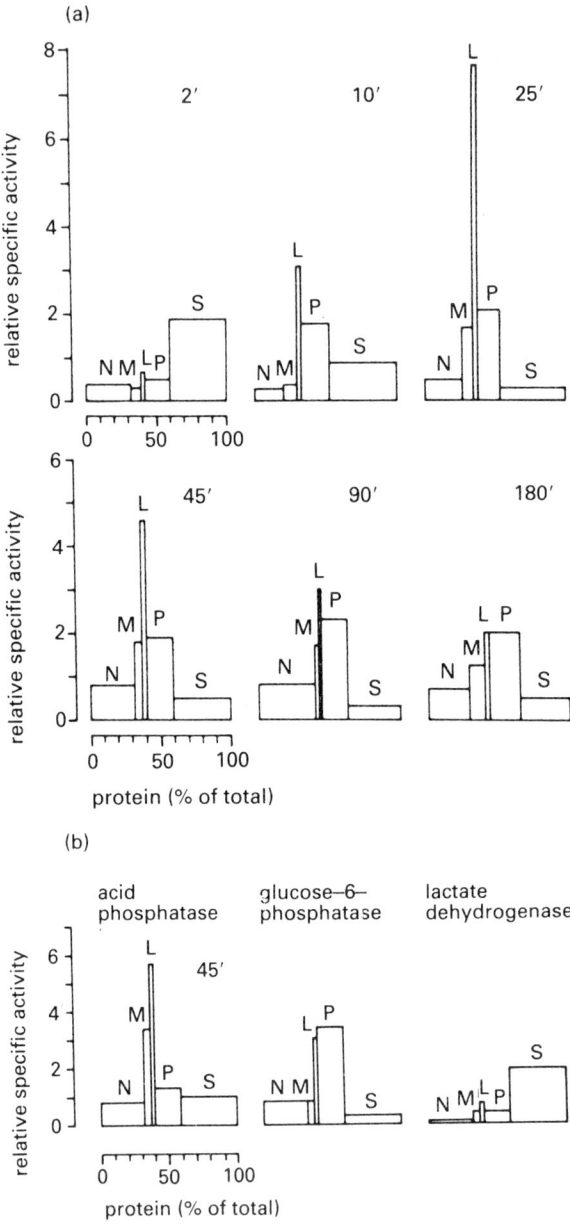

Fig. 8. Hepatic subcellular distribution of [3H]cholesteryl-oleate-labelled β-VLDL. (a) [3H]cholesteryl-oleate-labelled β-VLDL (50 mg apolipoprotein) was injected into anaesthestized rats. At the indicated times after injection, subcellular distribution of radioactivity was determined. N, nuclear fraction; M, mitochondrial fraction; L, lysosomal fraction; P. microsomal fraction; S, final supernatant. (b) Distribtion of the indicated marker enzymes 45 min after injection of β-VLDL.

Intracellular processing

In order to investigate the intracellular fate of carriers, the liver can be subjected to a subcellular fractionation. When the liver is subfractioned at various times after injection of β-VLDL (Fig. 8), it is clear that the radioactivity in the lysosomal fraction (L fraction) increases with time, subsequently followed by a decrease. This indicates that the particles are taken up by the liver cells and subsequently processed by a lysosomal route (De Water et al., 1990). Also, the hepatic processing of tris-gal–chol LDL and HDL appears to involve the lysosomal compartment.

The use of tris-gal–chol might find application in targeting drugs, hormones, or other material of interest to specific liver cell types. The use of liposomes as transport vesicles is hampered by the difficulty in targeting these vesicles rapidly to parenchymal liver cells. The incorporation of tris-gal–chol into HDL leads to a successful and rapid targeting to the asialoglycoprotein (galactose) receptor on hepatocytes. This property might be used to deliver any compound either covalently linked to the protein moiety or incorporated into the lipid core of HDL to the liver parenchymal cells.

Chemical modification of lipoproteins

The fate of the lipoproteins may also be changed upon a chemical modification of the apolipoproteins. For instance, acetylation of LDL leads to a rapid removal of LDL from serum (Table 1).

Table 1. Distribution of radioactivity between liver and serum 3, 10 and 30 min after intravenous injection of acetyl-LDL

Time after injection (min)	Radioactivity distribution (% of injected dose)	
	Liver	Serum
3		
10	83.4 ± 1.7	2.2 ± 0.2
30	18.0 ± 1.2	8.4 ± 0.3

Values are means of three different experiments.

Table 2. Relative contribution of the different liver cell types to the total liver uptake of asialofetuin, tris–gal–chol HDL, [^{14}C]sucrose-labelled LDL, acetylated LDL, chylomicrons and β-VLDL

Cell type	Asialofetuin	Tris–gal–chol HDL	Tris–gal–chol LDL	[^{14}C]sucrose-labelled LDL	Acetylated LDL	Chylomicrons	β-VLDL
Parenchymal cells (%)	82.5	98.0	7.7	29	38	65	96
Endothelial cells (%)	9.3	0.5	15.5	9	53	35	1
Kupffer cells (%)	8.2	1.5	76.8	62	9		3

The amount of radioactivity per mg cell protein in the isolated cell fractions was multiplied by the amount of protein that each cell type contributes to total liver protein. Lipoproteins (20 μg apolipoproteins) were mixed with 13 μg tris–gal–chol. The values are calculated from the mean of 3 independent experiments for each substrate.

Isolated endothelial cells contained more acetyl-LDL per mg of cell protein than Kupffer cells and hepatocytes (Table 2). This uptake is mediated by a highly active receptor (scavenger receptor) on the liver endothelial cells (Nagelkerke *et al.*, 1983). Morphological studies on the interaction of acetyl-LDL conjugated to 20 nm colloidal gold illustrate that the liver endothelial cells bind acetyl-LDL in coated pits, which is followed by rapid uptake (Mommaas-Kienhuis *et al.*, 1985). Uptake proceeds through small coated vesicles and finally degradation of the apoprotein occurs in the lysosomes.

Incorporation of (pro)drugs into lipoproteins
The apolar core of lipoproteins provides an ideal domain for highly lipophilic drugs. Drugs that are transported in the core of a lipoprotein carrier are protected from the environment during transport; also, the environment is protected from the drug. Furthermore, a drug that is located inside the lipid moiety of a lipoprotein carrier is not able to disturb the recognition of the (modified) apoprotein present on the surface of the particle. Amphiphilic compounds can also be incorporated into lipoproteins. Such compounds are not incorporated into the apolar core, but in the more amphiphilic phospholipid coat. An example is tris-gal–chol. The cholesterol moiety incorporates into lipoproteins, while the galactose residues protrude. A disadvantage of an amphiphilic compound is, however, that the compound is not shielded from the environment during transport and that it may affect the specific uptake of the carrier.

Some highly lipophilic drugs (e.g. porphyrin-containing compounds, diphenylhydantoin, reserpine and oestradiol) incorporate spontaneously into lipoproteins. However, most of the drugs that are currently used for the treatment of diseases are too hydrophilic. For incorporation into lipoproteins, these drugs have to be rendered more lipophilic by the coupling of hydrophobic residues. Such a derivatized compound can be referred to as a prodrug. Oleyl, retinyl and cholesteryl residues, which are naturally present in the lipid moieties of lipoproteins, are particularly suitable for this purpose. Other lipophilic groups may also be used. It has been shown, for instance, that coupling of a hexadecyl chain facilitates the incorporation of methotrexate and cytosine arabinoside into LDL and HDL.

Derivatization of the drug by the coupling of these hydrophobic 'anchors' will probably affect its pharmacological activity. It is therefore essential that, once inside the cell, the anchors can be removed to yield the original drug. The lysosomal compartment, the intracellular destination of most of the lipoprotein carriers discussed above, contains a wide array of hydrolytic enzymes. Linkages that are sensitive to lysosomal enzymes, such as ester and peptide bonds, are therefore very useful. When the hydrophobic anchors are released, the original drug has to diffuse to its intracellular target to be pharmacologically active. If the intracellular target is not located in the lysosomes, it is necessary that the drug is able to pass the lysosomal membrane. The ability of a compound to permeate the lysosomal membrane depends largely on its size. The lysosomal membrane is readily permeable for compounds with a molecular weight lower than about 200. In addition factors such as ionization, hydrophobicity and steric configuration may affect the penetration. Some compounds with molecular weights exceeding 200, for instance nucleosides, are able to pass lysosomal membranes because of the hydrophobic character of (part of) the molecule. Furthermore, in order to survive its (short) stay in the lysosomes, the original drug has to be sufficiently resistant to lysosomal hydrolases and the low lysosomal pH.

In conclusion, to use a (modified) lipoprotein carrier for the transport of a drug to its (intra)cellular target, the following conditions have to be met.

(1) The drug needs to possess a high affinity for the lipid moiety of the lipoprotein carrier, either on its own or after the attachment of hydrophobic residues.
(2) The (derivatized) drug should remain firmly associated with the carrier during transport in the circulation.
(3) If present, the hydrophobic anchor attached to the drug needs to be removed in the lysosomes.
(4) The original drug should be sufficiently stable in the lysosomes, and it should be able to diffuse from the lysosomal compartment to its intracellular targets.

Some potential applications
LDL-mediated delivery of cytotoxic agents to tumour cells
In vivo, only liver, and to a smaller extent endocrine glands, intestine and spleen, show substantial uptake of LDL. The expression of LDL receptors on the surface of a cell is regulated by its need for cholesterol. Tumour cells require large amounts of cholesterol for their replication, and uptake of LDL cholesterol from the circulation may meet these requirements. It has been found that a number of tumour cell lines are highly active in the uptake of LDL. The number of LDL receptors on normal cells is regulated by the metabolic state of the cell, and depends on the amount of intracellular cholesterol and the rate of intracellular cholesterol synthesis. The uptake of LDL by the liver, for instance, can be regulated by the diet. Dietary fat is transported to the liver by chylomicron remnants, which are taken up by parenchymal cells via the remnant receptor. It has been shown in hamsters that the receptor-dependent uptake of LDL by the liver can be reduced by 90% by feeding the animals a diet with a particular fat composition. Tumour cells lack many of the regulatory mechanisms present in normal cells, and in some tumour cells the regulation of the LDL receptor is lost too. Such tumour cells express a high number of LDL receptors under conditions where receptors in normal tissues are down regulated. Under these conditions, LDL loaded with a cytotoxic drug may selectively be delivered to tumour cells, whereas normal tissues are protected. Not only cytotoxic drugs but also photosensitive porphyrins (which incorporate easily into lipoproteins) may be delivered to tumour cells in this way. In the so-called photodynamic therapy, a porphyrin-loaded tumour is subsequently exposed to visible light. The phorphyrins act as photosensitizers and convert light energy to chemical energy, which results in severe biological damage. By selectively illuminating tumour tissue, an additional degree of specificity is obtained.

Solid tumours are usually poorly perfused, and therefore not readily accessible for LDL. Application of cytotoxic drug-loaded LDL in the treatment of cancer is probably most effective in combination with other therapies. Drug-loaded LDL may be used to eradicate residual tumour cells after elimination of the bulk of the tumour mass by surgery or radiotherapy.

Delivery of antiviral drugs to parenchymal liver cells
Tris-gal–chol-loaded HDL is taken up rapidly and very specifically via the galactose-specific receptors on parenchymal liver cells. The remnant receptor on this cell type mediates uptake of chylomicron remnants and β-VLDL. These (modified) lipoprotein particles might therefore be used to deliver drugs specifically to parenchymal liver cells. An attractive potential application is the delivery of antiviral drugs to parenchymal cells, in order to treat a viral infection such as hepatitis B. Drugs that are currently used for the treatment of hepatitis B, such as acyclovir and adenosine arabinoside, have a low specificity for the liver because less than 10% of the administered dose of these drugs is taken up by the liver of various species.

Targeting of immunomodulators, antivirals and antiparasitic drugs to Kupffer and endothelial cells
Tris-gal–chol-loaded LDL is taken up rapidly and selectively via the galactose-specific receptors on Kupffer cells, and this particle is therefore an attractive carrier for the specific delivery of drugs to this cell type. It could be particularly useful for the introduction into Kupffer cells of drugs that modulate the immunological activity of these cells. For instance, activation of Kupffer cells to a tumoricidal state might prevent the development of liver metastases, a serious clinical problem. Lipophilic derivatives of the immunomodulator muramyl dipeptide seem very suitable for this purpose. Preliminary experiments in our laboratory indicate that such compounds can indeed be incorporated into tris-gal–chol-loaded LDL and render Kupffer cells tumoricidal.

In addition, the particle may be used in the treatment of infections of Kupffer cells. For instance, Kupffer cells can be infected by a number of parasites (e.g. *Leishmania donovani* and malaria parasites), and it was reported recently that Kupffer and endothelial cells can be infected by the human immunodeficiency virus (HIV). Like antiviral drugs (see above), antiparasitic drugs such as primaquine have a low specificity for the liver. Tris-gal–chol-loaded LDL could, therefore, be applied for the selective delivery of antiviral and antiparasitic drugs to Kupffer cells. Acetylated LDL, on the other hand, could be used as a vehicle for the specific delivery of antiviral drugs to virus-infected endothelial liver cells.

CONCLUDING REMARKS
The ability to introduce rapidly chylomicrons (Groot *et al.*, 1981) and β-VLDL (de Water *et al.*, 1990) into parenchymal cells, acetylated LDL into endothelial cells (Naagelkerke *et al.* 1983), tris-gal-chol LDL into Kupffer cells (van Berkel *et al.*, 1985a) and tris-gal–chol HDL into parenchymal cells (van Berkel *et al.*, 1985b) clearly indicates that, in a complex tissue such as liver, successful targeting of lipoproteins to the cell of choice can be achieved. The efficiency and specificity of these uptake processes may be modulated by individual apolipoproteins or modification of surface characteristics. Provided that basic knowledge (especially receptor characteristics) is available, it can be speculated that similar approaches are possible for other cell types or tissues. It will be a challenge to apply these new strategies for site-specific drug delivery in which both industrial laboratories and university centres for biopharmaceu-

tical sciences may combine practical approaches with basic cellbiological achievements.

ACKNOWLEDGEMENTS

Martha Wieriks is thanked for the preparation of the manuscript and secretarial help. This research was partly supported by Grant 31.014 from the Dutch Heart Foundation.

REFERENCES

De Water, R., Hessels, E. M. A. J., Bakkeren, H. F. and van Berkel, Th. J. C. (1990) *Eur. J. Biochem.* **192** 419–425.
Groot, P. H. E., van Berkel, Th. J. C. and van Tol, A. (1981) *Metabolism* **30** 792–797.
Harkes, L. and van Berkel, Th. J. C. (1984) *Biochem. J.* **224** 21–27.
Kempen, H. J. M., Hoes, G., van Boom, J. H., Spanjer, H. H., de Lange, J., Langendoen, A. and van Berkel, Th. J. C. (1984) *J. Med. Chem.* **27** 1306–1312.
Mommaas-Kienhuis, A. M., Nagelkerke, J. F., Vermeer, B. J., Daems, W. Th. and van Berkel, Th. J. C. (1985) *Eur. J. Cell. Biol.* **38** 42–50.
Nagelkerke, J. F., Barto, K. P. and van Berkel, Th. J. C. (1983) *J. Biol. Chem.* **258** 12221–12227.
Van Berkel, Th. J. C., Kruijt, J. K., Spanjer, H. H., Nagelkerke, J. F., Harkes, L. and Kempen, H. J. M. (1985a) *J. Biol. Chem.* **260** 2694–2699.
Van Berkel, Th. J. C., Kruijt, J. K. and Kempen, H. J. M. (1985b) *J. Biol. Chem.* **260** 12203–12207.

3

Novel immunoliposome targeting system avoiding reticuloendothelial cell interactions

Atsuhide Mori, Dexi Liu and Leaf Huang

INTRODUCTION

Liposomes have attracted a considerable amount of interest for potential use as a drug delivery system owing to their suitable characteristics. They consist of one or more concentric phospholipid bilayers enclosing an aqueous space. They are biocompatible, biodegradable, and normally nonimmunogenic. More importantly, they are capable of loading both hydrophilic and hydrophobic drugs in the aqueous and bilayer phase, respectively. Drugs encapsulated in liposomes are protected from enzymatic degradation and other inactivation processes.

There are basically two different modes in liposome targeting: passive and active targeting. The former takes advantage of the fact that systemically injected liposomes are rapidly and efficiently taken up by phagocytic cells of the reticuloendothelial system (RES) located mainly in the liver and the spleen (for a review, see Hwang, 1987). This natural homing activity of liposomes provides an effective targeting system for the liver and the spleen, and various studies have been carried out with this targeting mode (for a review, see Alving, 1986). However, this predominant uptake of liposomes by the RES and a resulting rapid clearance from the circulation have been a major obstacle in any attempt to deliver liposomes to cells, tissues or organs other than the RES, which is referred to as 'active targeting'. One of the exciting approaches in the active targeting of liposomes takes advantage of a specific ligand-receptor interaction. Liposomes are covalently or noncovalently linked to a suitable ligand for the target specificity. Antibody-directed liposomes, or so-called 'immunoliposomes', have been extensively studied because of their high degrees of specificity and versatility (for a review, see Wright and Huang, 1989). A number of methods for covalent conjugation of antibody on the liposome surface have been developed. While the rationale of this approach has been well established in various *in vitro* systems, vigorous *in vivo* studies of immunoliposome targeting have been carried out only recently. Several studies have shown that considerable amounts of immunoliposomes also accumulate in the liver and the spleen, showing the difficulty arising from the vivid RES competition for liposomes uptake (for a review, see Peeters *et al.*, 1987). If the rate of immunoliposome binding to the target is less than the rate of uptake by the RES, little if any target binding would be expected.

One of the current efforts in the active targeting of liposomes is to overcome the above-described kinetic barrier by manipulating the liposomes characteristics such that the affinity of liposomes to the RES is reduced and the circulation time of liposomes is thus increased. In this chapter, we will first describe details of the construction and optimization of this novel type of liposome, and then describe our efforts to design immunoliposomes for efficient targeting based on the development of such long-circulating liposomes.

LIPOSOMES WITH REDUCED AFFINITY TO THE RETICULOENDOTHELIAL SYSTEM

The *in vivo* biodistribution of liposomes has been exhaustively studied in the last decade (for a review, see Senior, 1987). Many studies have been focused on the mechanism underlying the efficient uptake of liposomes by the RES. It is now generally understood that the mononucleophagocytes of the RES, principally the Kupffer cells of the liver and secondarily the splenic macrophages, are responsible for the clearance of liposomes from the circulation (Segal *et al.*, 1974; Scherphof *et al.*, 1986). In addition, the parenchymal cells of the liver are also involved in liposome uptake (Gregoriadis and Ryman, 1972). Furthermore, serum factor(s) (opsonins) coating the liposome surface are believed to promote the specific uptake of liposomes by the liver and the spleen, although these molecules have not been identified (Moghimi and Patel, 1989). These interactions obviously depend on the physical and chemical characteristics of the liposomes. Thus, our effort has been to optimize some variables in the construction of liposomes such that the affinity of the liposomes to the RES is reduced and the circulation time is prolonged. Two such variables, lipid composition and liposome size, have been optimized in this regard.

Optimization of lipid composition

Liposomes can be prepared from a variety of lipid components. Some parameters of liposomes, such as the bilayer rigidity and surface charge, depend largely on the lipid composition and also affect the stability of liposomes. The basic lipid composition of liposomes consists of a mixture of phospholipid and cholesterol (chol). Inclusion of chol results in an enhanced structural stability of liposomes in serum, resulting in a relatively prolonged circulation time as compared with the chol-free liposomes (Patel *et al.*, 1983). A major breakthrough, however, is the recent finding that inclusion of a glycolipid such as monosialoganglioside (GM_1), hydrogenated phosphatidylinositol, sulphatides (Allen and Chonn, 1987; Gabizon and Papahadjopoulos, 1988; Allen *et al.*, 1989; Liu and Huang, 1990) and amphipathic polyethyleneglycol (PEG) (Klibanov *et al.*, 1990, 1991; Blume and Cevc, 1990; Senior *et al.*, 1991) in the lipid composition results in a significantly prolonged circulation time of liposomes. Fig. 1 shows the activities of various PEGs conjugated to phosphatidylethanolamine (PEG–PEs) and GM_1 in prolonging the circulation time of liposomes. Liposomes used in this study were prepared, using the extrusion method, from phosphatidylcholine (PC) and chol (2:1, molar) also containing 6.3 mol.% of PEG–PE or GM_1. Inclusion of PEG–PE or GM_1 in the lipid composition results in a reduced clearance rate from the circulation with a

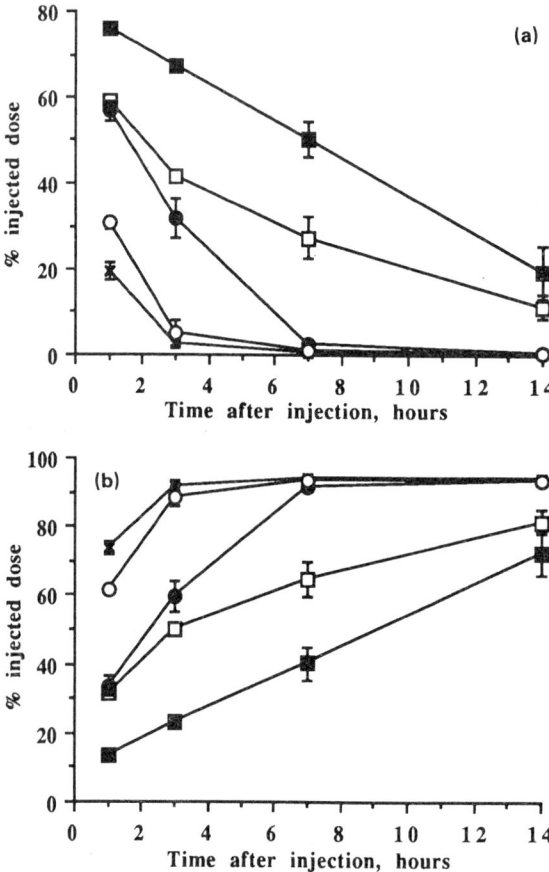

Fig. 1. Effect of PEG–PE and GM_1 on (a) blood clearance and (b) RES uptake of liposomes. Liposomes composed of PC and chol (2:1, molar) and also containing 6.3 mol.% of either PEG–PE or GM_1 were prepared by the extrusion method. Briefly, the solvent-free lipid mixture containing 1 mol.% of ^{111}In-labelled diethylenetriamine pentaacetic acid distearylamide comlex (DTPA–SA) as a lipid marker (Kabalka et al., 1987) was hydrated with phosphate-buffered saline (PBS) (pH 7.5) overnight. The liposome suspension was extruded several times through Nucleopore membranes to generate liposomes with about 200 nm in average diameter. The resulting ^{111}In-labelled liposomes (400 µg lipid) were injected i.v. into Balb/c mice. At indicated time intervals, percent injected dose of liposomes in blood, the RES (liver and spleen) was examined by ^{111}In radioactive counting. The total radioactivity in the blood was determined by assuming that the total volume of blood was 7.3% of the body weight. Bars represent S.D. ($n = 3$). X, PC–chol; O, PC–chol–PEG750–PE; ●, PC–chol–PEG2000–PE; ∎, PC–chol–PEG5000–PE; □, PC–chol–GM_1. (Data taken from Mori et al. (1991) with permission.)

concomitant decrease in the rate of RES uptake. The estimated half-life for liposome blood clearance increased from 0.5 h to 0.7 h, 1.7 h, 6.2 h, and 3.4 h by the inclusion of PEG750–PE, PEG2000–PE, PEG5000–PE, and GM_1, respectively. Thus, the activity of PEG–PE in prolonging the circulation time of liposomes is directly proportional to the polymer chain length: the longer the polymer chain, the higher the activity. Activities of the above amphiphiles in prolonging the circulation time of liposomes are concentration dependent, plateauing at 5 mol.% of the total lipid (except for PEG750–PE which plateaus at 10 mol.%).

The mechanism of action of the above amphiphiles in prolonging the circulation time of liposomes has not been fully elucidated. However, it has been postulated that an increased hydrophilicity (Senior *et al.*, 1991) and/or steric barrier on the liposome surface (Klibanov *et al.*, 1990, 1991; Blume and Cevc, 1990) may prevent or reduce interactions of liposomes with serum constituents, thus resulting in an enhanced stability of liposomes and a reduced rate of specific and/or nonspecific interaction with the RES. The 'steric barrier hypothesis' is supported by a study with a liposome agglutination assay to assess the degree of steric barrier produced on the liposome surface by PEG–PEs (Mori *et al.*, 1991). This assay takes advantage of the fact that the agglutination of liposomes containing biotinamidocaproyl-phosphatidylethanolamine (biotin-cap–PE), mediated by streptavidin, requires a close apposition of the neighbouring liposomes (Klibanov *et al.*, 1989). Thus, a decrease in the liposome turbidity compared with the control liposomes directly reflects the relative steric barrier activity on the liposome surface. It is clear from the data in Fig. 2 that the steric barrier activity of PEG–PE is directly proportional to the polymer chain length: the longer the polymer chain, the stronger the steric barrier, which is in turn directly proportional to the activity in prolonging the circulation time of liposomes. Thus, the mechanism by which PEG–PE reduces the RES uptake of liposomes can be attributed at least partially to the steric barrier presented by these polymers on the liposome surface. Also shown in Fig. 2 is that the steric barrier activity of PEG–PE is also concentration dependent: the higher the concentration of PEG–PE, the stronger the steric barrier activity. Other study using radiolabelled streptavidin showed that the inhibitory effect of PEG5000–PE on the binding of streptavidin to liposomes containing biotincap–PE is also concentration dependent (Klibanov *et al.*, 1991). However, no significant inhibitory effect was observed at low concentrations of PEG–PE, indicating that a protein molecule, i.e. streptavidin, is able to penetrate a relatively weak steric barrier. These results suggest two independent modes of action of PEG–PE. Firstly, the presence of PEG may increase the hydrophilicity of the liposome surface and reduce nonspecific interaction of liposomes with the RES. Secondly, the steric barrier of PEG may prevent opsonins from direct interaction with the liposomes and thus reduce specific interaction of liposomes with the RES. Maximal activity of PEG–PE in prolonging the circulation time of liposomes can be obtained when sufficient concentration and polymer chain length are used so that both specific and nonspecific interactions of liposomes with the RES are minimized. On the other hand, the mechanism of action of GM_1 is not obvious. It is unlikely that GM_1 prolongs the circulation time of liposomes entirely through the steric barrier mechanism. The steric barrier activity of GM_1 is weaker than that of PEG2000–PE; however, its activity in prolonging the circulation time of liposomes is greater than that of PEG2000-PE (Fig. 1). Allen et al. (1985) have shown that incorporation of gangliosides results in enhanced stability of liposomes in the presence of serum, as shown by the reduced leakage of aqueous markers from liposomes. The stabilizing effect of gangliosides depends on the number of sialic acid residues: the higher order the ganglioside, the greater the activity in enhancing the stability of liposomes. However, among various gangliosides, GM_1 is unique in terms of having a strong activity in prolonging the circulation time of liposomes; other gangliosides such as GD_{1a} and GT_{1b} exhibit only little or no activity (Allen, 1989). This and our results from the liposomes agglutination assay indicate that the stabilizing effect of GM_1 via the steric barrier provided by the oligosaccharide residues is probably not a major mechanism in prolonging the circulation time of liposomes.

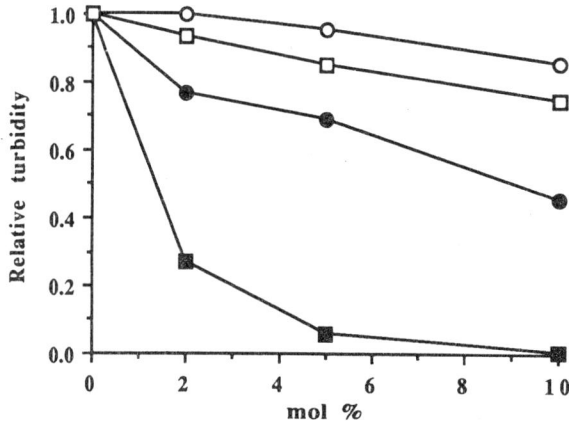

Fig. 2. Effect of increasing concentrations of PEG-PE and GM_1 on streptavidin-induced agglutination of liposomes containing biotin-cap-PE. Liposomes composed of PC and chol (1:1, molar) and also containing 2.5 mol.% of biotin-cap-PE and various amounts of PEG-PE or GM_1 were prepared by the extrusion method as described in Fig. 1. The agglutination was initiated by mixing the liposome suspension (60 γg phospholipid in 560 γl PBS, pH 7.5) with 10 γg streptavidin in a microcuvette. Increase in turbidity, monitored by optical density at 440 nm, was measured 12 min after incubation and was normalized with respect to the control liposomes composed of PC and chol. O, PC-chol-PEG750-PE; ●, PC-chol-PEG2000-PE; ■, PC-chol-PEG5000-PE; □, PC-chol-GM_1. (Data taken from Mori et al. (1991) with permission.)

Several studies have also shown the importance of bilayer rigidity in prolonging the circulation time of liposomes (Hwang, et al., 1980; Senior and Gregoriadis, 1982; Allen and Chonn, 1987; Allen et al., 1989; Gabizon and Papahadjopoulos, 1988). Allen and Chonn (1987) have shown that the use of phospholipids having a high melting temperature such as sphingomyelin and distearoylphosphatidylcholine (DSPC) leads to further increase in the circulation time of GM_1-containing liposomes. The mechanism of these phospholipids in improving the circulation time of GM_1-containing liposomes has been attributed to the increased bilayer rigidity, as a result of the diminished rotational and translational diffusions of the lipids at the physiological temperature, and thus the enhanced stability of liposomes. To test this hypothesis, we have compared the membrane rigidity between dioleoylphosphatidylethanolamine (DOPE)- and DSPC-based liposomes, as a model of the fluid and rigid liposomes, respectively. The membrane microviscosity was determined by measuring the fluorescence depolarization of a hydrophobic probe, diphenylhexatriene, incorporated into the lipid core of the liposome membrane (Shinitzky and Barenholz, 1978; Liu et al., 1989). As can be seen from the data in Table 1, DSPC-based liposomes have much higher microviscosities than DOPE-based liposomes in phosphate-buffered saline (PBS). However, the microviscosity of the liposome membrane changed significantly after the plasma treatment. The DOPE-based liposomes with low microviscosity in PBS showed increased microviscosity after the plasma treatment. Plasma treatment had also significantly decreased the microviscosities of DSPC-based 'rigid' liposomes. Thus, treatment of liposomes with plasma showed a 'buffer' effect on the microviscosity of liposomes; it made the originally large difference in microviscosity among the different lipid compositions much smaller. Furthermore, both GM_1-containing DOPE- and DSPC-based liposomes showed the prolonged circulation time irrespective of the large difference in their microviscosities. These results indicate that the membrane rigidity is not a strong requirement in liposome construction for the prolonged circulation.

Table 1. Effect of plasma exposure on liposome microviscosity

Composition (molar ratio)	Microviscosity (poise)	
	PBS	Human Plasma
DOPE–OA (10:5)	0.761 (0.038)	1.194 (0.115)
DOPE–OA–GM_1 (10:5:1)	0.807 (0.054)	1.290 (0.114)
DOPE–OA–DSPC (40:20:40)	2.929 (0.133)	2.632 (0.090)
DSPC–chol (10:5)	22.154 (0.340)	5.991 (0.125)
DSPC–chol–GM_1 (10:5:1)	19.029 (1.458)	6.312 (0.170)

Liposomes (10 mM) containing 0.25 mol.% diphenylhexatriene were incubated with equal volume of either PBS or human plasma for 1 h at 37°C, followed by chromatography on a BioGel A1.5M column. Fluorescence anisotropy was measured in five determinations, which was used to calculate the microviscosity according to Shinitzky and Barenholz (1978).

Optimization of liposome size
In addition to the lipid composition, liposome size also plays an important role in determining the biodistribution of liposomes. Our systematic biodistribution study using GM_1-containing liposomes with homogeneous size distribution showed that the activity of GM_1 in prolonging the circulation time is restricted to a relatively narrow size range (Liu et al., 1991b). Optimal liposome size for prolonged circulation ranges from 70 to 200 nm in average diameter (Fig. 3). The larger liposomes have an increased tendency to accumulate in the spleen (Klibanov et al., 1991; Liu et al., 1991a), whereas the smaller liposomes accumulate in the liver very efficiently (Liu et al., 1991b). In contrast, this size-dependent accumulation in the spleen and the liver is less profound for the liposomes containing no GM_1. The preferential accumulation of GM_1-containing large and small liposomes in the spleen and the liver, respectively, can be attributed to

the anatomical structures of these organs in addition to their lower affinity to the RES, in particular the Kupffer cells of the liver. Since GM_1-containing liposomes show the reduced affinity to the liver Kupffer cells, they have an increased chance to stay in the circulation. When liposomes are large enough (>300 nm in diameter), they are retained by the splenic sinusoidal filter, thus resulting in the enhanced accumulation in the spleen. On the other hand, sufficiently small liposomes (>70 nm in diameter) can extravasate to the liver parenchyma through the holes (approximately 100 nm in average diameter) located in the fenestrae of the liver sinus (Wisse, 1970), thus resulting in the enhanced accumulation in the liver. Thus, the mechanisms responsible for the biodistribution of small and large liposomes are basically different. The highest circulation level of GM_1-containing liposomes can be obtained using liposomes of appropriate size, i.e. between 70 and 200 nm in diameter; the total uptake of these liposomes by the spleen and the liver is minimized. Although we specifically discussed the importance of liposome size using GM_1-containing liposomes, it is likely that the activities of other amphiphiles such as amphipathic PEG in prolonging the circulation time of liposomes are also liposome size dependent.

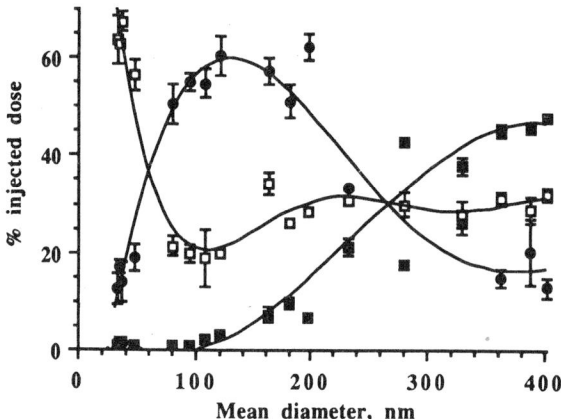

Fig. 3. Size-dependent biodistribution of GM_1-containing liposomes. ^{111}In-labelled liposomes composed of PC, chol and GM_1 (10:5:1, molar) with defined diameter were prepared by the extrusion method as described in Fig. 1. Liposomes (1 μmol lipid) were i.v. injected, and biodistribution was examined 4 h after injection. Data are expressed as per cent injected dose of liposomes in blood (●), spleen (■) and liver (□). Bars represent S.D. (n = 3). (Data taken from Liu et al. (1991b) with permission.)

Applications of long-circulating liposomes

The above-described development of long-circulating liposomes offers several potential applications which have been previously proven to be difficult. An immediate application is to deliver the liposomes to cells, tissues, or organs other than the RES. Gabizon and Papahadjopoulos (1988) have shown that GM_1-containing liposomes accumulate in an experimental solid tumour more efficiently than the conventional liposomes. This is presumably due to the ability of such long-circulating liposomes to extravasate the leaky vessels of the tumour. This hypothesis was supported by our finding that GM_1-containing liposomes with 90 or 190 nm average diameter showed much higher accumulation in the murine EMT-6 solid tumour than those with a diameter of 40 nm or greater than 200 nm (Liu et al., 1991b). These results clearly show the importance of prolonged circulation for the accumulation of liposomes in tumour. Consequently, the long-circulating liposomes would be expected to deliver cytotoxic drugs to tumours efficiently (Gabizon et al., 1989). Several preliminary studies have shown the improved therapeutic index of cytotoxic drugs using these liposomes (Gabizon, 1990; Martin et al., 1990; Papahadjopoulos, 1990). In addition to the above-discussed passive targeting of liposomes to the tumour, the efficiency of active targeting of liposomes via the ligand-receptor interaction, e.g. immunoliposome targeting, would also be enhanced by the prolonged circulation time of liposomes.

HIGHLY TARGETABLE IMMUNOLIPOSOMES

A pulmonary endothelial model for liposome targeting

One of the important factors for successful targeting of immunoliposomes *in vivo* is the choice of antibody–antigen system. Several variables including antibody specificity and affinity, antigen concentration on the target site(s), and accessibility of the antigen to the antibody depend on the individual system to be used and directly affect the feasibility of liposome targeting. Moreover, in view of the fact that liposomes are too large to penetrate most of the endothelial barrier of the vascular wall, i.v. injected immunoliposomes would be expected to interact efficiently with the target site only within the intravascular compartment. Considering these factors, the monoclonal antibody 34A (MoAb 34A) system is a nearly ideal model for the study of *in vivo* immunoliposome targeting. MoAb 34A is a rat IgG_{2a} which binds specifically with a glycoprotein antigen, gp112, expressed in high concentrations on the luminal surface of the capillary endothelial cells of the mouse lung (Rorvik et al., 1988; Kennel et al., 1988). For the preparation of immunoliposomes, we have developed a detergent-dialysis method (Holmberg et al., 1989). Antibody molecule is first conjugated to *N*-glutarylphosphatidylethanolamine (Weissig et al., 1986) in the presence of detergent. The resulting amphipathic antibody is then mixed with the lipid–detergent mixture, and the incorporation of antibody is achieved upon the removal of the detergent by dialysis. Fig. 4 shows the representative biodistribution of MoAb 34A bearing liposomes (34A-liposomes). The i.v. injected 34A-liposomes gain direct access to the lung target and accumulate primarily in the lung and secondarily in the liver, while liposomes without antibody molecules accumulate exclusively in the liver and the spleen and nothing is found in the lung (Hughes et al., 1989; Maruyama et al., 1990a; Holmberg et al., 1990). Lung binding of 34A-liposomes was completely blocked by a preinjection of free MoAb 34A, indicating that the binding of 34A-liposomes with the lung is via immunospecific interactions. We have thus used the MoAb 34A system to study various factors affecting the *in vivo* targeting of immunoliposomes. An earlier study showed that the efficiency of target binding of 34A-liposomes strongly depends on the antibody density of liposomes. The higher the antibody density, the higher the rate and extent of target binding of immunoliposomes.

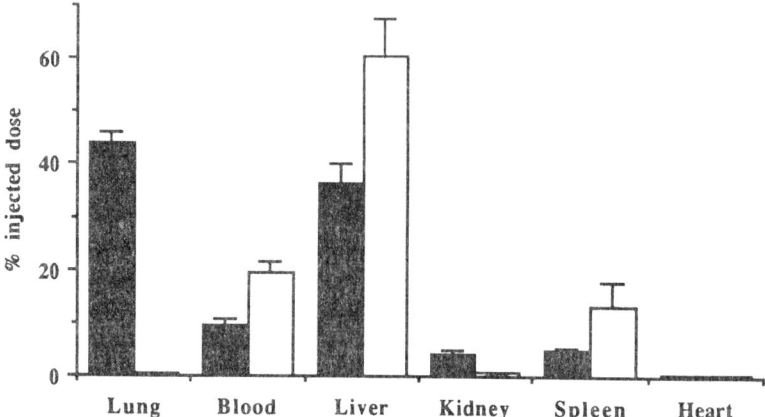

Fig. 4. Biodistribution of 34A-liposomes ad bare liposomes. Bare liposomes were prepared by the extrusion method as described in Fig. 1. Immunoliposomes composed of PC and chol (2:1 molar) were prepared by the detergent–dialysis method (Holmberg et al., 1989). Briefly, the lipid mixture containing 1 mol.% of ^{111}In-labelled DTPA–SA solubilized with octylglucoside in PBS (pH 7.5) was mixed with preconjugated antibody to NGPE at a lipid-to-antibody weight ratio of 1:4. The mixture was then dialysed against PBS for 16–20 h at 4°C. The resulting immunoliposomes were extruded several times through stacked 0.4 and 0.2 µm Nucleopore membranes, and the unbound antibody was then removed by chromatography on a BioGel A1.5M column. The antibody-to-lipid weight ratio of immunoliposomes was determined by the specific radioactivities of ^{125}I for the antibody and ^{111}In for the lipids. Liposomes (200 µg lipid) were i.v. injected, and biodistribution was examined 1 h after injection. Bars represent S.D. ($n = 3$). ■, 34A-liposomes with a antibody-to-lipid ratio of 1:18 and 194 nm in average diameter; □, bare liposomes with 201 nm average diameter.

Effect of prolonged circulation on target binding of immunoliposomes
Although 34A-liposomes bind significantly to the lung target, substantial accumulation of the immunoliposomes in the liver is also observed (Fig. 4). This and several other studies of immunoliposomes (Peeters et al., 1987) have shown the difficulty of in vivo immunoliposome targeting as a result of the high affinity of liposomes to the RES. Moreover, RES uptake of liposome is often facilitated via the Fc receptor mediated endocytosis owing to the presence of the antibody molecules on the liposomes (Aragnol and Leserman, 1986; Derksen et al., 1988; Peeters et al., 1987). Thus, it seems to be difficult to achieve an 'absolute targeting' of immunoliposomes in vivo. The rationale of our strategy is based on the development of liposomes with reduced affinity to the RES. By including a specific amphiphile such as GM_1 and PEG–PE in the lipid composition, immunoliposomes are allowed to circulate for a prolonged period of time so that they have an increased chance to interact with the target site. We have thus

examined the effects of these amphiphiles on target binding of immunoliposomes using the MoAb 34A system.

Effect of GM_1 on target binding of immunoliposomes

The 34A-liposomes used in this study were prepared from PC and chol (2:1 molar) also containing 6.3 mol.% of GM_1 (Maruyama et al., 1990b). Since GM_1 contains one negative charge per molecule, we have included the negatively charged phosphati-

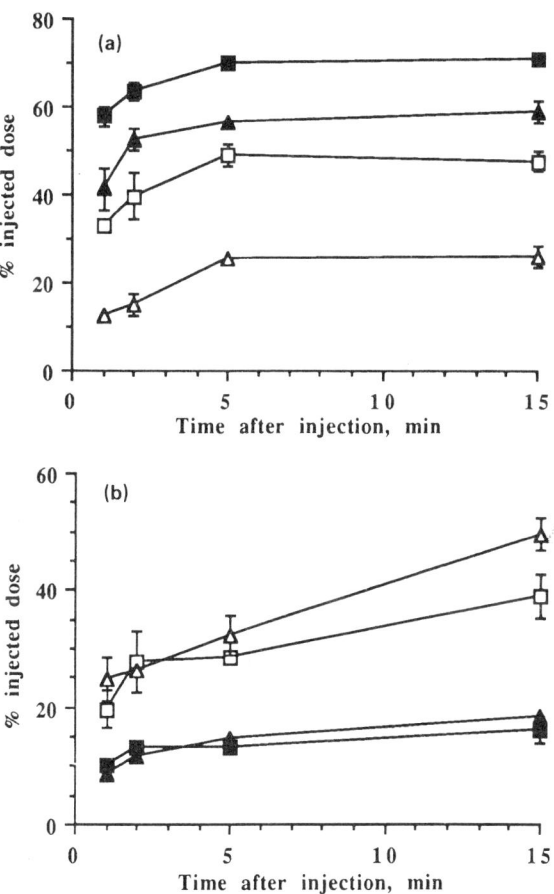

Fig. 5. (a) Lung and (b) liver uptake of 34A-liposomes containing GM_1 or PS. ^{111}In-labelled immunoliposomes containing 6.3 mol.% of either GM_1 or PS were prepared by the detergent–dialysis method as described in Fig. 4. Liposomes (200 μg lipid) were i.v. injected. Bars represent S.D. ($n = 3$). Lipid composition, antibody-to-lipid weight ratio and average diameter are as follows: ■, PC–chol–GM_1, 1:11, 297 nm; ▲, PC–chol–GM_1, 1:37, 292 nm; □, PC–chol–PS, 1:8, 253 nm; △, PC–chol–PS, 1:31, 255 nm. (Data taken from Maruyama et al. (1990b) with permision.)

dylserine (PS), which is known as an 'opsonin lipid' (Raz et al., 1981; Allen et al., 1988), in the control liposomes. It is clear from the data in Fig. 5 that 34A-liposomes containing GM_1 showed much more efficient target binding than those containing PS. In addition, the liver uptake rate of 34A-liposomes containing GM_1 was significantly lower than that of those containing PS. These results clearly indicate the importance of the lipid composition with reduced affinity to the RES in target binding of immunoliposomes. Also shown in Fig. 5 is the importance of antibody density of immunoliposomes. The 34A-liposomes with a higher antibody density showed more rapid and higher target binding than those with a lower antibody density irrespective of the lipid composition. One important observation in a separate experiment is that the 34A-liposomes containing GM_1 show much longer retention at the target site than those containing PS. Since PS-containing liposomes exhibit a high affinity to macrophages, this result suggests that circulating macrophages may be responsible for the removal of immunoliposomes from the lung target. Alternatively, released immunoliposomes could re-enter the circulation and rebind to the target if they are still in the circulation. GM_1-containing 34A-liposomes would have a greater chance of rebinding, owing to the lower affinity to the RES, than those containing PS.

Effect of PEG–PE on target binding of immunoliposomes
The 34A-liposomes used in this study were prepared from PC and chol (1:1 molar) also containing 7.0 mol.% of PEG–PE (Klibanov et al., 1991; Mori et al., 1991). Among various PEG–PEs tested PEG2000–PE showed the highest activity in enhancing the target binding of 34A-liposomes; its activity was comparable with that of GM_1, while PEG750–PE showed only a little activity (Table 2). In contrast, PEG5000–PE caused a significantly reduced target binding. These observations can be understood on the basis of the relative steric barrier activity of each PEG–PE species. As shown in Fig. 2, PEG5000–PE provides the highest steric barrier on the liposome surface which presumably prevents the antibody–antigen interaction, thus resulting in a decreased target binding of immunoliposomes. In contrast, the steric barrier activities of PEG750–PE and PEG2000–PE are not strong enough to interfere with the antibody–antigen interaction, resulting in an enhanced target binding of immunoliposomes according to their activities in prolonging the circulation time of liposomes. Another *in vivo* study using liposomes bearing the rabbit anti-myosin antibody showed that inclusion of PEG5000–PE at a lower concentration (4 mol.%) in the lipid composition results in a several-fold increase in the accumulation of immunoliposomes in the region of experimental myocardium infarction as compared with those containing no PEG5000–PE (Torchilin et al., 1991). This is presumably due to the low concentration of PEG5000–PE in the lipid composition which provides a weaker steric barrier and thus does not interfere with the target binding. These results suggest a rational strategy in using amphipathic PEG in the immunoliposome targeting. As can be seen in Fig. 2, the degree of steric barrier activity of amphipathic PEG is a function of both polymer chain length and concentration in the lipid composition. Thus, one can optimize target binding of immunoliposomes by altering these parameters such that the activity in prolonging the circulation time of liposomes is maximized, but the antibody–antigen interaction is not compromised.

Table 2. Effects of various PEG–PEs and GM_1 on target binding of immunoliposomes[a]

Lipid composition (molar ratio)	34A:lipid (by weight)	Average diameter (nm)	Percentage of injected dose[b]		
			Lung[c]	RES	Blood
PC–chol (1:1)	1:18.1	194	43.8 (2.2)[d]	41.3 (3.5)	9.5 (1.3)
	1:13.9	194	42.9 (3.2)[d]	41.9 (2.7)	12.5 (0.2)
PC–chol–GM_1 (1:1:0.15)	1:15.0	188	52.5 (2.9)[e]	35.9 (5.1)	6.3 (0.8)
PC–chol–PEG750PE (1:1:0.15)	1:16.9	192	47.1 (1.8)[f]	40.6 (4.6)	7.6 (0.3)
PC–chol–PEG2000PE (1:1:0.15)	1:17.7	176	52.6 (2.5)[g]	34.6 (1.5)	11.4 (1.1)
PC–chol–PEG5000PE (1:1:0.15)	1:15.0	163	21.5 (1.2)	21.1 (2.6)	55.0 (2.7)

[a] ^{111}In-labelled 34A-liposomes with the indicated lipid composition, antibody-to-lipid weight ratio, and average diameter were prepared by the detergent–dialysis method as described in Fig. 4. Liposomes (0.4 mg lipid) were i.v. injected, and the percentage injected dose in lung, RES (liver and spleen), and blood was measured 1 h after injection.
[b] Data are expressed as mean (S.D.), $n = 3$.
[c] Statistical analysis (Student's t test): ^{d} vs ^{e}, $p < 0.01$; ^{d} vs ^{f}, $p < 0.05$; ^{d} vs ^{g}, $p < 0.01$; ^{f} vs ^{g}, $p < 0.02$.
Data taken from Mori et al. (1991) with permission.

Optimization of *in vivo* immunoliposome targeting

Our studies in *in vivo* immunoliposome targeting using the MoAb 34A system indicate that accumulation of immunoliposomes at the target site is determined as a result of two kinetically competing processes: binding to the target site and uptake by the RES. The rate of target binding of immunoliposomes is directly proportional to the antibody density of liposomes, while uptake by the RES depends strongly on the lipid composition and, presumably, also the liposome size to be used. Consequently, general requirements for an efficient target binding of immunoliposomes are a sufficiently high antibody density and a reduced affinity to the RES. Maximum targeting of immunoliposomes to the target site can be achieved when these two variables are optimized.

Perspective in drug targeting with immunoliposomes

In order for drugs carried by immunoliposomes to be effective at the target cell, several consecutive events must take place. These include the binding of immunoliposome to the target cell, internalization of immunoliposome by the target cell, and release of the drug to the cytoplasmic compartment of the target cell to exert its functional activity.

In the previous section, we have described the construction and optimization of immunoliposomes for efficient target binding. It should be noted that the target antigen for the system used in this study is located at a readily accessible site, i.e. the vascular endothelial cell surface. For a much less accessible target site, the described immunoliposome formulations may not necessarily exhibit the same high degree of target binding. For example, the amount of blood circulating through a solid tumour is only a small fraction of the total. Furthermore, the morphology of tumour vasculature differs highly depending on the type, age, growth rate, and location of the tumour (for a review, see Jain, 1988). Thus, the targeting of liposomes to the tumour cell surface antigen in a solid tumour may require much stronger activity of liposomes to stay in the circulation.

The above-described strategy for efficient binding of immunoliposomes seems, however, to be effective only when the target cell is in the intravascular compartment or can be accessible through the leaky vasculature. Targeting of immunoliposomes to those localized outside the continuous vascular compartment, such as the neurons in the brain, is still limited by the inability of immunoliposomes to cross the continuous endothelial vascular wall. Although any practical strategy to overcome this anatomical barrier has not been proposed, one potential approach might be to take advantage of the transcytosis function of the endothelial cells. In transcytosis, certain ligand-receptor complexes are, upon endocytosis, transported across the endothelial cells (Mostov and Simister, 1985; Casanova *et al.*, 1990). When such a ligand is incorporated into the liposome membrane, the liposome might be transcytosed and reach the target cells localized in the other side of endothelium.

Once the immunoliposomes bind to the target cell, the next step is their internalization into the cell. Although there seem to be several mechanisms responsible for the liposome internalization, evidence suggests that receptor–mediated endocytosis is the major pathway, which in turn is a function of the target cell membrane. Thus, binding of immunoliposomes to the target cells does not necessarily result in their rapid internalization. Moreover, the destination of the internalized immunoliposomes via endocytosis is usually the lysosomes where the entrapped drugs as well as the antibody molecules and the lipids are degraded. To overcome these problems, various types of liposomes with a triggered release mechanism have been developed. The pH-sensitive immunoliposomes are designed to destabilize at mildly acidic pH as found in the endosomes (Connor and Huang, 1986; Collins and Huang, 1987; Wang and Huang, 1987). The target-sensitive immunoliposomes, on the other hand, are designed to release their contents upon binding to the target cell via bilayer destabilization (Ho *et al.*, 1986). Finally, the temperature-sensitive immunoliposomes release their contents at the cell surface upon heating to their characteristic transition temperature (Sullivan and Huang, 1986). The effectiveness of these novel types of immunoliposome for cytoplasmic delivery has been well proven in various *in vitro* systems. However, the results of *in vivo* studies have indicated their rapid clearance from the circulation (Connor *et al.*, 1986). Although attempts have been made to improve the circulation time of these liposomes by inclusion of a specific amphiphile such as GM_1 and PEG–PE in the lipid composition, these modifications often resulted in a reduced sensitivity to the appropriate environmental change (Liu and Huang, 1990). Thus, the development of immunoliposomes having both reduced affinity to the RES and a target-triggered release mechanism would be one of our future goals.

ACKNOWLEDGEMENT

The original work of this laboratory was supported by National Institutes of Health Grants CA 24553 and AI 29893.

REFERENCES

Allen, T. M. (1989) Stealth™ liposomes: avoiding reticuloendothelial uptake. In: *Liposomes in the Therapy of Infectious Diseases and Cancer.* Alan R. Liss, New York, pp. 405–415.
Allen, T. M. and Chonn, A. (1987) Large unilamellar liposomes with low uptake into the reticuloendothelial system. *FEBS Lett.* **223** 42–46.
Allen, T. M., Ryan, J. L. and Papahadjopoulos, D. (1985) Gangliosides reduce leakage of aqueous-space markers from liposomes in the presence of human plasma. *Biochim. Biophys. Acta* **818** 205–210.
Allen, T. M., Williamson, P. and Schlegel, R. A. (1988) Phosphatidylserine as a determinant of reticuloendothelial recognition of liposome models of the erythrocyte surface. *Proc. Natl. Acad. Sci. USA* **85** 8067–8071.
Allen, T. M., Hansen, C. and Rutledge, J. (1989) Liposomes with prolonged circulation times: factors affecting uptake by reticuloendothelial and other tissues. *Biochim. Biophys. Acta* **981** 27–35.
Alving, C. R. (1986) Delivery of liposome-encapsulated drugs to macrophages. In: Ihler, G. M. (ed.) *Methods of Drug Delivery.* Pergamon, Oxford, pp. 281–300.
Aragnol, D. and Leserman, L. (1986) Immune clearance of liposomes inhibited by an anti-Fc receptor antibody *in vivo. Proc. Natl. Acad. Sci. USA* **83** 2699–2703.

Blume, G. and Cevc, G. (1990) Liposomes for the sustained drug release *in vivo*. *Biochem. Biophys. Acta* **1029** 91–97.

Casanova, J. E., Breitfeld, P. P., Ross, S. A. and Mostov, K. E. (1990) Phosphorylation of the polymeric immunoglobulin receptor required for its efficient transcytosis. *Science* **248** 742–745.

Collins, D. and Huang, L. (1987) Cytotoxicity of diphtheria toxin A fragment to toxin-resistant murine cells delivered by pH-sensitive immunoliposomes. *Cancer Res.* **47** 735–739.

Connor, J. and Huang, L. (1986) pH-sensitive immunoliposomes as an efficient and target-specific carrier for antitumor drugs. *Cancer Res.* **46** 3431–3435.

Connor, J., Norley, N. and Huang, L. (1986) Biodistribution of pH-sensitive immunoliposomes. *Biochim. Biophys. Acta* **884** 474–481.

Derksen, J. T. P., Morselt, H. W. M. and Scherphof, G. L. (1988) Uptake and processing of immunoglobulin-coated liposomes by subpopulations of rat liver macrophages. *Biochim. Biophys. Acta* **971** 127–136.

Gabizon, A. (1990) A new generation of anthracycline-loaded liposomes with improved localization in tumors. In: *Abstracts of Conference on Liposomes in Drug Delivery: 21 Years On, School of Pharmacy, London, December 12–15, 1990*.

Gabizon, A. and Papahadjopoulos, D. (1988) Liposome formulations with prolonged circulation time in blood and enhanced uptake by tumors. *Proc. Natl. Acad. Sci. USA* **85** 6949–6953.

Gabizon, A., Shiota, R. and Papahadjopoulos, D. (1989) Pharmacokinetics and tissue distribution of doxorubicin encapsulated in stable liposomes with long circulation times. *J. Natl. Cancer Inst.* **81** 1484–1488.

Gregoriadis, G. and Ryman, B. E. (1972) Fate of protein-containing liposomes injected into rats. An approach to the treatment of storage diseases. *Eur. J. Biochem.* **24** 485–491.

Ho, R. J. Y., Rouse, B. T. and Huang, L. (1986) Target-sensitive immunoliposomes: preparation and characterization. *Biochemistry* **25** 5500–5506.

Holmberg, E., Maruyama, K., Litzinger, D. C., Wright, S., Davis, M., Kabalka, G. W., Kennel, S. J. and Huang, L. (1989) Highly efficient immunoliposomes prepared with a method which is compatible with various lipid compositions. *Biochem. Biophys. Res. Commun.* **165** 1272–1278.

Holmberg, E., Maruyama, K., Kennel, S., Klibanov, A., Torchilin, V., Ryan, U. and Huang, L. (1990) Target-specific binding of immunoliposomes *in vivo*. *J. Liposome Res.* **1** 393–406.

Hughes, B. J., Kennel, S., Lee, R. and Huang, L. (1989) Monoclonal antibody targeting of liposomes to mouse lung *in vivo*. *Cancer Res.* **49** 6214–6220.

Hwang, K. J. (1987) Liposome pharmacokinetics. In: Ostro, M. J. (ed) *Liposomes: From Biophysics to Therapeutics* Dekker, New York, pp. 109–156.

Hwang, K. J., Luk, K.-F. S. and Beaumier, P. L. (1980) Hepatic uptake and degradation of unilamellar sphingomyelin/cholesterol liposomes: a kinetic study. *Proc. Natl. Acad. Sci. USA* **77** 4030–4034.

Jain, R. K. (1988) Determinants of tumor blood flow: a review. *Cancer Res.* **48** 2641–2658.

Kabalka, G., Buonocore, E., Hubner, K., Moss, T., Norley, N. and Huang, L. (1987) Gadolinium-labeled liposomes: targeted MR contrast agents for the liver and spleen. *Radiology* **163** 255–258.

Kennel, S. J., Lankford, T., Hughes, B. and Hotchkiss, J. A. (1988) Quantitation of a murine lung endothelial cell protein, P112, with a double monoclonal antibody assay. *Lab. Invest.* **59** 692–701.

Klibanov, A. L., Bogdanov, A. A. J., Torchilin, V. P. and Huang, L. (1989) Biotin-bearing pH-sensitive liposomes: high-affinity binding to avidin layer. *J. Liposome Res.* **1** 233–244.

Klibanov, A. L., Maruyama, K., Torchilin, V. P. and Huang, L. (1990) Amphipathic polyethyleneglycols effectively prolong the circulation time of liposomes. *FEBS Lett.* **268** 235–237.

Klibanov, A. L., Maruyama, K., Beckerleg, A. M., Torchilin, V. P. and Huang, L. (1991) Activity of amphipathic poly(ethylene glycol) 5000 to prolong the circulation time of liposomes depends on the liposome size and is unfavourable for immunoliposome binding to target. *Biochim. Biophys. Acta* **1062** 142–148.

Liu, D. and Huang, L. (1990) pH-sensitive, plasma-stable liposomes with relatively prolonged residence in circulation. *Biochim. Biophys. Acta* **1022** 348–354.

Liu, D., Zhou, F. and Huang, L. (1989) Characterization of plasma-stabilized liposomes composed of dioleoylphosphatidylethanolamine and oleic acid. *Biochem. Biophys. Res. Commun.* **162** 326–333.

Liu, D., Mori, A. and Huang, L. (1991a) Large liposomes containing ganglioside GM_1 accumulate effectively in spleen. *Biochim. Biophys. Acta,* **1066** 159–165.

Liu, D., Mori, A. and Huang, L. (1991b) Role of liposome size and RES blockage in controlling biodistribution and tumor uptake of GM_1-containing liposomes. *Biochim. Biophys. Acta* **1104** 95–101.

Martin, F., Woodle, M., Redemann, C., Lasic, D., Newman, M., Allen, T., Mayhew, E., Gabizon, A. and Papahadjopoulos, D. (1990) Polyethylene glycol containing stealth liposomes. In: *Abstracts of Conference on Liposomes in Drug Delivery: 21 Years On, School of Pharmacy, London, December 12–15, 1990.*

Maruyama, K., Holmberg, E., Kennel, S. J., Klibanov, A., Torchilin, V. P. and Huang, L. (1990a) Characterization of *in vivo* immunoliposome targeting to pulmonary endothelium. *J. Pharm. Sci.* **79** 978–984.

Maruyama, K., Kennel, S. J. and Huang, L. (1990b) Lipid composition is important for highly efficient target binding and retention of immunoliposomes. *Proc. Natl. Acad. Sci. USA* **87** 5744–5748.

Moghimi, S. M. and Patel, H. M. (1989) Differential properties of organ-specific serum opsonins for liver and spleen macrophages. *Biochim. Biophys. Acta* **984** 379–383.

Mori, A., Klibanov, A. L., Torchilin, V. P. and Huang, L. (1991) Influence of the steric barrier activity of amphipathic poly(ethyleneglycol) and ganglioside GM_1 on the circulation time of liposomes and on the target binding of immunoliposomes *in vivo*. *FEBS Lett.,* **284** 263–266.

Mostov, K. E. and Simister, N. E. (1985) Transcytosis. *Cell* **43** 389–390.

Papahadjopoulos, D. (1990) Stealth liposomes: prolonged circulation time in blood, improved accumulation in tumors and increased therapeutic index. In: *Abstracts of*

Conference on Liposomes in Drug Delivery: 21 Years On, School of Pharmacy, London, December 12–15, 1990.
Patel, H. M., Tuzel, N. S. and Ryman, B. E. (1983) Inhibitory effect of cholesterol on the uptake of liposomes by liver and spleen. *Biochim. Biophys. Acta* **761** 142–151.
Peeters, P. A. M., Storm, G. and Crommelin, D. J. A. (1987) Immunoliposomes *in vivo*: state of the art. *Adv. Drug Deliv. Rev.* **1** 249–266.
Raz, A., Bucana, C., Fogler, W. E., Poste, G. and Fidler, I. J. (1981) Biochemical, morphological, and ultrastructural studies on the uptake of liposomes by murine macrophages. *Cancer Res.* **41** 487–494.
Rorvik, M. C., Allison, D. P., Hotchkiss, J. A., Witschi, H. P. and Kennel, S. J. (1988) Antibodies to mouse lung capillary endothelium. *J. Histochem. Cytochem.* **36** 741–749.
Scherphof, G. L., Spanjer, H. H., Dijkstra, J., Derksen, J. T. P. and Roerdink, F. H. (1986) Participation of Kupffer cells and hepatocytes in hepatic uptake and processing of liposomes. In: Yati, K. (ed.) *Medical Application of Liposomes*. Japan Scientific Societies Press, New York, pp. 43–54.
Segal, A. W., Willis, E. J., Richmond, J. E., Slavin, G., Black, C. D. V. and Gregoriadis, G. (1974) Morphological observations on the cellular and subcellular destination of intravenously administered liposomes. *Br. J. Exp. Pathol.* **55** 320–327.
Senior, J. (1987) Fate and behavior of liposomes *in vivo*: a review of controlling factors. *Crit. Rev. Drug Carrier Syst.* **3** 123–193.
Senior, J. and Gregoriadis, G. (1982) Is half-life of circulating liposomes determined by changes in their permeability? *FEBS Lett.* **145** 109–114.
Senior, J., Delgado, C., Fisher, D., Tilcock, C. and Gregoriadis, G. (1991) Influence of surface hydrophilicity of liposomes on their interaction with plasma protein and clearance from the circulation: studies with poly(ethylene glycol)-coated vesicles. *Biochim. Biophys. Acta* **1062** 77–82.
Shinitzky, M. and Barenholz, Y. (1978) Fluidity parameters of lipid regions determined by fluorescence polarization. *Biochim. Biophys. Acta* **515** 367–394.
Sullivan, S. M. and Huang, L. (1986) Enhanced delivery to target cells by heat-sensitive immunoliposomes. *Proc. Natl. Acad. Sci. USA* **83** 6117–6121.
Torchilin, V. P., Klibanov, A. L., Huang, L., O'Donnell, S., Nossif, N. D. and Khaw, B. A. (1992) Targeted accumulation of polyethylene glycol-coated immunoliposomes in infarcted rabbit myocardium. *FASEB J.* **6** 2716–2719.
Wang, C.-Y. and Huang, L. (1987) pH-sensitive immunoliposomes mediate target-cell-specific delivery and controlled expression of a foreign gene in mouse. *Proc. Natl. Acad. Sci. USA* **84** 7851–7855.
Weissig, V., Lasch, J., Klibanov, A. L. and Torchilin, V. P. (1986) A new hydrophobic anchor for the attachment of proteins to liposomal membranes. *FEBS Lett.* **202** 86–90.
Wisse, E. (1970) An electron microscopic study of the fenestrated endothelial lining of rat liver sinusoids. *J. Ultrastruct. Res.* **31** 125–150.
Wright, S. and Huang, L. (1989) Antibody-directed liposomes as drug-delivery vehicles. *Adv. Drug Deliv. Rev.* **3** 343–389.

Part II
Gastrointestinal and buccal routes

4

Structure and barrier function of the epithelium of gastrointestinal and oral mucosa

C. A. Squier

INTRODUCTION

The alimentary canal is lined with a moist mucosa that extends from the lips to the anus. The function of this lining is to form a barrier layer that will protect the deeper tissue layers from physical and chemical damage and limit the entry of microorganisms. On the other hand, absorption of digested foodstuffs and of water across certain areas of the intestinal mucosa is essential if the body is to obtain nutrients and to avoid dehydration. The ease with which substances can penetrate this mucosa has been exploited for the delivery of drugs in almost every region between the oral cavity and the rectum. This chapter will examine the barrier function of the oral and gastro-intestinal mucosa in relation to its structure so as to stimulate the development of improved strategies for the rational delivery of therapeutic compounds across these tissues.

The barrier function of mucosa is everywhere fulfilled by three important components; a surface layer of mucin, the cells of the superficial lining epithelium, and the intercellular elements of the epithelium. Differences in permeability are a reflection of differences in these components in different regions. Measurements of diffusion or permeability constants to water give an estimate of the relative efficiency of the barrier in different regions. From an examination of such data (Table 1), it is evident that the permeability of oral mucosa is an order of magnitude greater than that of skin although there are significant differences between different oral regions. The permeability of the gastro-intestinal mucosa is one to one and a half orders of magnitude greater than that of oral mucosa, but considerable differences are also seen between regions. However, there are also considerable differences in the surface areas across which absorption might occur in each of these regions. Skin has an area estimated at 1.8 m^2, whereas the infoldings and microvilli of the small intestine provide a total area of about 350 m^2 (values calculated from Selkurt, 1982). On the other hand, the surface of oral mucosa amounts to only 0.02 m^2 (Collins and Dawes, 1987).

Table 1. Permeability constants (K_p) to water for skin and different regions of oral and gastrointestinal mucosa

Region	Value ($K_p \times 10^7$ cm/min)	References
Skin (human)	44	Lesch et al. (1989)
Oral mucosa (human)		
Palatal mucosa	470	
Buccal mucosa	579	Lesch et al. (1989)
Floor of mouth mucosa	973	
Stomach (dog)	24000	Altamirana and Martinoya (1966)
Small intestine (human)		
Jejunum	8400	Soergel et al. (1968)
Ileum	10200	
Large intestine (dog)	37800	Grim (1962)

MUCUS AND THE LUMINAL ENVIRONMENT

The moist surface of mucosa is a result of the secretions of glandular cells in, or beneath, the tissue. These secretions are different in composition and consistency between different regions; saliva in the oral cavity is a mobile and slightly acidic fluid with low enzymatic activity. Gastrointestinal secretions can be viscous, contain high levels of enzyme activity and show considerable variation in pH in different regions, as illustrated in Fig. 1. The thickness of the mucous layer coating the tissue surface also varies, ranging from 70 µm in the oral mucosa (Collins and Dawes, 1987) to almost 200 µm in the intestine (Winne and Verheyen, 1990). This layer has important barrier functions: it limits bacterial colonization of the mucosal surface by restricting adhesion sites as well as by binding secretory immunoglobulins (Butler, 1987); it protects the tissue from enzymatic and acid attack, particularly when damaged (Wallace and Whittle 1986); it acts as a lubricant, thus reducing abrasion. There is some debate as to the extent that a mucin layer restricts diffusion at the mucosal surface and so contributes to the permeability barrier of the tissue. Winne and Verheyen (1990) have shown that the contribution of mucin to the diffusional barrier increases as that of the epithelium decreases (Fig. 2) so that it may represent over 20% of the diffusional barrier to small molecules. However, an unstirred fluid layer at the tissue surface may also restrict diffusion (Thomson and Dietschy, 1984) and it is difficult to distinguish between these effects. It is likely that only the diffusion of large molecules and particles is impeded by a mucin coating. Treatment of the surface of oral mucosa with 0.1% sodium dodecyl sulphate significantly increases the permeability to water although there is no overt cellular damage to the epithelium; this effect may represent the loss of an adherent surface layer of mucin (Romanowski et al., 1987).

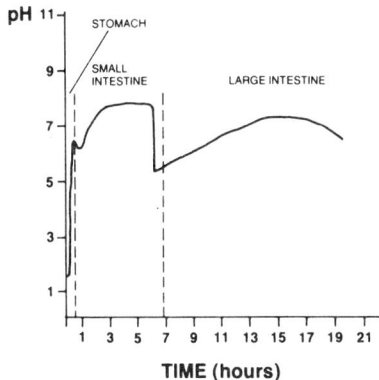

Fig. 1. Profile of luminal pH at different locations in the gastrointestinal tract. (Modified from Davis (1989)).

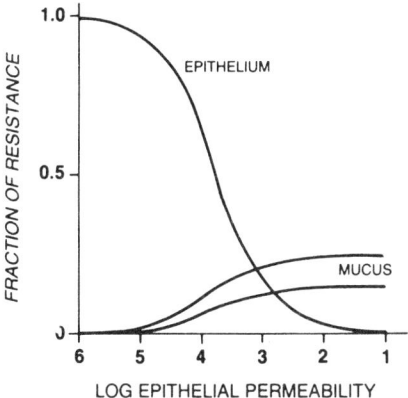

Fig. 2. Graph showing the increasing contribution of mucin to diffusional resistance as that of the intestinal epithelium decreases. (Modified from Winne and Verheyen (1990)).

THE EPITHELIAL BARRIER

Two main types of epithelia line the alimentary canal; stratified squamous and simple epithelium. The oral cavity and oesophagus are lined by stratified squamous epithelium which shows a keratinized surface layer (Fig. 3(a)), like that of skin, over the gingiva, hard palate and dorsum of tongue, but has a nonkeratinized surface elsewhere (Fig. 3(b)). The oral epithelium shows differences in thickness which tend to be inversely related to the rate of epithelial replacement or turnover time (Table 2). The remainder of the gastrointestinal tract is lined by a simple cuboidal or columnar epithelium (Fig. 4) which not only is much thinner but also turns over much faster than stratified squamous epithelium. All epithelia rest on a basal lamina which separates them from the underlying connective tissue elements. The basal lamina, although a complex macromolecular structure, is only likely to act as a barrier to large proteins (Wolff and Honigsmann, 1971) and immunoglobulin complexes (Tolo, 1974).

48   The epithelium of gastrointestinal and oral mucosa   [Ch. 4

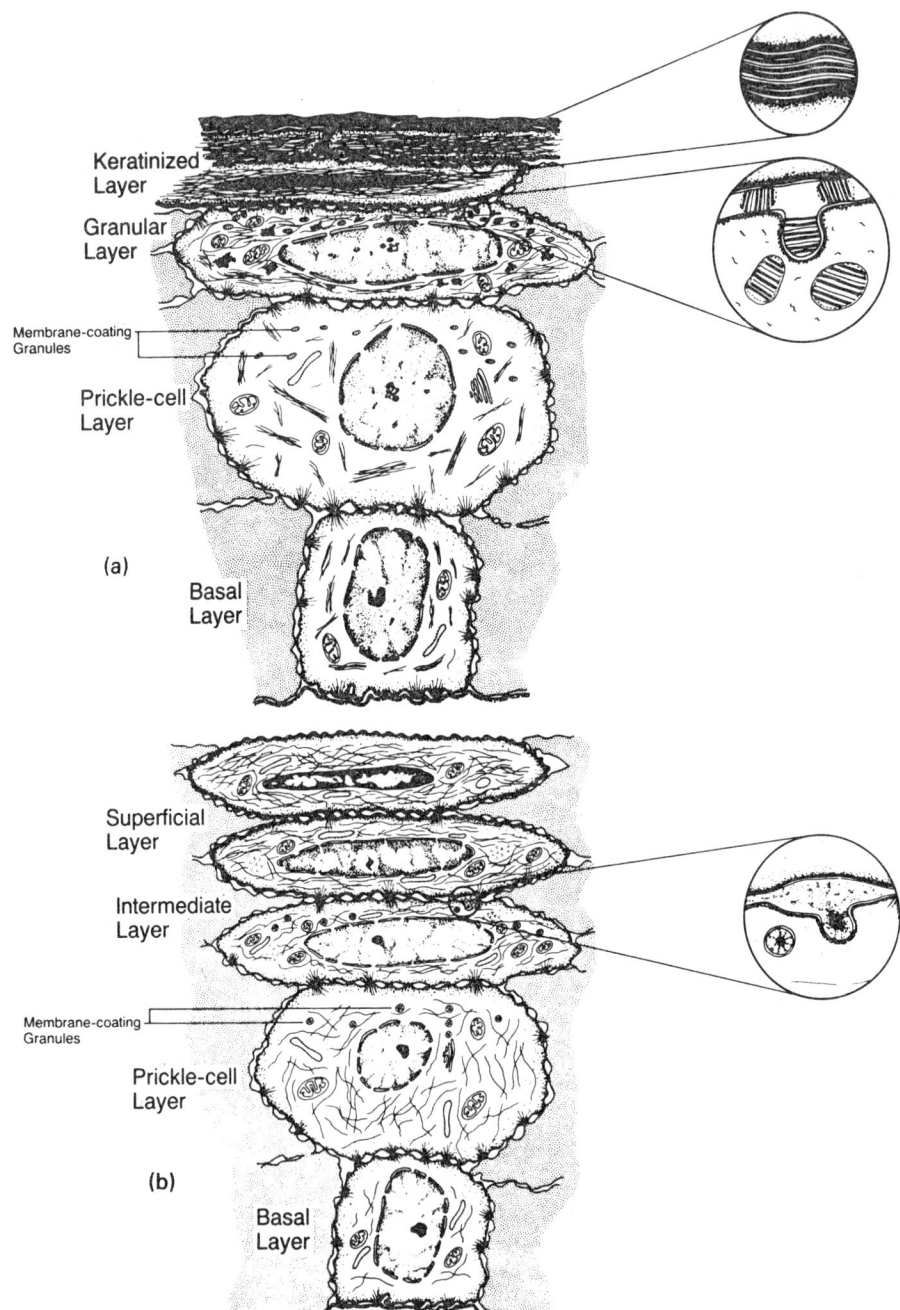

Fig. 3. (a) Diagram of a keratinized stratified squamous epithelium; inserts show the intercellular events after extrusion of the contents of the membrane coating granules. (b) Diagram of a nonkeratinized stratified squamous epithelium; inset shows extrusion of the membrane coating granules. (From Squier (1991).)

Table 2. Thickness and turnover times of epithelium from human skin and oral and intestinal mucosa

	Mean thickness (μm)[a]	Median turnover time (days)[b]
Skin		
Epidermis	120	27
Oral mucosa		
Palatal mucosa	310	24
Buccal mucosa	580	14
Floor of mouth mucosa	190	20
Intestine		
Small intestine	35	4
Large intestine	25	

[a]From Schroeder (1981).
[b]From Squier et al. (1976).

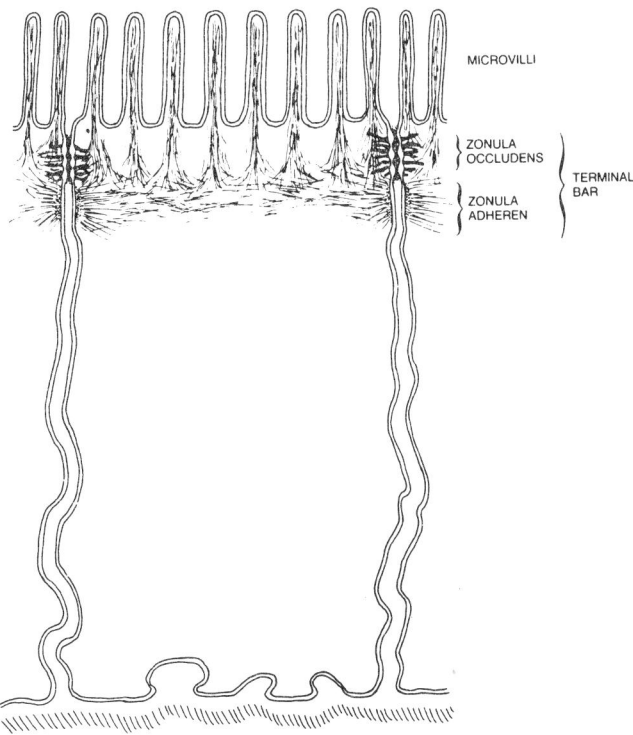

Fig. 4. Diagram of an epithelial cell (enterocyte) from intestinal mucosa. There is an extensive apical cytoskeletal network which is associated with the zonula adhaerens; some filamets (heavy lines) connect with the tight junction (zonula occuludens).

Oral and oesophageal epithelium

The barrier function of stratified squamous epithelium resides principally in the superficial cell layers (Squier, 1990). There is little evidence for transcellular (intracellular) passage of compounds across oral stratified squamous epithelium (Squier, 1991; Wertz and Squier, 1991) and the majority of substances are believed to penetrate paracellularly (intercellularly; Squier and Lesch 1988), as claimed for epidermis (Nemanic and Elias, 1980; Williams and Elias, 1987). Such a route will limit contact with intracellular hydrolytic enzymes, such as the peptidases that have been identified in mucosal homogenates (Stratford and Lee, 1986). The major junctional attachment between the epithelial cells is the desmosome, which does not impede intercellular diffusion; tight junctions (macula occludens) are rare in oral and oesophageal epithelia, and active transport is probably of minor significance. Belt-like zonula occludens, characteristic of intestinal epithelium, have never been described in these stratified epithelia.

In keratinized oral epithelium, the intercellular barrier consists of oriented arrays of neutral lipids, with a large proportion of ceramides. It is believed that these are formed by hydrolysis of glucosylceramides which are extruded into the intercellular space as lamellae by the membrane coating granules at the junction of the granular and keratinized layer (see Fig. 3(a)). There are slight differences in the composition of barrier lipids between keratinized oral epithelium (gingiva and palate) and epidermis, and the relative amount of ceramides present correlates well with the permeability differences to water (Table 3; Squier *et al.*, 1991).

Table 3. Water permeability and lipid content of skin and oral mucosa (from Squier *et al.*, 1991)

	Skin	Gingiva	Palate	Buccal mucosa	Floor of mouth
Water permeability[a] ($K_p \times 10^7$ cm/min ($\pm$ SEM))	62 ± 5	364 ± 18	412 ± 27	634 ± 19	808 ± 52 [a]
Epidermal–epithelial lipid content (mg/g tissue)					
Total phospholipids	37.8	27.0	30.5	42.7	57.6
Total glycosylceramides	8.5	2.8	3.6	18.4	7.5
Ceramides	25.3	4.8	2.7	0.9	1.0
Total nonpolar lipids	49.7	18.1	27.4	23.5	45.7
Total lipids	122.4	55.7	65.5	94.3	116.0

[a] All values significantly different ($p < 0.05$) from one another except for gingiva and palate.

The barrier in nonkeratinized oral epithelium appears to be derived from a population of granules which, although homologous in location and behaviour with those of keratinized tissue, have a different morphology (see Fig. 3(b)). The lipid barrier in nonkeratinized oral epithelium (buccal mucosa and floor of mouth) contains only very small amounts of ceramides but larger quantities of glycosylceramides (Table 3). The mixture of lipids in these epithelia seems to be incapable of forming the organized intercellular laminae present in keratinized tissues and persists as an amorphous material. This is unlikely to represent such an effective barrier as the oriented ceramides of keratinized epithelium and may explain the greater water permeability of these regions. Given the striking morphological similarities between nonkeratinized oral and oesophageal epithelium, including the presence of identical membrane coating granules (Hopwood et al., 1978), it is likely that the tissues have similar structural barriers and permeability properties. Although small proteins such as ovalbumin (Squier, 1991) and dextrans as large as 70 kDa (Tolo and Jonsen, 1975) have been shown to cross oral mucosa, it is unlikely that there is penetration of the tissue by larger particles, and pinocytosis does not occur in the surface cells, which probably have minimal metabolic capability.

Gastro-intestinal epithelium

The gastro-intestinal tract is lined by a simple epithelium consisting of a single layer of columnar cells, sometimes called enterocytes, attached to one another by a complex, apical, junctional region (Fig. 4). This consists of two bands girding the circumference of the cells; the most apical is a region of intimate membrane contact which obliterates the intercellular region and forms the zonula occludens or tight junction. Distal to this is a belt-like desmosome attachment, the zonula adhaerens, into which are inserted actin microfilaments of the cytoskeleton; this system is often called the terminal web. The apical membrane of the enterocyte is thrown into a series of microvilli, representing the microscopical brush border, into which penetrate actin filaments. It has been suggested that the actin filaments of the cytoskeleton may be linked to the membranes of the tight junction (Madara, 1987).

The presence of the apical tight junctions around the enterocytes of the gastro-intestinal epithelium restricts the paracellular pathway across the tissue to small molecules and ions, approximately 85% of which may diffuse by this route (Madara, 1990). Larger molecules such as amino acids, sugars and fatty acids may either diffuse across the apical membrane or be actively transported into the cell and subsequently reach the intercellular region via the lateral or basal cell membrane of the enterocyte (Fig. 5). Recently, it has been suggested that the tight junctions may play a more active role in the uptake of solutes than had previously been suspected (Madara, 1990). As molecules such as glucose are actively transported across the apical cell membrane of the enterocyte there is contraction of the peripheral actin cytoskeleton which exerts tension on the membranes of the tight junctions as a result of the interconnecting actin filament system. Consequently, these junctions become 'leaky', allowing quantities of water and larger molecules to cross the epithelium by the paracellular pathway. Absorption promoters are also believed to act by increasing the leakiness of the tight junctions (Tomita et al., 1988).

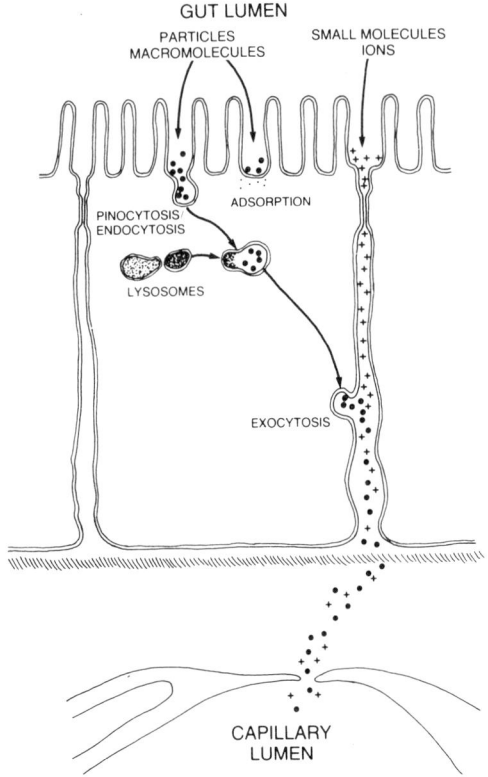

Fig. 5. Diagram of the transcellular and paracellular pathways across intestinal epithelium.

Penetration of proteins; macromolecules and particles
Particles such as viruses and large proteins enter the enterocyte in vesicles derived from the apical membrane and may subsequently be extruded into the intercellular space distal to the junctional complex (see Fig. 5; Worthington and Syrotuck, 1976). Such a process is well documented in neonate intestine where two mechanisms have been proposed (O'Hagan et al., 1987). The first involves a receptor-mediated process in which clathrin-coated vesicles transport ingested particles to the basolateral cell membrane where they are released extracellularly. An alternative process involves the uptake of particles by pinocytosis without the involvement of receptors. These vesicles enter the lysosomal system of the enterocyte where the contents may be digested; for horseradish peroxidase, there is between 67% and 97% degradation by this process (O'Hagan et al., 1987). This latter mechanism is believed to persist in adult intestinal epithelium when the receptor-mediated process is no longer active. Quantitatively, these mechanisms account for only a small proportion of total uptake across the intestinal barrier.

Apart from enterocytes, several other cell types may transport materials across the intestinal mucosa. Paneth cells are exocrine glandular cells that have an ability to phagocytose bacteria, and M (membranous epithelial) cells are found in the region of the gut containing abundant lymphoid tissue (the Peyers patches). M cells are able to take up antigens, viruses and even bacteria which are subsequently presented to cells of the lymphocyte series so as to initiate an immune response to a foreign antigen (Walker, 1987). However, although uptake of particles by these means may be important for applications such as vaccination, they are quantitatively insignificant in terms of bulk transport across the intestinal barrier.

Although a lining epithelium forms a continuous covering over the underlying tissues, large particles such as pollen and starch grains have been shown to enter the intestinal mucosa through gaps between the cells where desquamation is occurring at the tips of the intestinal villi (Fig. 6). This process has been called persorption (Volkheimer *et al.*, 1969) but probably has limited quantitative significance as a means of particle uptake.

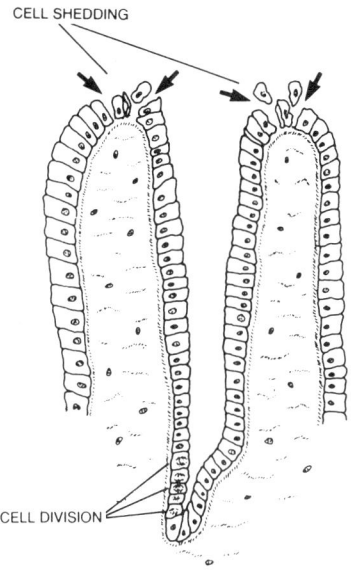

Fig. 6. Diagram to show persorption in the intestinal epithelium. Cell division occurs at the base of the villous crypts and cells are desquamated at the tips of the villi, giving rise to discontinuities (arrows) through which particles may enter the mucosa.

CONCLUSIONS - IMPLICATIONS FOR DRUG DELIVERY

The structural and functional correlates of mucosal permeability described above have some important implications for drug delivery. The gastro-intestinal mucosa, because of its lower diffusional resistance and larger surface area, permits greater uptake of exogenous substance than oral and, probably, oesophageal mucosa. However, the luminal environment of the gastro-intestinal tract places extreme demands on drug formulation. The acid environment of the stomach necessitates compounds with a pK_a close to 3 to obtain optimal absorption, and digestive enzymes in the intestine complicate the delivery of small proteins and polypeptides. Similarly, if these compounds are absorbed transcellularly they may encounter significant levels of intracellular peptidase activity in the gastric and intestinal mucosa (Stratford and Lee, 1986). Finally, it is difficult to provide controlled release of compounds at these sites as accessibility is limited. The limitations to drug delivery across the oral mucosa as a result of its superior barrier properties are, to some extent, offset by the advantages of the oral environment. Digestive enzymes are present in negligible amounts in saliva and the majority of compounds probably traverse the epithelial barrier by a paracellular route, thus avoiding intracellular proteolytic enzymes. The oral pH is close to neutrality (6.1-7.8) and slow release devices can be attached to those oral regions that have a relatively large and accessible surface, such as the buccal mucosa. Optimal drug delivery via the alimentary canal will thus depend not only on the structure and functional state of the barrier tissues to be traversed but also on the nature and dose form of the therapeutic compound and its desired mode of action.

ACKNOWLEDGEMENTS

This work was supported by NIH Grant R01 DE07930. I am grateful to Dr P. W. Wertz for reviewing the manuscript, to Sherrie Sheldon for typing it, and to Mr J. Herd for preparing the illustrations.

REFERENCES

Altamirana, M. and Martinoya, C. (1966) The permeability of gastric mucosa of dogs. *J. Physiol. (London)* **84** 771–790.

Butler, J. E. (1987) Basic concepts of secretory immunity and its relationship to mucosal disease, in: *Oral Mucosal Diseases: Biology, Etiology and Therapy* (Mackenzie, I.C., Squier, C. A. and Dabelsteen, E. (eds.)) Chapter 7, 28–35, Laegeforeningens forlag, Denmark.

Collins, L. M. C. and Dawes, C. (1987) The surface area of the adult human mouth and the thickness of the salivary film covering the teeth and oral mucosa. *J. Dent. Res.* **66** 1300–1302.

Davis, S. S. (1989) Small intestine transit. In: Hardy, J. G., Davis, S. S. and Wilson, C. G. (eds) *Drug Delivery to the Gastrointestinal Tract.* Ellis Horwood, Chichester, Chap. 4, pp. 49–61.

Grim, E. (1962) Water and electrolyte flux rates in the duodenum, jejunem, ileum and colon and effects of osmolarity. *Am. J. Dig. Dis.* **7** 17–27.

Hopwood, D., Logan, K. R. and Bouchier, I. A. D. (1978) The electron microscopy of oral human oesophageal epithelium. *Virchows Arch. B.* **26** 345.

O'Hagan, D. T., Palin, K. J. and Davis, S. S. (1987) Intestinal absorption of proteins and macromolecules and the immunological response. *CRC Crit. Rev. Ther. Drug Carrier Syst.* **4** 197–220.

Lesch, C. A., Squier, C. A., Cruchley, A., Williams, D. M. and Speight, P. (1989) The permeability of human oral mucosa and skin to water. *J. Dental Res.* **68** 1345.

Madara, J. L. (1987) Intestinal absorptive cell TJ's are linked to cytoskeleton. *Am. J. Physiol.* **253** C171–C175.

Madara, J. L. (1990) Pathobiology of the intestinal epithelial barrier. *Am. J. Pathol.* **137** 1273–1281.

Nemanic, M. K., and Elias, P. M. (1980) *In situ* precipitation: a novel cytochemical technique for visualization of permeability pathways in mammalian stratum corneum. *J. Histochem. Cytochem.* **28** 673.

Romanowski, A. R., Lesch, C. and Squier, C. A. (1987) Contribution of salivary mucins to the oral mucosal permeability barrier. *J. Dent. Res.* **66** 1054 (abstract).

Schroeder, H. E. (1981) *Differentiation of Human oral Stratified Epithelia.* p. 33, S. Karger, Basel.

Selkurt, E.E. (1982) *Basic Physiology for the Health Sciences.* Little Brown, Boston, MA, Chap. 12, pp. 468–511.

Soergel, K. H., Whalen, G. E. and Harris, J. A. (1968) Passive movement of water and sodium across the human small intestinal mucosa. *J. Appl. Physiol.* **24** 40–48.

Squier, C. A., Johnson, N. W. and Hopps, R. M. (1976) *Human oral Mucosa: Development, Structure and Function.* p. 20, Blackwell Scientific, Oxford.

Squier, C. A. (1991) The permeability of oral mucosa. *Crit. Rev. Oral Biol. Med.* **2** 13–32.

Squier, C. A. and Lesch, C. A. (1988) Penetration pathways of different compounds through epidermis and oral epithelia. *J. Oral Pathol.* **17** 512.

Squier, C A., Cox, P. and Wertz, P. W. (1991) Lipid content and water permeability of skin and oral mucosa. *J. Invest. Dermatol.* **96** 123–126.

Stratford, R. E. and Lee, V. H. L. (1986) Aminopeptidase activity in homogenates of various absorptive mucosae in the albino-rabbit: implication in peptide delivery. *Int. J. Pharm.* **30** 73–82.

Thomson, A. B. R. and Dietschy, J. M. (1984) The role of the unstirred water layer in intestinal permeation. In: Csaky, T. Z. (ed.) *Pharmacology of Intestinal Permeation II.* Springer, Berlin, Chap. 21, pp. 165–269.

Tolo, K. (1974) Penetration of human albumin through oral mucosa of guinea pigs immunized to this protein. *Arch. Oral Biol.* **19** 259.

Tolo, K. and Jonsen, J. (1975) *In vitro* penetration of tritiated dextrans through rabbit oral mucosa. *Arch. Oral Biol.* **20** 419–422.

Tomita, M., Shiga, M., Hayashi, M. and Awazu, S. (1988) Enhancement of colonic drug absorption by paracellular permeation route. *Pharm. Res.* **5** 341–345.

Volkheimer, G., Schulz, F. F., Lindenau, A. and Beitz, U. (1969) Persorption of metallic iron particles. *Gut* **10** 32–33.

Walker, W. A. (1987) Role of the mucosal barrier in antigen handling by the gut. In: Brostoff, J. and Challacombe, S. J. (eds) *Food Allergy and Intolerance.* Bailliere Tindall, London, Chap. 11, pp. 209–222.

Wallace, J. C. and Whittle, B. J. R. (1986) The role of extracellular mucus as a protective cap over gastric mucosal damage. *Scand . J. Gastroenterol.* **21** 79–84.

Wertz, P. W. and Squier, C. A. (1991) Cellular and molecular basis of barrier function in oral epithelium. *CRC Crit. Rev. Ther. Drug Carrier Syst.* **8** 237–269.

Willias, M. L. and Elias, P. M. (1987) The extracellular matrix of stratum corneum: role of lipids in normal and pathological function. *CRC Crit. Rev. Ther. Drug Carrier Syst.* **3** 95–122.

Wine, D. and Verheyen, W. (1990) Diffusion coefficient in mature mucus gel of rat small intestine. *J. Pharm. Pharmacol.* **42** 517.

Wolff, K. and Honigsman, H. (1971) Permeability of the epidermis and the phagocyte activity of keratinocytes. *J. Ultrastruct. Res.* **36** 176.

Worthington, B. S. and Syrotuck, J. (1976) Intestinal permeability to large particles in normal and protein deficient adult rats. *J. Nutr.* **106** 20.

5

Buccal drug delivery: mucoadhesion requirements and transmucosal transport barriers

H. E. Boddé, M. E. de Vries, C.-M. Lehr, J. A. Bouwstra, J. C. Verhoef, M. Ponec, W. H. M. Craane-van Hinsberg and H. E. Junginger

PART I: INTERFACIAL ENERGY AND MOLECULAR MOBILITY ASPECTS

In recent years, there has been increasing interest among pharmaceutical scientists and developers in bioadhesive drug delivery systems (BDDSs). The possible advantages of such delivery systems rely on a prolonged residence time at the site of absorption and an improved contact to the absorbing biological membrane. Both effects may lead to a prolonged or improved bioavailability of the drug being delivered. Successful development of bioadhesive drug delivery systems would be impossible without thorough knowledge of adhesive properties. In this section, a scientific basis is given for understanding the adhesion of polymers to biological surfaces, the buccal mucosa in particular, and some criteria for bioadhesion are pointed out. The following definitions are important.

- **Bioadhesion:** the molecular force exerted across the interface between a biological (here, human epithelial) surface and a polymeric drug carrier, that resists interfacial separation.
- **Mucoadhesion:** a special case of bioadhesion, in which the mucous gel layer acts as an intermediate between the adherent and the epithelial surface.

According to the so-called adsorption–interpenetration theory (Kaelble, 1971), adhesion may be described generally as a two-step phenomenon. The first step (which will always take place in any adhesive event) is mutual adsorption of the adherents; the second step (which may or may not take place) is interfacial interpenetration. This chapter focuses on the first and decisive adsorption step. Furthermore, we may discern surface energy and molecular mobility criteria for mucoadhesion. Reviews on the physicochemical aspects of bioadhesion have been written by, for example, Kaelble (1971), Peppas and Buri (1985) and Gu *et al.* (1988).

Surface energy criteria for adhesion

The interfacial free energy between two phases γ may be regarded as being composed of two parts: a **polar** contribution corresponding to polar interactions (ion–ion, ion–dipole and dipole–dipole interactions), and a **dispersive** contribution corresponding to so-called London dispersion interactions (these operate between any molecules by virtue of their polarizability, whether they have a permanent dipole moment or not):

$$\gamma = \gamma^p + \gamma^d \tag{1}$$

where p and d denote polar and dispersive contributions, respectively (Owens and Wendt, 1969).

In many cases, the adhesion between mucoadhesive polymers and mucosal surfaces takes place in the presence of a third interstitial (liquid) phase, e.g. gastric juices, saliva. Hence we have to take into account the possible interactions between both the adherent and the substrate, and the surrounding medium, and introduce a third phase into the formulas (Sacher, 1988).

In order to reach an unambiguous criterion for bioadhesion (Lehr et al., 1990), we propose that the mucoadhesive interface should be completely described in terms of three spreading coefficients:

$$S_P = \gamma_{ML} - \gamma_{PM} - \gamma_{PL} \tag{2}$$

$$S_M = \gamma_{PL} - \gamma_{PM} - \gamma_{ML} \tag{3}$$

$$S_L = \gamma_{PM} - \gamma_{PL} - \gamma_{ML} = -2\gamma_G \tag{4}$$

Here, the subscripts M, L and P refer to 'mucus', 'liquid' and 'polymer' and the corresponding interfaces. S_P reflects the tendency of the polymer to spread on the mucus, S_M describes the spreading of the mucus on the polymer and S_L describes spreading of the liquid on the mucus in the presence of the polymer. γ_G is the so-called Griffith fracture energy. In each of these cases, spreading would be favoured only if the corresponding spreading coefficient is positive ($S > 0$). Few attempts have been made in the past to find an unambiguous fracture–bonding criterion for such a three-phase system. Based on the Griffith fracture energy, Kaelble (1971) derived an expression to predict adhesion failure in the presence of a liquid (denoted by subscript L) which would flow into the 'crack' forming between adherent polymer P and mucosal substrate M.

Writing the Griffith fracture energy as a function of the polymer properties, we obtain

$$\gamma_G = k - \alpha_P(\alpha_L - \alpha_M) - \beta_P(\beta_L - \beta_M) \tag{5}$$

with

$$k = \alpha_L^2 + \beta_L^2 - \alpha_M\alpha_L - \beta_M\beta_L$$

For simplicity, the square roots of the γ^d and γ^p are replaced by the appropriate symbols α and β, respectively. According to Kaelble (1971), adhesion is expected when γ_G becomes positive. This criterion alone, however, would ignore the spreading coefficients S_P and S_M of the polymer and the mucosa. It is therefore considered to be insufficient and an alternative is needed. As demonstrated by Lehr et al. (1990), the spreading coefficients of the mucosa and polymer according to Eqs (2) and (3) can be rewritten as a function of surface energy parameters of all three phases involved in mucoadhesion, yielding

$$S_P/2 = -\alpha_P^2 - \beta_P^2 - \alpha_M\alpha_L - \beta_M\beta_L + \alpha_P(\alpha_L + \alpha_M) + \beta_P(\beta_L + \beta_M) \quad (6)$$

and

$$S_M/2 = -\alpha_M^2 - \beta_M^2 + \alpha_M\alpha_L + \beta_M\beta_L - \alpha_P(\alpha_L - \alpha_M) - \beta_P(\beta_L - \beta_M) \quad (7)$$

Again, taking α_M, β_M, α_L, β_L as constants, both spreading coefficients can be interpreted as functions of the polymer parameters α_P, β_P. In addition to a positive Griffith fracture energy (i.e. $S_L < 0$), a further necessary condition for mucoadhesion is either $S_M > 0$ or $S_P > 0$.

In order to quantify the expected mucoadhesive performance of candidate polymers, it would be desirable to unify the three spreading criteria as defined by Eqs (2)–(4) to one single parameter. Lehr et al. (1990) have proposed a new criterion, called the combined spreading coefficient S_c which is given by the geometric mean of the Griffith fracture energy γg and the polymer spreading criterion S_P:

$$S_c = \gamma_G^{0.5} S_P^{0.5} \quad (8)$$

This quantity should be a good predictor of mucoadhesive performance in a given situation (Lehr et al., 1990; Boddé et al., 1991).

A computer simulation was used to investigate the behaviour of S_c as a function of the polymer properties α_P and β_P. The properties of mucosa and liquid were kept constant. This simulation yielded a three-dimensional plot as shown in Fig. 1. Positive S_c values lie on the surface of an asymmetric paraboloid and thus all adhesive polymers

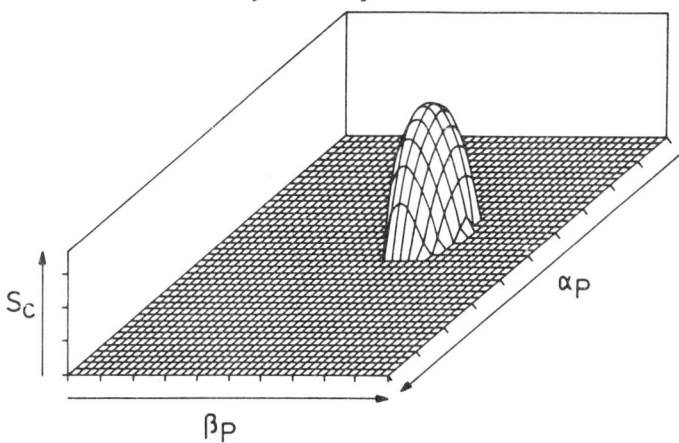

Fig. 1. Three-dimensional plot of S_c as a function of polymer parameters α_P and β_P (Lehr et al., 1991).

have (α_P, β_P) values within it. Other polymers lead to imaginary S_c values, plotted as $S_c = 0$. These polymers are not expected to have mucoadhesive properties.

The system polycarbophil–pig intestinal mucosa was used to test the predictive value of S_c. Three different aqueous test media were used as interstitial fluids. The contact angle values needed to calculate S_c were measured as described by Lehr *et al.* (1990), principally following the approach described by Andrade *et al.* (1979). In short, with each liquid two experiments were done with a mucosal tissue specimen and another two with a polymer film specimen. All specimens were equilibrated with the liquid and mounted submerged and horizontally. A small air bubble or a droplet of *n*-octane respectively was 'snapped' from a microsyringe onto the lower surface of the specimen and contact angles were measured. By combining the water and octane data, dispersive γ_{SV}^d and polar γ_{SV}^p components of the free surface energies for the various sample-liquid systems were calculated.

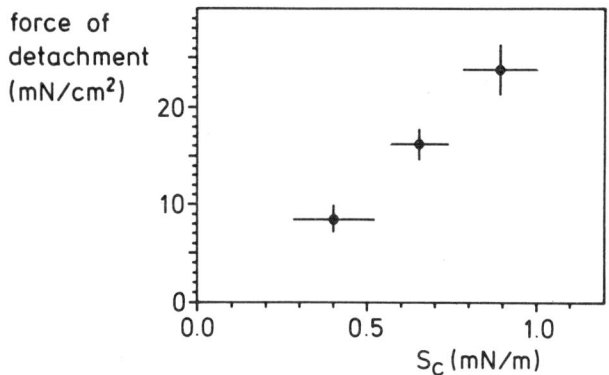

Fig. 2. Correlation between combined spreading coefficient and force of detachment (Lehr *et al.*, 1991), measured in the polycarbophil–pig intestinal mucosa system, using three different aqueous buffers.

The force of detachment was measured in the same three test media. Fig. 2 shows the results. There is a good correlation between the S_c values and the force of detachment, i.e. the mucoadhesive performance.

Molecular properties favouring the bioadhesion of polymers
In a recent study, an attempt was made to estimate both thermodynamic and kinetic factors in bioadhesion by systematically varying the properties of the adhesive, using synthetic polybutylacrylate–acrylate copolymers for buccal adhesive drug carriers (de Vries *et al.*, 1988). The butylacrylate moiety was chosen to modulate the **fluidity** (or molecular mobility) of the polymers, the acrylate to control the **polarity** (here, hydrogen-bonding capacity) and hence the surface properties of the polymers. It was assumed that a sufficient degree of fluidity would be needed to ensure favourable kinetic conditions (polymer segment mobility) for polymer–mucus adsorption and polymer–mucus interpenetration.

It was expected that an optimal balance between the two properties (**fluidity and polarity**) could be found by making use of a combination of methods, i.e. (1) glass transition measurements, (2) water contact angle measurements and (3) fracture (peel and shear) tests. A homologous series of acrylic acid (AA)–butylacrylate (BuAA) copolymers, ranging from 0% BuAA to 100% BuAA, and containing various amounts of the crosslinker ethyleneglycol–dimethacrylate (EGDMA) was synthesized and subjected to the aforementioned tests. Porcine buccal mucosa was used as substrate for the fracture test. The results are shown synoptically in Fig. 3.

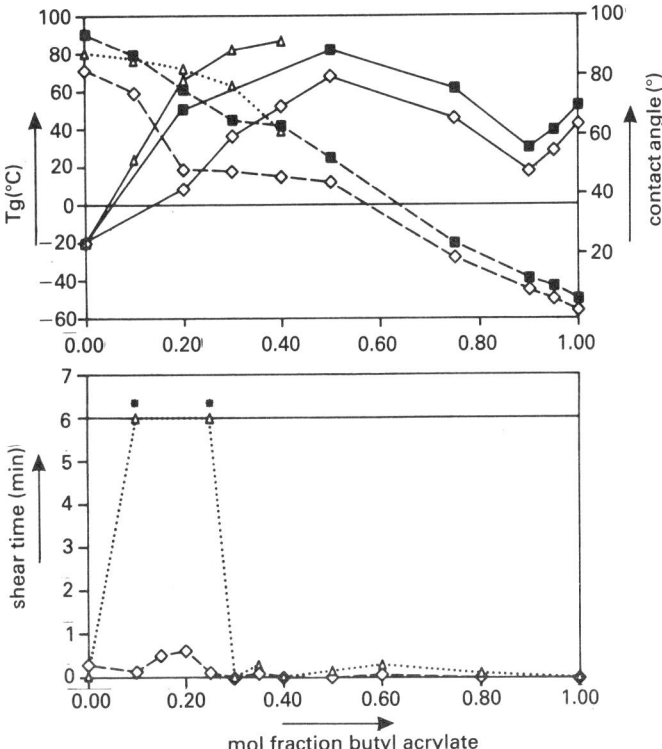

Fig. 3. Water contact angles, glass transition temperatures and shear adhesion on porcine buccal mucosa of polyAABuAA copolymer films with various crosslinker (XL) contents. In the upper plot, the continuous lines correspond to water contact angles and the interrupted lines to glass transition temperatures. ◊, no XL; ■, 0.5 mol.% XL; △, 1 mol.% XL.

An optimal mucoadhesive range appears to exist in the range between 0.1 and 0.3 BuAA (mole fraction). This probably arises from the interplay between fluidity and polarity. At low BuAA content the fluidity is insufficient (high T_g), and at intermediate BuAA content (0.3–0.5 mole fraction of BuAA) the polarity is insufficient. Upon increasing the BuAA content above a mole fraction of 0.5, T_g passes through the experimental temperature, leading to a sudden increase in fluidity, so that the still present AA residues can more easily reorient themselves towards the polymer mucus interface. This may explain why the contact angle decreases beyond a BuAA mole fraction of 0.5.

Conclusions of Part I

In developing mucoadhesive polymers for drug delivery a number of considerations should be borne in mind. Firstly, it is preferable to have criteria based on easily measurable parameters predictive for bioadhesiveness. The concept of the 'combined spreading coefficient' may provide one such criterion, which can be measured or calculated from literature data. Secondly, the choice of basic components has to meet requirements related to both surface polarity and molecular mobility of the polymer. In addition, the internal cohesion is an important factor, which can be controlled by varying the degree of crosslinking. Although surface energy parameters clearly play a decisive role in determining whether a stable adhesive bond can be formed, the mobilities of the molecules at the interface will chiefly control the rate at which this bond will be formed, and thereby modulate the adhesive process.

PART II: BUCCAL MUCOSA AS A PERMEABILITY BARRIER TO DRUGS

In a cross-section of buccal mucosa an upper layer of squamous epithelium can be distinguished, which is, at the proximal end, bound to a connective tissue layer called the lamina propria. The two layers are separated by the so-called basal lamina (Fig. 4).

This section deals with the question as to which part(s) of the buccal epithelium contribute(s) significantly to the permeability barrier for drugs.

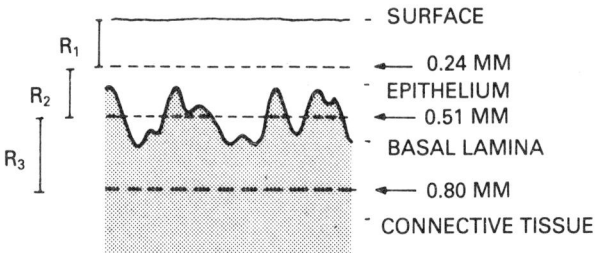

Fig. 4. Schematic cross-section of porcine buccal mucosa, in which the effect of dermatomizing at various depths is illustrated.

In order to localize the absorption barrier within the buccal mucosa Squier and Hall (1985a,b) visualized horse radish peroxidase (HRPO) transport. HRPO appeared intercellularly in the upper third part of porcine oral mucosae, corresponding to the presence of intercellular glycoproteinaceous material, extruded by membrane coating granules. It was concluded that these organelles play a major role as a barrier system. Similar results were found for rabbit buccal mucosa (Squier, 1973; Squier and Rooney, 1976; Dowty et al., 1990; Knuth et al., 1990). However, it has to be noted that the HRPO visualization technique probably revealed HRPO binding tissue components rather than a (major) permeation barrier; rabbit buccal epithelium has been reported to appear para-keratotic (Squier, 1973).

The basal lamina has been reported to act as a barrier to the passage of several high molecular weight compounds (Brandtzaeg and Tolo, 1977).

In this study an attempt was made to localize the permeability barrier within porcine buccal mucosa. In earlier experiments the epithelial layer of porcine buccal tissue was separated from the underlying tissue by a chemical splitting procedure (Le Brun et al., 1989). In the present study it was decided to separate the epithelium from the underlying tissue mechanically using a dermatome; this mechanical slicing method made it possible to use epithelial tissue layers with varying thickness (see Fig. 5). The barrier

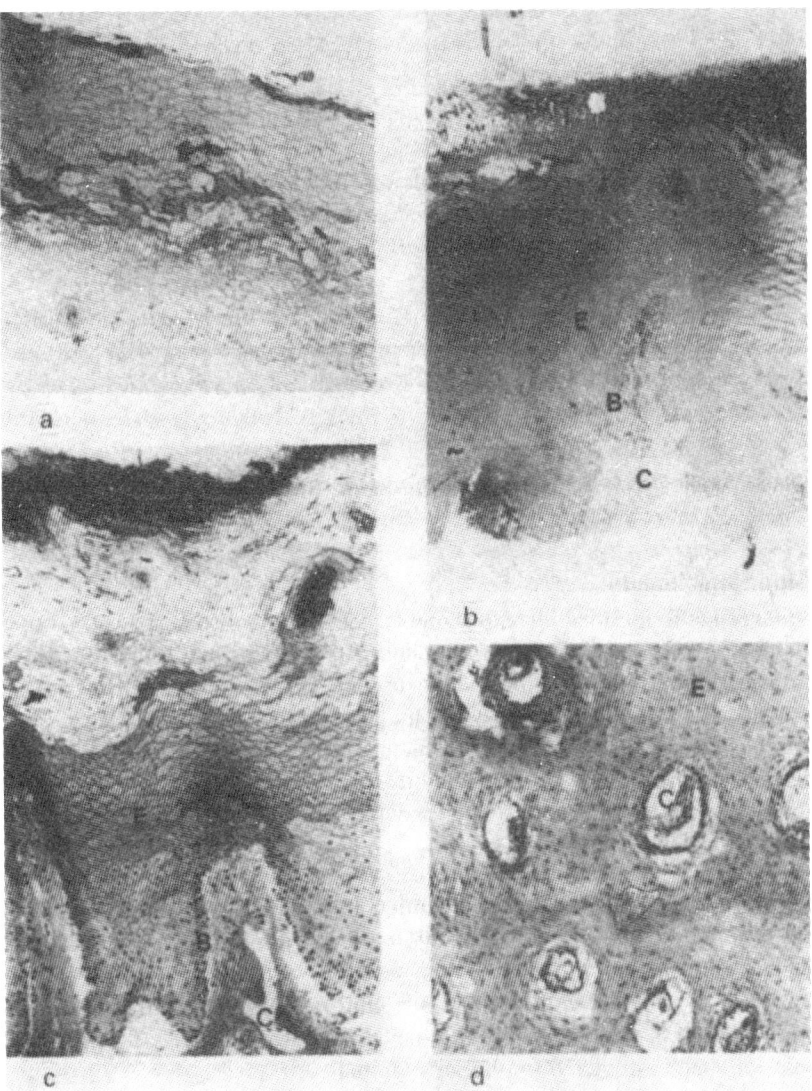

Fig. 5. Photomicrographs of porcine buccal mucosa that has been dermatomed at (a) 0.24 mm, (b) 0.51 mm and (c) 0.8 mm. (d) Photomicrograph of a horizontal section of porcine buccal mucosa which has been cut at 0.5 mm.

properties of the buccal mucosa were studied from three different samples by investigating (1) *in vitro* drug permeation kinetics (2) electrical resistance and (3) tissue morphology.

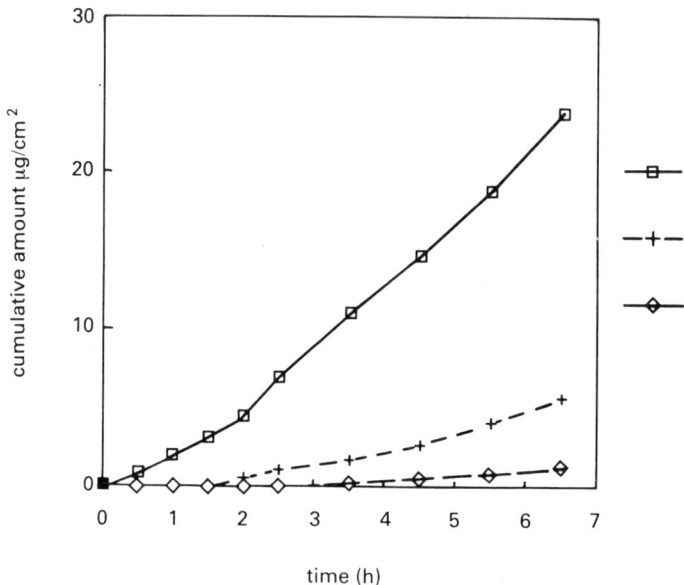

Fig. 6. Results of an acebutolol diffusion experiment: effect of dermatomizing tissue of one animal at 0.24 mm (□), 0.51 mm (+) and 0.8 mm (◊).

Diffusion experiments

As model drugs for permeation experiments, acebutololhydrochloride and bupranololhydrochloride were used. These compounds are the least and most lipophilic ones, respectively, among a series of β-blockers used in a former study (Le Brun *et al.*, 1989). Their molecular weights and pK_a values are comparable.

Fresh buccal tissue (from 40–70 kg castrated male pigs) was dermatomed at 0.24, 0.51 and 0.80 mm and used within 3 h upon slaughter. For diffusion studies the mucosal membranes were sandwiched between dialysis membranes and placed in Ussing chambers. For details see de Vries *et al.* (1991). A set of flux curves of acebutolol is shown in Fig. 6. It is apparent that the flux decreases with increasing tissue thickness. Results from different pigs showed a similar trend but the variability in the absolute value was rather large. Presumably, this is due to the fact that the tissue was not completely viable anymore. Although the tissue had been kept in Krebs buffer and was fed with oxygen, viability of different tissue samples must have decreased to a different extent. Therefore, it was decided to calculate the relative diffusion resistance (R_{rel}) for each pair of tissue samples from the same animal:

$$R_{rel} = \frac{R_x}{R_{0.8}} \tag{9}$$

where $R_{0.8}$ and R_x are the diffusion resistance (reciprocal permeabilities, in s cm^{-1}) of epithelial membranes dermatomed at thicknesses of 0.8 mm and x (mm) respectively, from the same animal. In this way results from different pigs could be compared. The results of these calculations are plotted vs tissue thickness in Fig. 7(a), from which it is evident that the effect of increasing the membrane thickness is similar for different

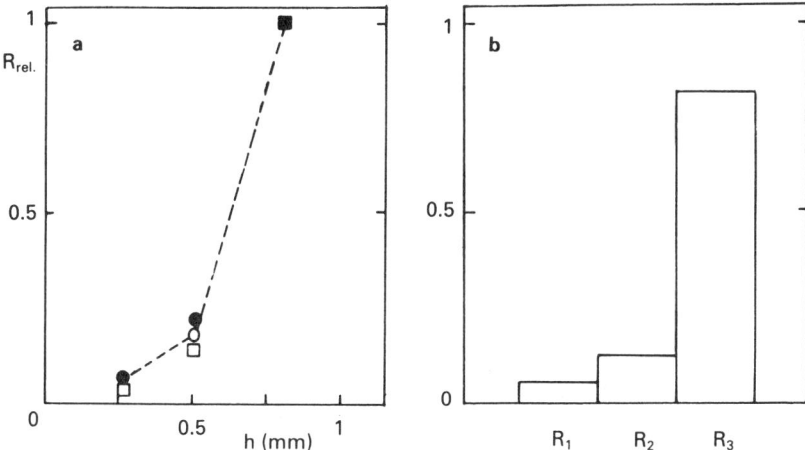

Fig. 7. (a) Plot of R_{rel} vs tissue thickness for three pigs for acebutolol. (b) Plot of R_1, R_2 and R_3 for acebutolol (mean values, calculated from (a)).

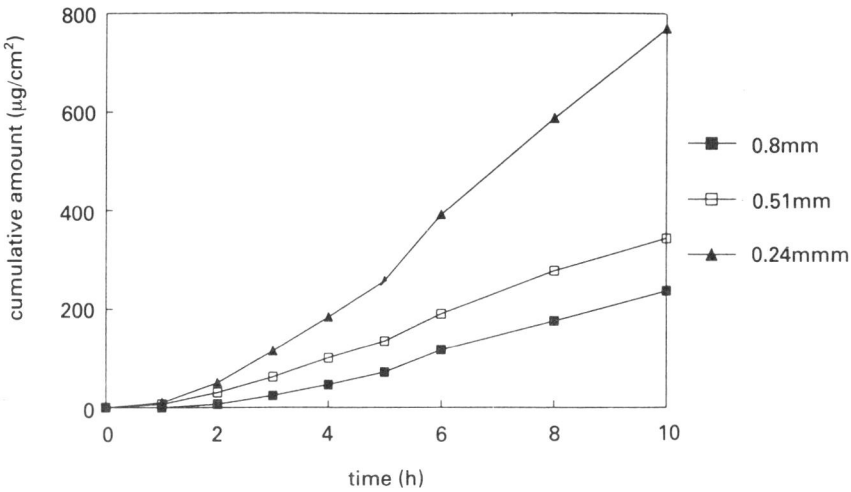

Fig. 8. Results of a bupranolol diffusion experiment: effect of dermatoming tissue of one animal at 0.24 mm (▲), 0.51 mm (□) and 0.8 mm (■).

animals. It is noteworthy that the diffusional resistance increases non-linearly with increasing tissue thickness. Fig. 7(b) shows the separately calculated diffusion resistances R_1, R_2 and R_3. In Fig. 8 a set of flux curves of bupranolol is shown. The absolute permeability for bupranolol was larger than for acebutolol. Moreover, a similar non-linear relationship was observed, as with acebutolol.

Electrical resistance

Buccal epithelium samples were clamped in Ussing chamber. The chambers were filled with Krebs buffer (pH 7.4) and provided with Ag–AgCl electrodes, positioned on either side of the mucosal slab. The electrical resistance across the membranes was measured using a pulsed current source in combination with a home-made computer-controlled resistance measurement unit (Craane-Van Hinsberg *et al.*, 1991). The resistance was calculated as the quotient of the voltage amplitude and current amplitude. See for details de Vries *et al.* (1991). The results of the electrical resistance measurements are shown in Fig. 9. From the right-hand part of the plot it appears that the thickest tissue corresponds to a relatively high resistance and that resistance is not linearly proportional to tissue thickness (i.e. dermatomizing depth). The left-hand part of the plot shows that, irrespective of the splitting method used, the resistance of the residual epithelium is much smaller than of intact (i.e. untreated) tissue.

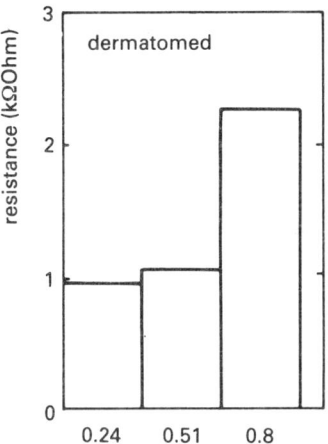

Fig. 9. Electrical resistance of epithelial slabs plotted vs tissue thickness and vs splitting procedure.

Morphological studies

For morphological studies, dermatomed tissue samples were processed for standard light microscopy (de Vries *et al.*, 1991). Subsequently, the sections were thawed, treated with acetone, rinsed with PBS, and incubated. For basal lamina visualization, cryosections were stained for collagen VII using an immunofluorescent technique (Leigh *et al.*, 1987). For details see also de Vries *et al.* (1991). Figs 5(a)–(c) show photomicrographs of dermatomed buccal mucosae, cut at 0.24 mm, 0.51 mm and 0.8 mm, respectively. As evident from these figures tissue layers of different compositions are obtained. Dermatoming at 0.24 mm yields samples which consist of epithelial cells only. Tissue cut at 0.51 mm shows cross-sectioned papillae and some connective tissue whereas the thickest tissue samples contained the entire epithelium with intact papillae and thus the complete basal lamina. Fig. 5(d) represents a horizontal section of an 0.51 mm thick sample; the relatively tight epithelial cells surround 'holes' of loose connective tissue at the sites where the papillae have been cross-sectioned.

Fig. 10 shows a light-microscopic image of an FITC-immunolabelled cross-section of intact buccal mucosa. The immuno-labelled collagen VII reflects the location of the basal lamina.

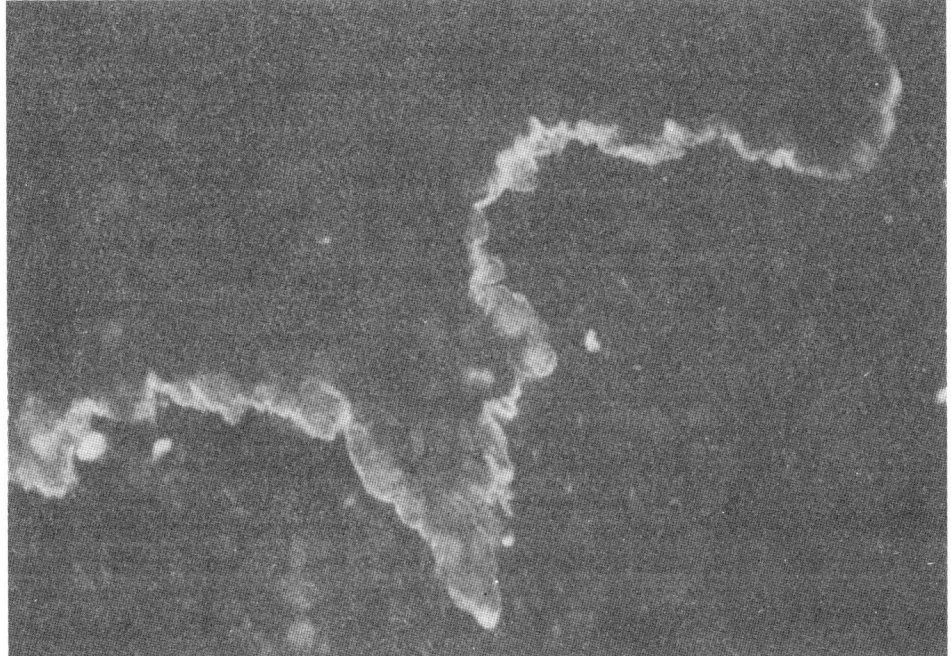

Fig. 10. Photomicrograph of FITC collagen VII antibody labelled porcine buccal mucosa, showing the location of the basal lamina in intact mucosa.

General remarks on Part II

When R_{rel} is plotted vs h, the tissue thickness, it can be seen that reducing the thickness of the membrane by a factor of 2 does not result in a reduction of the diffusion resistance by the same factor (Fig. 7(a)). Hence, a relatively large absorption barrier has to be present in the thickest dermatomed tissue. This point is illustrated more clearly when the separate diffusion resistances are considered (see Fig. 7(b)). Once again, it is evident that R_3, representing the contribution of the 'deepest' tissue layer as a diffusion barrier, is much larger than R_1 or R_2, underlining the aforementioned non-linearity.

Permeability data for bupranolol show a similar non-linearity between R and h. However, when the diffusion resistances for acebutolol are compared with those for bupranolol by calculating their ratio ($R_{AcBu} = R_{Ac}/R_{Bu}$) at various tissue thicknesses, a remarkable difference is noticed (Fig. 11). Apart from the observation that the diffusion resistance for bupranolol is much smaller than for acebutolol, indicating that the buccal mucosa is more permeable for lipophilic compounds, the ratio R_{Ac}/R_{Bu} appears to decrease with increasing tissue thickness. This observation suggests that a relatively hydrophilic barrier is present in the deeper tissue layers as compared to the upper mucosal layer.

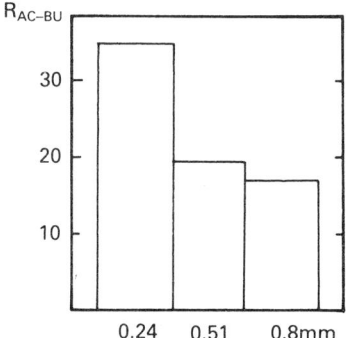

Fig. 11. Ratio of diffusion resistances for acebutolol and bupranolol (R_{Ac-Bu}) at various tissue thicknesses.

The results of the electrical resistance measurements on dermatomed tissue layers show a similar non-linearity with increasing tissue thickness as those of the diffusion experiments, indicating that the major absorption barrier for small ions might be the same as for the β-blockers (which are ionic at pH 7.4).

From the morphological investigations it is observed that by dermatoming porcine buccal mucosa at 0.8 mm tissue slabs are obtained that contain both the complete epithelium and the intact (i.e. not cross-sectioned) basal lamina, which separates the epithelium from the underlying connective tissue. Dermatoming at 0.24 or 0.51 mm yields slabs containing epithelium only or epithelium with a cross-sectioned (i.e. damaged) basal lamina as well, respectively. Since it is unlikely that the loose, hydrophilic connective tissue acts as a barrier, these findings together with the results of the flux and electrical resistance measurements strongly suggest that the basal lamina presents a major barrier to absorption.

Although experiments of Squier and Hall (Squier, 1973; Squier and Hall, 1985a,b) showed that the water-soluble HRPO, when injected subepithelially, passes the basal lamina easily, our results correlate well with their findings in stripping experiments. Upon stripping porcine buccal mucosa the permeability of the tissue did not increase, indicating that the permeability barrier remained intact.

Comparison of the diffusion resistances for acebutolol and bupranolol suggests that there must be a relatively hydrophilic barrier in the deeper tissue layers; this again supports the notion that the basal lamina, being mainly proteinaceous (Squier and Rooney, 1976), is the rate-limiting barrier to drug transport.

ACKNOWLEDGEMENTS

We are grateful to Dr L. Jager from the Dutch National Veterinary Institute in Lelystad (The Netherlands) and Dr A. Pijpers from the faculty of Veterinary Medicine of the State University of Utrecht (The Netherlands) for providing us with fresh porcine tissue. Furthermore, we want to thank Dr I. Leigh for kindly providing us with human collagen VII antibody.

REFERENCES

Alfano, M. C., Drummond, J. F. and Miller, S. A. (1975) Localization of rate-limiting barrier to penetration of endotoxin through non-keratinized oral mucosa in vitro. *J. Dent. Res.* **54** 1143–1148.

Alfano, M. C., Chasens, A. I. and Masi, C. W. (1977) Autoradiographic study of the penetration of radiolabeled dextrans and inulin through non-keratinized oral mucosa in vitro. *J. Periodont. Res.* **12** 368–377.

Andrade, J. D., King, R. N., Gregonis, D. E. and Coleman, D. L. (1979) Surface characterization of poly(hydroxyethyl methacrylate) and related polymers. I. Contact angle methods in water. *J. Polym. Sci., Polym. Symp.* **66** 313–336.

Boddé, H. E., Lehr, C.-M., de Vries, M. E., Bouwstra, J. A and Junginger, H. E. (1991) Bioadhesive polymers – surface energy and molecular mobility considerations. *Biofouling* **4** 163–169.

Brandtzaeg, P. and Tolo, K. (1977) Mucosal penetrability enhanced by serum-derived antibodies. *Nature (London)* **266** 262–263.

Craane-Van Hinsberg, W. H. M., Boddé, H. E., Verhoef, J., Bax, L. J. and Junginger, H. E. (1991) Evaluation of a pulsed current and high frequency voltage sampling system designed to study transdermal peptide iontophoresis and skin impedance. *Proc. Int. Symp. Control. Release Bioact. Mater.* **18** 107–108.

Dowty, M. E., Irons, B. K., Knuth, K. E. and Robinson, J. R. (1990) Characterization of transport pathways of thyrotropin releasing hormone in rabbit buccal mucosa. *Proc. Int. Symp. Control. Release Bioact. Mater.* **17** 226–227.

Gu, J. M., Robinson, J. R. and Leung, S. H. S. (1988) Binding of acrylic polymers to mucin/epithelial surfaces: structure/property relationships, *CRC Crit. Rev. Ther. Drug Carrier Syst.* **5** 21–67.

Kaelble, D. D. (ed.) (1971) *Physical Chemistry of Adhesion*, Wiley-Interscience, New York.

Knuth, K. E., Dowty, M. E. and Robinson, J. R. (1990) Biochemical characterization of rabbit buccal mucosa. *Proc. Int. Symp. Control. Release Bioact. Mater.* **17** 297–298.

Le Brun, P. P. H., Fox, P. L. A., de Vries, M. E. and Boddé, H. E. (1989) In vitro penetration of some β-adrenoreceptor blocking drugs through porcine buccal mucosa. *Int. J. Pharm.* **49** 141–145.

Lehr, C.-M., Bouwstra, J. A., Boddé, H. E., Spies, F., Van Munsteren, C., Vermeij-Keers, C. and Junginger, H. E. (1990) Surface energy analysis and visualization studies on mucoadhesion. *Proc. Int. Symp. Control. Release Bioact. Mater.* **17** 91–92.

Leigh, I. N., Purkis, P. E. and Bruckner-Studerman (1987) LH-7.2 monoclonal antibody detects tight-VII collagen in the sublamina densa zone of ectodermally-derived epithelia, including skin. *Epithelia* **1** 17–29.

Owens, D. K. and Wendt, R. C. (1969) Estimation of the surface free energy of polymers. *J. Appl. Polym. Sci.* **13** 1741–1747.

Peppas, N. A. and Buri, P. A. (1985) Surface, interfacial and molecular aspects of polymer bioadhesion on soft tissues. *J. Control. Release* **2** 257–275.

Sacher, E. (1988) The determination of the surface tensions of solid forms. In: Ratner, B. D. (ed.). *Surface Characterization of Biomaterials*. Elsevier, Amsterdam, pp. 53–64.

Squier, C. A. (1973) The permeability of keratinized and non-keratinized oral epithelium to horseradish peroxidase. *J. Ultrastruct. Res.* **43** 160–177.

Squier, C. A. and Hall, B. K. (1985a) The permeability of skin and oral mucosa to water and horseradish peroxidase as related to the thickness of the permeability barrier. *J. Invest. Dermatol.* **84** 176–179.

Squier, C. A. and Hall, B. K. (1985b) *In vitro* permeability of porcine oral mucosa after epithelial separation, stripping and hydration. *Arch. Oral Biol.* **30** 485–491.

Squier, C. A. and Rooney, L. (1976) The permeability of keratinized and non-keratinized oral epithelium to lanthanum *in vivo*. *J. Ultrastruct. Res.* **54** 286–295.

de Vries, M. E., Boddé, H. E., Busscher, H. J. and Junginger, H. E. (1988) Hydrogels for buccal drug delivery; properties relevant for muco-adhesion. *J. Biomed. Mater. Res.* **22** 1023–1032.

de Vries, M. E., Boddé, H. E., Verhoef, J., Ponec, M., Craane, W. H. M. and Junginger, H. E. (1991) Localization of the permeability barrier inside porcine buccal mucosa: a combined *in vitro* study of drug permeability, electrical resistance and tissue morphology. *Int. J. Pharm.* **76** 25–35.

6

Colloidal drug delivery systems for gastrointestinal application

Jean-Philippe Devissaguet, Hatem Fessi, Nazih Ammoury and Gillian Barratt

INTRODUCTION
Colloidal drug delivery systems (CDDSs) are particulate or vesicular dosage forms in the nanometre size range. They include liposomes, niosomes®, nanospheres and nanocapsules. Biphasic (O-W) or triphasic (W-O-W) emulsions of the same size will not be considered here. Their size avoiding any risk of mechanical embolism following intravenous injection, CDDSs were initially designed, and were studied, as drug carriers for targeting purposes. The assumption was the expected ability of CDDSs to concentrate the drug at the therapeutic target and/or divert if from the toxicological one. Some interesting results have been obtained with drugs possessing a narrow therapeutic margin such as anticancer drugs. In addition, CDDSs were shown to be able to act as sustained-release dosage forms when injected subcutaneously.

However, the oral route of administration has the advantage of convenience, versatility and safety, and is preferred whenever the physicochemical properties of a drug allow adequate systemic bioavailability. Many drugs are rendered ineffective after oral administration because of their chemical lability or susceptibility to enzymes in luminal fluids, or because of their hydrophilic character and ionizability at all pH values, or because of their high molecular weight or insolubility. It was therefore tempting to test the effectiveness of CDDSs either to protect drugs from luminal degradation or to transfer them from the mucosal to the serosal side of the gastrointestinal barrier. In addition, the transfer of the drug-loaded carrier could avoid any intracellular degradation if drug release occurred in the blood or lymph. Candidate drugs for entrapment in CDDS were peptides (hormones, enzymes, clotting factors, etc.), quaternary ammoniums, hydrophilic antibiotics (gentamycin, etc.), all of them exhibiting poor or unpredictable oral bioavailability.

Nevertheless, since the discovery of liposomes in the 1960s most of the studies involving CDDSs have examined parenteral routes. Their use as oral delivery systems only started in 1976 and has not been completely investigated. Furthermore, nanospheres and nanocapsules were developed in the 1980s and most of the available literature concerns liposomes rather than these more promising tools.

LIPOSOMES, NIOSOMES, NANOSPHERES AND NANOCAPSULES AS DRUG DELIVERY SYSTEMS

Liposomes

Liposomes are vesicular CDDSs. They consist of one (or more) concentric spheres of lipid bilayer(s) surrounding aqueous compartment(s). Small unilamellar liposomes can be as small as 20 nm in diameter. Large multilamellar liposomes can be as large as 10 µm. Large unilamellar or oligolamellar liposomes usually range from 100 to 500 µm. Liposomes can be prepared by various methods, not discussed here (see Weiner *et al.* (1989) or Martin (1990). Amphiphilic lipids are needed to obtain liposomes: natural phospholipids, such as phosphatidylcholine, or synthetic, such as dipalmitoylphosphatidylcholine, prepared from saturated, more stable, fatty acids. Lipids must have tensioactive properties with a polar (hydrophilic) moiety and a non-polar (lipophilic) moiety. Entrapment of drugs (Table 1) within liposomes depends on the physicochemical properties of the substance: hydrophilic drugs will be entrapped in the aqueous compartment(s) of liposomes, while lipophilic drugs will be included within the bilayer(s), amphiphilic drugs being partitioned at the interface of the components of the liposomal structure. Drugs entrapped in the aqueous phase are released by diffusion through the bilayer(s), while lipophilic drugs are released following partition between the surrounding medium and the bilayer(s).

Table 1. Liposomally entrapped drugs tested for gastrointestinal application

Drug	References
Hydrophilic	
Insulin	Patel and Ryman (1976, 1977a,b), Dapergolas and Gregoriadis (1976, 1977), Patel *et al.* (1978, 1982), Hashimoto and Kawada (1979) Tragl *et al.* (1979), Weingarten *et al.* (1981), Kawada *et al.* (1981), Arrieta-Molero *et al.* (1982), Shenfield and Hill (1982), Dobre *et al.* (1983)
Glucose oxidase	Dapergolas *et al.* (1976)
d-Tubocurarine	Dapergolas and Gregoriadis (1977)
Angiotensin II	Papaioannou *et al.* (1978)
1-β-D-Arabinofuranosylcytosine	Rustum *et al.* (1979)
Gentamycin	Morgan and Williams (1980)
Factor VIII	Hemker *et al.* (1980), Kirby and Gregoriadis (1984)

Table 1. (continued)

Drug	Reference
Factor IX	Ueno *et al.* (1982a)
Heparin	Ueno *et al.* (1982b)
Cysteamine	Jaskierowicz *et al.* (1985)
Lipophilic	
Vitamin K	Nagata *et al.* (1984)
Dolichol	Kimura *et al.* (1989)
Indomethacin	Soehngen *et al.* (1988)

Niosomes

Niosomes are structurally related to liposomes and probably have similar properties. They are prepared from synthetic amphiphilic lipids and their proprietary name derived from 'non-ionic' surfactants (see Florence and Baillie (1989)).

Nanospheres

Nanospheres are a solid spherical matrix. The size of nanospheres, depending on the method of preparation, ranges from 50 nm to 500 nm in diameter. They are usually prepared from polymeric materials but they also can be obtained from other macromolecular materials such as proteins, polyosides. Polymeric nanospheres can be prepared either by polymerization of monomers (latex) or from preformed polymers (pseudolatex). For drug delivery purposes (Table 2) biodegradable polymers are preferred: poly(alkylcyanoacrylate) for latex (Couvreur *et al.*, 1984) or poly(lactide) and poly(lactide-coglycolide) for pseudolatex (Fessi *et al.*, 1987a) are examples of such materials. To prepare protein nanospheres, the raw material, i.e. albumin or gelatin, must be modified chemically or physically in order to obtain stable, water-insoluble colloids: heat denaturation (Kramer, 1974) or salt desolvation followed by covalent cross-linkage (Marty *et al.*, 1978) are generally used. Drug attachment to nanospheres can be either by superficial adsorption or by embedding within the matrix, leading to different release-time profiles and mechanisms. Release by diffusion through, or bioerosion of, the matrix may occur when the drug is entrapped in the core of nanospheres.

Table 2. Drug-loaded nanospheres tested for gastrointestinal application

Drug	Reference
Insulin	Couvreur *et al.* (1980), Opfenheim *et al.* (1982), Michel *et al.* (1991a)
Vincamine	Maincent *et al.* (1986)
Antigens	Cox and Taubman (1984), O'Hagan *et al.* (1989a,b), Eldridge *et al.* (1990)

Nanocapsules

Nanocapsules are vesicular polymeric CDDSs. Their size is between 100 nm and 400 nm in diameter. They are made from a central oily core surrounded with a thin polymeric wall. The nanocapsule can be obtained either by interfacial polymerization of alkylcyanoacrylate monomers (Al Khouri Fallouh et al., 1986) or following interfacial deposition of any preformed polymer (Fessi et al., 1987b). Nanocapsules with an aqueous central core are not easily prepared (El Samaligy et al., 1986). Drug entrapment in nanocapsules (Table 3) is therefore essentially limited to lipophilic chemicals either as a solution in a biocompatible solvent or as a pure, preferably fluid, entity. One of the advantages of nanocapsules is their high loading capacity (drug:polymer ratio) as compared with nanospheres. The release properties of nanocapsules depend on the partition coefficient of the entrapped drug between the oily core and the suspending medium. The permeability characteristics of the polymeric wall seem to have little or no influence on the release rate; this may be due to the thickness, a few nanometres, of this barrier.

Table 3. Drug-loaded nanocapsules tested for gastrointestinal application

Drug	Reference
Indomethacin	Andrieu et al. (1986, 1989), Gursoy et al. (1989), Ammoury et al. (1990a,b, 1991), Ammoury (1990)
Insulin	Damgé et al. (1988, 1990), Michel et al. (1991b)
Lipiodol®	Aprahamiam et al. (1987), Damgé et al. (1991)

CDDS pharmaceutics

For therapeutic purposes, liposomes, niosomes, nanospheres and nanocapsules are suspended in an aqueous medium. Their small size allows physically stable dispersions to be obtained. When drug leakage is suspected, liposomes, niosomes and nanospheres can be advantageously freeze dried. Nanocapsules are usually destroyed by such a treatment and, fortunately, do not need it. Since the oral route of administration implies the contact of CDDSs with various biological environments, stability represents an important property of the dosage form. Liposomes and niosomes are more or less stable *in vitro* and in biological fluids, depending on the composition and the number of bilayers. Nanospheres and nanocapsules are more stable than liposomes and niosomes, depending on the rate of biodegradation of the matrix or of the wall.

ORAL DELIVERY BY LIPOSOMES

Published results

Bangham et al., (1965) first suggested that liposomes may protect the entrapped drug from digestive degradations. They were followed by Sessa and Weissman (1970), who furthermore suggested an increase of absorption. In 1973 two patents from Inchema (1973) and Bayer (1973) claimed that liposomally entrapped insulin could induce hypoglycaemic shock in mice following oral administration. In 1976, two groups (Patel and Ryman, 1976; Dapergolas and Gregoriadis, 1976) again attempted to deliver insulin orally by liposomes and reported positive results in rats rendered diabetic. Thereafter, controversial literature emerged until 1988 debating the various influences of the physiopathological status of subjects (normal or diabetic), of the lipids used to prepare liposomes, etc (Patel and Ryman, 1977a,b; Dapergolas and Gregoriadis, 1977; Patel *et al.*, 1978; Hashimoto and Kawada, 1979; Tragl *et al.*, 1979; Weingarten *et al.*, 1981; Kawada *et al.*, 1981; Patel *et al.*, 1982; Arrieta-Molero *et al.*, 1982; Shenfield and Hill, 1982; Dobre *et al.*, 1983; Das *et al.*, 1988) (Table 4).

Table 4. *In vivo* results following gastrointestinal administration of liposomally entrapped insulin

Animal species	Physiopathological condition	Insulin dose (UI)	Results[a]	Experimental data[b]	References
Rat	Normal	5–12	–	G	Patel *et al.* (1976, 1977a,b)
Rat	Diabetic	5–12	+	G	Patel *et al.* (1976, 1977a,b)
Rat	Normal	1–35	+	G(+), I(+)	Dapergolas and Gregoriadis (1976, 1977)
Rat	Diabetic	1–35	+	G(+), I(+)	Dapergolas and Gregoriadis (1976, 1977)
Man	Normal	80–90	+/–	G(–), I(+)	Patel *et al.* (1978)
Rat	Diabetic	20	+/–	G	Hashimoto and Kawada (1979)
Rat	Diabetic	10/kg	+	G	Tragl *et al.* (1979)
Rat	Diabetic	20–40/kg	–[c]	G	Weingarten *et al.* (1981)
Rat	Diabetic	15–30	+/–	G(–), I(+)	Kawada *et al.* (1981)
Dog	Diabetic	50–100	+/–	G(–), I(+)	Patel *et al.* (1982)
Rat	Diabetic	5/kg	+/–	G	Arrieta-Molero *et al.* (1982)
Rabbit	Diabetic	5/kg	+/–	G	Arrieta-Molero *et al.* (1982)
Rat	Normal and Diabetic		+/–	G	Shenfield and Hill (1982)
Rat	Normal	5/kg	+/–	G	Dobre *et al.* (1983)

[a] –, no pharmacological response; +, reduction of blood glucose and/or enhancement of plasma insulin concentrations; +/– some responders in the test group, or contradiction between no reduction of blood glucose and increase of plasma insulin concentrations.
[b] G, blood glucose level; I, denotes plasma insulin concentration.
[c] No hypoglycaemia following intragastric administration but reduced blood glucose following intrabuccal administration.

During the same period many other drugs were also studied, either hydrophilic (glucose oxidase (Dapergolas *et al.*, 1977; *d*-tubocurarine (Dapergolas and Gregoriadis 1977); angiotensin II (Papaioannou *et al.*, 1978); 1-B-D arabinofuranosylcytosine (Rustum *et al.*, 1979); gentamycin (Morgan and and Williams, 1980); factor VIII (Hemker et al., 1980 ; Kirby and Gregoriadis, 1984); factor IX (Ueno *et al.*, 1982a); heparin (Ueno *et al.*, 1982b); cysteamine (Jaskierowicz *et al.*, 1985) or lipophilic (vitamin K) (Nagata *et al.*, 1984); dolichol (Kimura *et al.*, 1989)).

The overall results of those numerous *in vivo* studies indicate that liposomal entrapment does not facilitate the gastrointestinal absorption of drugs normally not absorbed when orally administered in conventional dosage forms. When liposomal entrapment appears to facilitate absorption, it is only to a small extent and, moreover, in an unpredictable manner. Thus, variations in response to oral liposome therapy renders problematic any human application and highlights questions.

- Are liposomes stable in the gastrointestinal tract?
- Are liposomes able to protect the entrapped drug from the luminal environment (low gastric pH, enzymes)?
- Are intact liposomes absorbed by the epithelial cells and then transferred to the serosal side of the barrier?
- Do liposomes protect the entrapped drug during intracellular transfer and release it in the blood stream or in the lymph?
- Do the lipid composition, the number of bilayers and the superficial charge have an influence on these properties?

Given the number of variables and the complexity of the system, *in vivo* experiments were not capable of answering the questions. *In vitro* and *in situ* studies allowing more specific answers were then started.

Fate of liposomes and liposomally entrapped drugs following oral administration
The stability of different lipidic compositions was tested under gastrointestinal conditions: low pH and pepsin for the gastric environment, bile salts and lipases for the intestinal one (Op Dem Kamp *et al.*, 1974; Richards and Gardner, 1978; Rowland and Woodley, 1980; Chiang and Weiner, 1987).

All these studies clearly demonstrated that liposomes were not likely to be stable in the gastrointestinal tract, particularly in the presence of bile salts. It is obvious that drug entrapped in the aqueous compartment(s) of liposomes would be released if the physical structure of the carrier is disrupted. Structural lability of liposomes in the intestinal fluids, following the bile salt secretion in the duodenal segment, would result in loss of the carrier function.

The stability of liposomal entrapped drugs may involve two aspects: one is the leakage of the free drug, the other its protection from degradation by the carrier. Assuming the integrity of the liposomal structure, the leakage of a hydrophilic drug will be governed by the rate of diffusion through a given lipidic bilayer and by the number of bilayers. Thus, unilamellar liposomes entrapping a drug of low molecular weight should be less stable than a multilamellar vesicle entrapping macromolecules. The protection of an entrapped drug from luminal degradation relies firstly on the physical integrity of the liposomes and secondly on the impermeability of the bilayers to the aggressive species of the gastrointestinal fluids. Thus a pH-dependent attack is possible, but an enzymatic attack is more unlikely as long as the bilayers remain intact. Weingarten *et al.* (1985) have shown that liposomally entrapped insulin resisted the proteolytic activity of pepsin, trypsin and α–chymotrypsin for more than 30 min whereas free insulin did not.

As previously stated, reports of the pharmacological activity following oral administration of liposomally entrapped drugs, when similar doses of the free drug remained ineffective, imply that some absorption could occur and lead to an effective systemic drug level. Assuming an increased stability of the entrapped drug and, at least, some persistence of intact liposomal structures in the luminal fluids, one might ask whether, and how, the carrier can be taken up by epithelial cells and transferred to the serosal side. Using *in vitro* techniques, such as the everted intestinal sac or loop, and *in situ* techniques, such as infusion through isolated vascularly perfused intestinal segments, both avoiding the presence of destabilizing bile salts and enzymatic activity (lipases), various kinds of liposome structures and compositions have been tested. Drugs or markers, poorly or not absorbed in their free form, were used as indicators of passage (Bridges *et al.*, 1978; Whitmore and Wheeler, 1979 Seiden and Lichtenberg, 1979; Rowland and Woodley, 1981a–c; Schwinke *et al.*, 1984a,b; Hashida *et al.*, 1984; Kimura *et al.*, 1984; Patel *et al.*, 1985; Weiner and Chiang, 1988) (Table 5). From those studies it can be concluded that endocytosis of liposomes by the intestinal cells, if it occurs at all, is a rare event. When endocytosis did seem to take place it was followed by digestion of liposomes, thus releasing the drug or marker intracellularly. No transfer

Table 5. *In vitro* (everted intestinal sac) and *in situ* (isolated vascularly perfused intestinal segment) studies of the absorption of liposomally entrapped markers

Marker	Technique	Result	Reference
^{125}I-PVP	*In vitro*	+	Bridges *et al.* (1978)
^{23}Na	*In vitro*	–	Whitmore and Wheeler (1979)
^{14}C-cholesterol	*In vitro*	+/–	Seiden and Lichtenberg (1979)
^{14}C-DPC			
^{3}H-inulin	*In situ*	–	Schwinke *et al.* (1984a,b)
^{14}C-PEG 4000			
^{14}C-glucose		+/–	
Carboxyfluorescein	*In situ*	+/–	Hashida *et al.* (1984)
Carboxyfluorescein	*In vitro*	+/–	Kimura *et al.* (1984)
^{14}C-inulin	*In situ*		Patel *et al.* (1985)
^{125}I-PVP			
^{14}C-glucose	*In vitro*	–	Weiner and Chaing (1988)
Carboxyfluorescein			
^{3}H-PEG 4000	*In situ*	–	Weiner and Chaing (1988)
^{3}H-glucose			

of intact liposomes to the serosal side of the barrier, or to the venous effluent was observed.

Conclusion and perspectives

A consensus view of available data leads to the following conclusions.

- Liposome entrapment may protect some labile drugs from luminal enzymatic degradation, but only while the physical structure of the bilayered system is preserved.
- Physical stability of liposomes in luminal fluids is related to the lipid composition, the number of bilayers and the superficial charge, but they are always more or less sensitive to bile salts.
- If liposomes escape destruction, only a small proportion can be taken up by digestive cells and, if so, will be digested and will release their contents intracellularly.
- Some superficial adsorption of carriers onto the mucus or brush border may also occur, which may possibly facilitate the transfer of small amounts of the free drug from liposome into the cells.
- Although positive pharmacological responses have been observed after oral administration of liposomally entrapped drugs ineffective in their free form, poor bioavailability and large variability preclude major therapeutic developments.

However, in addition to this pessimistic prospect, it should be mentioned that liposome entrapment may ensure the protection of gastrointestinal mucosae from the ulcerative effects of orally administered non-steroidal anti-inflammatory drugs, such as indomethacin (Soehngen *et al.*, 1988).

If intact liposomes cannot gain access to lymph or blood it is obvious that oral administration of liposomal entrapped drugs will not affect the disposition kinetics of these drugs, assuming that they are absorbed. Oral administration of liposomes for targeting purposes is therefore out of the question. However, a possible area for future research may be found in the stable liposome-like structures obtained with polymerizable lipids (Johnston *et al.*, 1980; Juliano *et al.*, 1984) which do not seem to have been tested by the oral route. Furthermore, although the uptake of particulate materials into Peyer's patches has been repeatedly reported, similar work with liposomes has not, to our knowledge, been carried out.

ORAL DELIVERY BY NIOSOMES

Structural analogies between niosomes and liposomes suggest that both types of vesicles should lead to comparable results following the oral administration of entrapped drugs. An unknown but conclusive parameter could be the stability of niosomes in the presence of bile salts and/or lipases. The only reported data concerning oral delivery by niosomes concerned methotrexate in mice (Azmin *et al.*, 1985). Niosome-entrapped methotrexate produced significantly higher serum, liver and brain concentrations than free drug in aqueous solution, even in the presence of 6% polysorbate 80.

ORAL DELIVERY BY NANOSPHERES

Drug delivery by orally administered particulates in the nanometre range, i.e. nanospheres, has only recently emerged as a potential therapeutic strategy. As previously mentioned, the amount of data available, compared with the liposome literature, is restricted. In contrast, because of the stability of polymeric particles, their transfer through the intestinal barrier has been described and will be discussed further below.

Published results

The drug for which oral delivery by nanospheres was first attempted was, of course, insulin: Couvreur *et al.* (1980) tried to promote insulin absorption following its adsorption on poly(alkylcyanoacrylate) nanospheres but failed to obtain a hypoglycaemic response in rats rendered diabetic. Oppenheim *et al.* (1982) used a different approach and prepared nanospheres directly from insulin by desolvation and cross-linking with glutaraldehyde: blood glucose levels were reduced following oral administration of high doses (35 to 75 mg per 100 g body weight) to mice and rats. Recent data from Michel *et al.* (1991a) indicate that reproducible hypoglycaemia could be obtained in rats rendered diabetic, following the oral administration of insulin-loaded nanospheres of poly(alkylcyanoacrylate) dispersed in an oily phase with deoxycholate and poloxamer; reduction of blood glucose level was about 50% and lasted for one week.

Vincamine-loaded nanoparticles of poly(alkylcyanoacrylate) were studied in rabbits following intravenous and oral administration, by Maincent *et al.* (1986). Compared with an aqueous solution of vincamine, it was shown that nanospheres were able to enhance the oral bioavailability as reflected by plasma concentration–time profiles. Taking into account the proportion of the drug loaded in the carriers and free in the suspending medium, and assuming stability of the drug–carrier association in the luminal fluids, a 350% increase of the systemic bioavailability was calculated to be specifically attributable to the vincamine-loaded nanospheres. In order to explain this result the authors suggested that the carrier might possess bioadhesive properties resulting in an increased contact with the gut wall and facilitating the transfer of vincamine from the nanospheres to the absorptive cells. Protection by the carrier against luminal degradation of the drug was also assumed.

Another interesting approach has been the use of larger particles, i.e. microspheres, to deliver antigens to the gut. Cox and Taubman (1984) demonstrated the efficacy of non-biodegradable poly(acrylamide) 1–3 μm microspheres in enhancing the immune response to an orally administered antigen. O'Hagan *et al.* (1989b) and Eldridge *et al.* (1990) confirmed the potential of 1–10 μm microspheres for oral delivery of antigens. This potential was extended to biodegradable poly(alkylcyanoacrylate) 100 nm nanospheres by O'Hagan *et al.* (1989a).

Fate of nanospheres and entrapped drugs following oral administration

Stability of nanospheres in the gastrointestinal fluids has not been specifically studied. Solid polymeric, or cross-linked proteic, structures, even if biodegradable, should ensure a better stability than would liposomes or niosomes in the presence of an acidic environment, of bile salts and of enzymes. However, the capacity of nanospheres to protect drugs might be quite different according to whether they were embedded within the matrix or adsorbed on the surface. It is quite obvious that superficial desorption could occur in the intestinal fluids, while the macromolecular network of the matrix could protect the entrapped material, at least from enzymes of high molecular weight, as long as bioerosion does not occur. The major question to ask is, therefore, are nanospheres able to cross the gastrointestinal barrier and to deliver their drug content to the blood or to the lymph or, even, to the target organs?

Translocation of particles
Translocation of particles is a controversial area, generally viewed with scepticism by many as the wall of the mammalian gastrointestinal tract is assumed to be an impermeable barrier, because of tight junctions, i.e. zona occludens, between the epithelial absorptive cells, i.e. enterocytes. The uptake and transport of solid particulates across the gastrointestinal epithelium may have, apart from drug delivery, important toxicological, immunological and pathological consequences as the diet allows ingestion of various mineral, vegetal or animal dusts, fibres and cell fragments. Related interesting topics are the translocation of bacteria or viruses (see Wells *et al.*, 1988a) and macromolecule absorption (see Weiner, 1988). Therefore, considerable efforts have been made to elucidate the mechanism(s) of translocation of solid particulates through the gastrointestinal barrier and to quantify it (see Volkheimer, 1977; Le Fevre and Joel, 1977; O'Hagan, 1990).

Many particulate materials, of various sizes and compositions, have been tested, including asbestos fibres (Pontefract and Cunningham, 1973; Cook, 1983), methylmethacrylate microspheres and nanospheres (Juhlin, 1959; Nefzger *et al.*, 1984), polystyrene nanospheres (Sanders and Ashworth, 1961; Jani *et al.*, 1989, 1990), polystyrene microspheres (Le Fevre *et al.*, 1989; Alpar *et al.*, 1989); the materials tested ranged from 7 nm colloidal silver particles (Cardell *et al.*, 1967) to 110 μm starch granules (Volkheimer and Schulz, 1968).

There is now much evidence that uptake and transfer of solid materials can and do occur, by and through the intestinal barrier. Thus, particle translocation may have pharmaceutical implications, not only for drug delivery purposes, but also because many excipients of orally administered conventional dosage forms are unsoluble, micro- or nanosized, particulate materials such as titanium or silicium oxides, aluminium and some calcium salts, etc. The use of coating materials such as aqueous dispersion of latex, i.e. acrylate derivatives (Eudragit^R) or aqueous dispersion of pseudo-latex, i.e. cellulose derivatives (Aquacoat^R) may also be involved.

Possible mechanisms of translocation
Mechanisms proposed for the translocation of particulates across the intestine include endocytosis by enterocytes, a paracellular pathway, phagocytosis and transport by intestinal macrophages and uptake into Peyer's patches.

- Only very small particles, up to 200 nm but preferably between 20 and 50 nm, seem to be endocytosable by the absorptive cells of the intestine. Particles would be then included in cytoplasmic vesicles and discharged in the serosal spaces to gain access

to the mesenteric lymph or blood (Barrnet, 1959; Sanders and Ashworth, 1961; Matsumo et al., 1983).
- The passage of particles between the absorptive cells, called persorption by Volkheimer, seems rather less likely than the intracellular route if the barrier of tight junctions has not been disrupted, either by natural desquamation of mature cells or by chemical treatment including alcoholic beverages and absorption enhancers (see Muranishi, 1987; Lee 1990), particularly those affecting the Ca^{2+}-dependent cell adhesion molecule uvomurolin.
- The phagocytic uptake of particles by intestinal macrophages has been demonstrated by Wells et al. (1988b) in isolated jejunal loops of dogs and ileal loops of rats. Intralysosomial localization of particles, eventually followed by digestion for biodegradable materials, and further migration of macrophages to the mesenteric lymph nodes seem to preclude any release of substantial amounts of unchanged drug in the blood stream. Thus, sufficient systemic bioavailability would be unlikely after uptake of drug-loaded nanospheres by intestinal macrophages.
- The uptake of particulate materials into Peyer's patches or into isolated lymphoid follicles has been repeatedly reported (Le Fevre et al., 1977; Le Fevre and Joel, 1984; Le Fevre et al., 1989; Jani et al., 1989; Pappo and Ermak, 1989; Eldridge et al., 1990). Subsequent passage of particles into mesenteric lymph nodes, and even the lymph nodes surrounding the lungs, or into remote body sites, organs and fluids, seems to be attributable to an uptake by macrophages. It is generally accepted that the M cells, which have been ascribed an antigen-sampling function, are implicated in the uptake of particles. The uptake by M cells has been demonstrated in rats (Seifert et al., 1983) and in rabbits (Pappo and Ermak, 1989) with particles less than 1 µm in diameter. M cells are particularly abundant in rabbit Peyer's patches where the rate of uptake of particles was about ten-fold the rate in murine Peyer's patches. Using the gut loop technique, Pappo and Ermak (1989) reported as many as 2000 particles per mm of Peyer's patch lymphoepithelial dome and estimated an average rate of transport of 2 µm/min and the total uptake to be about 5% of the administered dose of polystyrene particles (600–750 nm diameter).

Rate of translocation
Considering potential therapeutic applications following oral administration, the rate of translocation of drug-loaded nanospheres is of special interest and should be high enough to allow the systemic delivery of pharmacological doses during the time of residence in the gastrointestinal tract. From this fundamental point of view none of endocytosis by enterocytes, paracellular passage or phagocytosis by intestinal macrophages would provide a sufficient rate of translocation to ensure activity following a single administration. Translocation via the uptake in Peyer's patches is certainly the most rapid process and has been proved to allow substantial passage following chronic administration.

Quantitation of translocation of particles through the intestinal barrier has been studied (Le Fevre et al., 1989; Jani et al., 1990; Ebel, 1990) and the influence of particle size and surface properties tested. More studies will be necessary to determine the optimal characteristics for oral drug delivery. However, Jani et al. (1990) have already shown that the total uptake following chronic oral gavage could be as much as 30% of the administered dose if 50 nm particles are used, but is reduced to 10% of the dose with 300 nm particles and to less than 5% with 1 µm particles. Similar size-related uptake profiles were observed by Jani et al. (1990) in the organs where particles could be detected, i.e. liver and spleen, and in the blood. It was also demonstrated that hydrophobic particles were taken up by Peyer's patches and transported to liver and spleen to a larger extent than ionizable (carboxylated) ones (Jani et al., 1989). Eldridge et al. (1990) have shown that particles consisting of cellulose derivatives were taken up into mouse Peyer's patches slightly or not at all, whereas hydrophobic materials such as polystyrene or poly(methylmethacrylate) underwent larger absorption. It should be mentioned that neither Jani nor Eldridge specified the presence, and if any the nature, of stabilizing excipient(s) in the colloidal suspensions tested. The influence of such chemicals, surfactants or others, on the surface properties of particles may have some consequence on absorption characteristics as they have on the *in vivo* distribution of particles after parenteral administration (Tomlinson, 1987; O'Mullane et al., 1990). The influence of stabilizing agents on the permeability of the intestinal barriers to particulate materials should be also considered and would certainly need more specific studies.

ORAL DELIVERY BY NANOCAPSULES

Published results

Like nanospheres, nanocapsules have only recently been developed and tested for oral drug delivery. Poly(isobutylcyanoacrylate) nanocapsules were first studied (Andrieu et al., 1986, 1989; Gursoy et al., 1989), which was then followed by the study of poly(d,l-lactide) nanocapsules (Ammoury et al., 1990a,b, 1991), both loaded with indomethacin as a model drug. In comparison with an aqueous solution of indomethacin, both types of nanocapsules exhibited similar drug plasma concentration-time profiles and similar pharmacological activity following oral administration to rats. Moreover, both types of nanocapsules revealed a remarkable capacity to protect the gastrointestinal mucosae from the ulcerative effects of indomethacin at oral doses as large as 10 mg/kg for 3 consecutive days (Ammoury, 1990). This protection, also observed with indomethacin-loaded liposomes, was quite surprising as the pharmacological effects of systemic origin were preserved.

Insulin-loaded poly(alkylcyanoacrylate) nanocapsules were demonstrated to be ineffective at reducing glycaemia following oral administration to normal rats. However, they were capable of reducing hyperglycaemia in a reproducible manner in rats rendered diabetic, and also in normal rats after oral loading with glucose (Damgé et al., 1988). This result was confirmed following specific intraluminal injections of insulin-loaded nanocapsules in isolated intestinal segments of rats rendered diabetic (Michel et al., 1991b). A rank order of absorptive sites was established as follows: ileum > jejunum ≥ duodenum > colon. One astonishing aspect of the data from Damgé et al. (1988) and Michel et al. (1991b) is the 2-day lag time preceding the hypoglycaemic response to insulin-loaded nanocapsules, followed by a maintained efficiency for up to 20 days. It was also surprising that the duration of the effect was correlated with the insulin dose, while there was no relationship observed between the peak of hypoglycaemia and the dose. These results may suggest some bioadhesive properties for poly(alkylcyanoacrylate) nanocapsules inducing prolonged retention of the carrier and sustained uptake in the gastrointestinal tract. In this case we must assume that nanocapsules and their insulin loading remain stable in the intestinal fluids for several days. Damgé et al. (1990) have shown that nanoencapsulation could protect insulin from proteolytic degradation *in vitro*: 75% of the initial insulin was preserved following 30 min incubation at 37°C of nanocapsules in the presence of pepsin, trypsin or a-chymotrypsin, while free insulin was largely degraded. It should be mentioned that the delayed action and long-lasting hypoglycaemic effect following oral administration of insulin-loaded nanocapsules were not observed after subcutaneous injection of the same nanocapsules. The subcutaneous route provided a classical sustained release time profile with a hypoglycaemic effect not exceeding one day (Damgé et al., 1988). Another unanswered question concerning insulin nanocapsules is the capacity of a hydrophilic drug to be entrapped in the oily core of the carrier. Moreover, the formation of the polymeric wall of the nanocapsules used by Damgé and coworkers involved an anionic interfacial polymerization of alkylcyanoacrylate monomers, very sensitive to basic groups such as amino groups, and Gallardo et al. (1989) have shown that cross-reaction between the drug content and the alkylcyanoacrylate monomer could occur during the preparation of nanocapsules. Therefore it cannot be excluded that insulin may be covalently linked to the wall of poly(alkylcyanoacrylate) nanocapsules. It should be mentioned here that all attempts to entrap insulin into nanocapsules prepared from preformed polymers, i.e. poly(*d,l*-lactide), were unsuccessful in our laboratory.

Fate of nanocapsules and entrapped drugs following oral administration
Repeated experiments have demonstrated the effectiveness of insulin-loaded nanocapsules following oral administration to hyperglycaemic animals. The question again arises of the translocation of nanocapsules through the gastrointestinal barrier, and of their capacity to deliver their drug-content either at the site of administration or to the blood. Aprahamian et al. (1987) have demonstrated that poly(alkylcyanoacrylate) nanocapsules, loaded with an iodine marker (Lipiodol[R])for X-ray microprobe analysis in a scanning electron microscope, were able to cross the jejunal barrier of dog and to gain access to the blood capillaries and the lymph ducts. This passage was confirmed for the ileal barrier of rat (Damgé *et al.*, 1991). In both dog and rat studies nanocapsules were not detected within enterocytes but only between them. In accordance with the size of Lipiodol-loaded nanocapsules (200–300 nm) and previously mentioned size restrictions for nanospheres, this suggests that endocytosis by absorptive cells is unlikely. From the data derived from the dog study, the paracellular pathway was evoked by Aprahamian *et al.* (1987). In the rat study Damgé *et al.* (1991) demonstrated that the Peyer's patches and M cells should play a major role in the translocation of Lipiodol-loaded nanocapsules.

As nanocapsules and nanospheres seem to follow parallel mechanisms of translocation through the gut wall, it can be assumed that both carriers will have the same rate of passage. *In vitro* studies using indomethacin have shown that drug release involves partition between the oily core and the surrounding medium of nanocapsules, with a minor role of the polymeric wall (Ammoury, 1990). This might not be the same with drugs of high molecular weight, whose release would require the disruption of the biodegradable polymeric barrier. Little is known about the *in vivo* release of drugs entrapped in nanospheres or in nanocapsules and more studies are needed. However, the release mechanisms would be different for a drug embedded within the polymeric network of the matrix of nanospheres and a drug entrapped in the lipidic core of nanocapsules, isolated from the surrounding fluid by a polymeric barrier a few nanometres thick.

CONCLUDING REMARKS AND PROSPECTS

Liposomes, niosomes, nanospheres and nanocapsules were expected to be able to enhance significantly the systemic bioavailability of some poorly absorbed or labile drugs following oral administration. These colloidal drug delivery systems have been tested in various experimental conditions *in vivo, in situ* and *in vitro*, by numerous research groups, using different model drugs. Positive pharmacological results have been obtained, but most often with a poor reproducibility. Quantitative studies have shown that some enhancement of the oral bioavailability could be obtained, but in all cases the overall absorption remained a low proportion of the administered dose. It is now well established that liposomes, and probably niosomes, are not stable enough to resist luminal and/or intracellular degradation, and that nanospheres and nanocapsules are the most promising candidates for gastrointestinal application. Nanospheres and nanocapsules have been proved able to cross the intestinal barrier by different mechanisms, from which the uptake by the gut-associated lymphoid tissue was the most efficient. However, the studies quantifying the uptake of particles by the intestinal mucosae have demonstrated that pharmacological doses are unlikely to be delivered in a reproducible manner following a single oral administration.

Among positive results allowing potential therapeutic developments, the use of antigen-loaded colloidal carriers could be the most promising as the colloidal carriers seem to target the Peyer's patches and because the systemic bioavailability is not a critical parameter. Also to be considered is the protection, by liposomes and nanocapsules, of the gastrointestinal mucosae from the ulcerative effects of non-steroidal anti-inflammatory drugs. The reproducible hypoglycaemic effect of orally administered insulin-loaded nanocapules is also a very interesting result, but the time–response profile observed in rats precludes any applicability to the treatment of human diabetes if this profile is maintained in man. Further studies will be necessary to elucidate the mode of action of insulin-loaded nanocapsules, and to optimize their time–response profile.

If stable colloidal carriers, i.e. nanospheres or nanocapsules, are taken up by the gastrointestinal mucosae and discharged to the lymph or blood, even in a very low proportion of the administered dose, their physiological fate will also need more studies. Moreover, long-term application of colloidal carriers in man would involve the use of biodegradable materials and knowledge of their rate of degradation will be needed in order to avoid any accumulation in the body.

REFERENCES

Al Khouri Fallouh, N., Roblot-Treupel, L., Fessi, H., Devissaguet, J. P. and Puisieux, F. (1986) Development of a new process for the manufacture of polyisobutylcyanoacrylate nanocapsules. *Int. J. Pharm.* **28** 125–132.

Alpar, H. O., Field, W. N., Hyde, R. and Lewis, D. A. (1989) The transport of microspheres from the gastro-intestinal tract to inflammatory air pouches in the rat. *J. Pharm. Pharmacol.* **41** 194–196.

Ammoury, N. (1990) Etude physicochimique et biologique de vecteurs colloïdaux vésiculaires d'indométacine-acide polylactique. *PhD Thesis.* Paris-Sud.

Ammoury, N., Fessi, H., Devissaguet, J. P., Puisieux, F. and Benita, S. (1990a) *In-vitro* release pattern of indomethacin from poly(*d,l*-lactide) nanocapsules. *J. Pharm. Sci.* **79** 763–767.

Ammoury, N., Fessi, H., Devissaguet, J. P., Allix, M., Plotkine, M. and Boulu, R. G. (1990b) Effect on cerebral blood flow of orally administered indomethacin-loaded poly(isobutylcyanoacrylate) and poly(*d,l*-lactide) nanocapsules. *J. Pharm. Pharmacol.* **42** 558–561.

Ammoury, N., Fessi, H., Devissaguet, J. P., Dubrasquet, M. and Benita, S. (1991) Jejunal absorption, pharmacological activity and pharmacokinetic evaluation of poly(*d,l*-lactide) and poly(isobutylcyanoacrylate) nanocapsules in rats. *Pharm. Res.* **8** 101–105.

Andrieu, V., Dubrasquet, M., Fessi, H. and Devissaguet, J. P. (1986) Etude pharmacocinétique, biopharmaceutique et de tolérance digestive et dispersions colloïdales d'indométacine. *Proc. 4th Int. Conf. Pharm. Technol.*, Vol. 4. APGI, Paris, pp. 166–174.

Andrieu, V., Fessi, H., Dubrasquet, M., Devissaguet, J. P., Puisieux, F. and Benita, S. (1989) Pharmacokinetic evaluation of indomethacin nanocapsules. *Drug Des. Deliv.* **4** 295–302.

Aprahamian, M., Michel, C., Humbert, W., Devissaguet, J. P. and Damgé, C. (1987) Transmucosal passage of polyalkylcyanoacrylate nanocapsules as a new drug carrier in the small intestine. *Biol. Cell* **61** 69–76.

Arrieta-Molero, J. F., Aleck, K., Sinha, M. K., Browscheidle, C. M., Shapiro, L. J. and Sperling, M. A. (1982) Oral administered liposome-entrapped insulin in diabetic animals. A critical assessment. *Hormone Res.* **16** 249–256.

Azmin, M. N., Florence, A. T., Handjani-Vila, R. M., Stuart, J. F. B., Vanlerberghe, G. and Whittaker, J. S. (1985) The effect of non-ionic surfactant vesicle (niosome) entrapment on the absorption and distribution of methotrexate in mice. *J. Pharm. Pharmacol.* **37** 237–242.

Bangham, A. D., Standish, M. M. and Watkins, J. C. (1965) Diffusion of univalent ions across the lamellae of swollen phospholipids. *J. Mol. Biol.* **13** 238–252.
Barrnet, R. J. (1959) The demonstration with the electron microscope of the end products of the histochemical reactions in relation with the fine structure of cells. *Exp. Cell Res. Suppl.* **7** 65–89.
Bayer (1973) *Belgian Patent* 796,610.
Bridges, J. F., Millard, P. C. and Woodley, J. F. (1978) The uptake of liposome-entrapped ^{125}I-labelled poly(vinyl-pyrrolidone) by rat jejunum *in-vitro*. *Biochim. Biophys. Acta* **544** 448–451.
Cardell, R., Badenhausen, S. and Porter, X. (1967) *J. Cell. Biol.* **24** 123–155.
Chiang, C. M. and Wiener, N. (1987) Gastrointestinal uptake of liposomes. I. *In-vitro* and *in-situ* studies. *Int. J. Pharm.* **37** 75–85.
Cook, P. M. (1983) Review of published studies on gut penetration by ingested asbestos fibres. *Environ. Health Perspect.* **53** 121–130.
Couvreur, P., Lenaerts, V., Kante, B., Roland, M. and Speiser, P. (1980) Oral and parenteral administration of insulin associated to hydrolysable nanoparticles. *Acta Pharm. Technol.* **26** 220–222.
Couvreur, P., Grislain, L., Lenaerts, V., Brasseur, F., Guiot, P. and Biernacki, A. (1984) Biodegradable polymeric nanoparticles as drug carrier for antitumor agents. In: Guiot, P. and Couvreur, P. (eds) *Polymeric Nanoparticles and Microspheres.* CRC Press, Boca Raton, FL, pp. 27–93.
Cox, D. S. and Taubman, M. A. (1984) Oral induction of the secretory antibody response by soluble and particulate antigens. *Int. Arch. Allergy Appl. Immunol.* **75** 126–131.
Damgé, C., Michel, C., Aprahamian, M. and Couvreur, P. (1988) New approach for oral administration of insulin with polyalkylcyanoacrylate nanocapsules as drug carrier. *Diabetes* **37** 246–251.
Damgé, C., Michel, C., Aprahamian, M., Couvreur, P. and Devissaguet, J. P. (1990) Nanocapsules as carriers for oral delivery of peptides. *J. Control. Release* **13** 233–239.
Damgé, C., Defontaine, M., Aprahamian, M., Michel, C., Humbert, W. and Devissaguet, J. P. (1991) Preferential uptake of nanocapsules through Peyer's patches in the rat. *Proceed. of the 18th Symp. Control. Release Bioact. Mater., Amsterdam*, pp. 349–350
Dapergolas, G. and Gregoriadis, G. (1976) Hypoglycaemic effect of liposome-entrapped insulin administered intragastrically into rats. *Lancet* **ii** 824–827.
Dapergolas, G. and Gregoriadis, G. (1977) Effect of liposomal lipid composition on the fate and effect of liposome-entrapped insulin and *d*-tubocurarine. *Biochem. Soc. Trans.* **5** 1383–1386.
Dapergolas, G., Neerunjum, E. D. and Gregoriadis, G. (1977) Penetration of target areas in the rat by liposome-associated bleomycin, glucose-oxidase and insulin. *FEBS Lett.* **63** 235–239.
Das, N., Basu, M. K. and Das, M. K. (1988) Oral application of insulin encapsulated liposomes. *Biochem. Int.* **16** 983–989.

Dobre, V., Georgescu, D., Simionescu, L., Aman, U., Stroescu, V. and Motas, C. (1983) The entrapment of biologically active substances into liposomes. I. Effects of oral administration of liposomally entrapped insulin in normal rats. *Rev. Roum. Biochim.* 20 15–29.

Ebel, J. D (1990) A method for quantifying particle absorption from the mouse small intestine. *Pharm. Res.* 7 848–851.

El Samaligy, M. S., Rohdewald, P. and Mahmoud, H. A. (1986) Polyalkylcyanoacrylate nanocapsules. *J. Pharm. Pharmacol.* 38 216–218.

Eldridge, J. H., Hammond, C. J., Meulbroek, J. A., Staas, J. K., Gilley, R. M. and Tice, T. R. (1990) Controlled vaccine release in the gut associated lymphoid tissue. I. Orally administered biodegradable microspheres target the Peyer's patches. *J. Control. Release* 11 205–214.

Fessi, H., Devissaguet, J. P., Puisieux, F. and Thies, C. (1987a) Procédé de préparation de systémes colloïdaux dispersibles d'une substance sous forme de nanoparticules. *Eur. Pat. Appl. 87402997.8.*

Fessi, H., Puisieux, F. and Devissaguet, J. P. (1987b) Procédé de préparation de systémes colloïdaux dispersibles d'une substance sous forme de nanocapsules. *Eur. Pat. Appl. 87402998.6.*

Florence, A. T. and Baillie, A. J. (1989) Non-ionic surfactant vesicles — alternatives to liposomes in drug delivery? In: Prescott, L. F. and Nimmo, W. S. (eds) *Novel Drug Delivery.* Wiley, Chichester, pp. 281–296.

Gallardo, M. M., Roblot-Treupel, L., Mahuteau, J., Genin, I., Couvreur, P., Plat, M. and Puisieux, F. (1989) Nanocapsules et nanosphéres d'alkylcyanoacrylate interactions principe actif/polymére. *Proc. 5th Int. Conf. Pharm. Technol.,* Vol. 4. APGI, Paris, pp. 36–45.

Gursoy, A., Eroglu, L., Ulutin, S., Tasyurek, M., Fessi, H., Puisieux, F. and Devissaguet, J. P. (1989) Evaluation of indomethacin nanocapsules for their physical stability and inhibitory activity on inflammation and platelet aggregation. *Int. J. Pharm.* 52 101–108.

Hashida, N., Murakami, M., Yoshikawa, H., Takada, K. and Muranishi, S. (1984) Intestinal absorption of carboxyfluorescein entrapped in liposomes in comparison with its administration with lipid-surfactant mixed micelles. *J. Pharm. Dyn.* 7 195–203.

Hashimoto, A. and Kawada, J. (1979) Effects of oral administration of positively charged insulin liposomes on alloxan diabetic rats. *Endocrinol. Jpn.* 26 337–344.

Hemker, H. C., Hermens, W. T., Muller, A. D. and Zwall, R. F. (1980) Oral treatment of haemophilia A by gastrointestinal absorption of factor VIII entrapped in liposomes. *Lancet* 1 70–71.

Inchema (1973) *German Patent 2,249,552.*

Jani, P., Halbert, G. W., Langridge, J. and Florence, A. T. (1989) Uptake and translocation of latex nanospheres and microspheres after oral administration to rats. *J. Pharm. Pharmacol.* 41 809–812.

Jani, P., Halbert, G. W., Langridge, J. and Florence, A. T. (1990) Nanoparticle uptake by the rat gastrointestinal mucosa: quantitation and particle size dependency. *J. Pharm. Pharmacol.* 42 821–826.

Jaskierowicz, D., Genissel, F., Roman, V., Berleur, F. and Fatome, M. (1985) Oral administration of liposome-entrapped cysteamine and the distribution pattern in blood, liver and spleen. *Int. J. Radiat. Biol.* **47** 615–619.
Johnston, D. S., Sanghera, S., Pons, M. and Chapman, D. (1980) Phospholipid-polymers: synthesis and spectral characteristics. *Biochim. Biophys. Acta* **602** 57–69.
Juhlin, L. (1959) Absorption of solid spherical particles through the intestinal mucosa. *Acta Physiol. Scand.* **47** 365–369.
Juliano, R. I., Hsu, M. J., Regen, S. L. and Singh, M. (1984) Photopolymerized phospholipid vesicles. *Biochim. Biophys. Acta* **770** 109–114.
Kawada, J., Tanaka, N. and Nozaki, Y. (1981) No reduction of blood glucose in diabetic rats after oral administration of insulin liposomes prepared under acidic conditions. *Endocrinol. Jpn.* **28** 235–238.
Kimura, T., Higaki, K. and Sezaki, H. (1984) Transmucosal passage of liposomally entrapped drugs in the small intestine. *Pharm. Res.* **1** 221–224.
Kimura, T., Takeda, K., Kageyu, A., Toda, M., Kurosaki, Y. and Nakayama, T. (1989) Intestinal absorption of dolichol from emulsions and liposomes in rats. *Chem. Pharm. Bull.* **37** 463–466.
Kirby, C. J. and Gregoriadis, G. (1984) Preparation of liposomes containing factor VIII for oral treatment of haemophilia. *J. Microencaps.* **1** 33–45.
Kramer, P. (1974) Albumin microspheres as vehicles for achieving specificity in drug delivery. *J. Pharm. Sci.* **63** 1646–1647.
Lee, V. H. L. (1990) Protease inhibitors and penetration enhancers as approaches to modify peptide absorption. *J. Control. Release* **13** 213–223.
Le Fevre, M. E. and Joel, D. D. (1977) Intestinal absorption of particulate matter. *Life Sci.* **21** 1403–1408.
Le Fevre, M. E. and Joel, D. D. (1984) Peyer's patch epithelium: an imperfect barrier. In: Schiller, C. M. (ed.) *Intestinal Toxicology*. Raven Press, New York, pp. 45–56.
Le Fevre, M. E., Joel, D. D., Laissue, J. A., El-Aasser, M.S. and Vanderhoff, J. W. (1977) Stability of ^{125}I label after intragastric or intravenous administration of radioiodinated latexes to mice. *J. Reticuloendothel. Soc.* **22** 189–198.
Le Fevre, M. E., Boccio, A. M. and Joel, D. D. (1989) Intestinal uptake of fluorescent microspheres in young and aged mice (42825). *Proc. Soc. Exp. Biol. Med.* **190** 23–27.
Maincent, P., Le Verge, R., Sado, P., Couvreur, P. and Devissaguet, J. P. (1986) Disposition kinetics and oral bioavailability of vincamin-loaded polyalkycyanoacrylate nanoparticles. *J. Pharm. Sci.* **75** 955–958.
Martin, F. J. (1990) Pharmaceutical manufacturing of liposomes. In: Tyle, P. (ed.) *Specialized Drug Delivery Systems*. Drugs and the Pharmaceutical Sciences, Vol. 41, Dekker, New York, pp. 267–316.
Marty, J. J., Oppenheim, R. C. and Speiser, P. (1978) A new colloidal drug delivery system. *Pharm. Acta Helv.* **53** 17–23.
Matsumo, K., Schaffner, T., Gerber, H. A., Ruchti, C. C., Hess, M. W. and Cottier, H. (1983) Uptake by enterocytes and subsequent translocation to internal organs, e.g. the thymus, of Percoll microspheres administered per os to suckling mice. *J. Reticuloendothel. Soc.* **33** 263–273.

Michel, C., Roques, M., Couvreur, P., Vranckx, H., Balschmidt, P. and Damgé, C. (1991a) Isobutylcyanoacrylate nanoparticles as a drug carrier for oral administration of insulin. Personal communication.

Michel, C., Aprahamian, M., Defontaine, L., Couvreur, P. and Damge, C. (1991b) The effect of site of administration in the gastrointestinal tract on the absorption of insulin from nanocapsules in diabetic rats. *J. Pharm. Pharmacol.* **43** 1–5.

Morgan, J. R. and Williams, K. E. (1980) Preparation and properties of liposome-associated gentamycin. *Antimicrob. Agents Chemother.* **17** 544–548.

Muranishi, S. (1987) Absorption barriers and absorption promoters in the intestine. In: Breimer, D. D. and Speiser, P. (eds) *Topics in Pharmaceutical Sciences 1987*. Elsevier, Amsterdam, pp. 445–455.

Nagata, M., Yotsuyanagi, T., Nonomura, H. and Ikeda, K. (1984) Coagulation recovery after warfarin-induced hypoprothrombinaemia by oral administration of liposomally-associated vitamin K1 to rabbits. *J. Pharm. Pharmacol.* **36** 527–533.

Nefzger, M., Kreuter, J., Voges, R., Liehl, E. and Czok, R. (1984) Distribution and elimination of polymethylmethacrylate nanoparticles after peroral administration to rats. *J. Pharm. Sci.* **73** 1309–1311.

O'Hagan, D. T. (1990) Intestinal translocation of particulates — implications for drug and antigen delivery. *Adv. Drug Deliv. Rev.* **5** 265–285.

O'Hagan, D. T., Palin, K. and Davis, S. S (1989a) Poly(butyl-2-cyanoacrylate) particles as adjuvants for oral administration. *Vaccine* **7** 213–216.

O'Hagan, D. T., Palin, K., Davis, S. S., Artursson, P. and Sjoholh, I. (1989b) Microparticles as potentially orally active immunological adjuvants. *Vaccine* **7** 421–424.

O'Mullane, J. E., Petrak, K., Hutchinson, L. E. F. and Tomlinson, E. (1990) The effect of adsorbed coats of poloxamers 237 and 338 on the *in vitro* aggregation and *in vivo* distribution of polystyrene latex (PSL) particles. *Int. J. Pharm.* **63** 177–180.

Op Dem Kamp, J. A. F., De Geir, J. and Van Deenen, L. L. M. (1974) Hydrolysis of phosphatidylcholine liposomes by pancreatic phospholipases A2 at the transition temperature. *Biochim. Biophys. Acta* **543** 253–256.

Oppenheim, R. C., Stewart, N. F., Gordon, L. and Patel, H. M. (1982) The production and evaluation of orally administered insulin nanoparticles. *Drug Dev. Ind. Pharm.* **8** 531–546.

Papaioannou, S., Yang, P. C. and Novotney, R. (1978) Encapsulation of angiotensin II in liposomes: characterization *in-vitro* and *in-vivo*. *Clin. Exp. Hypertension* **1** 407–422.

Pappo, J. and Ermak, T. H. (1989) Uptake and translocation of fluorescent latex particles by rabbit Peyer's patches follicle epithelium: a quantitative model for M cell uptake. *Clin. Exp. Immunol.* **76** 144–148.

Patel, H. M. and Ryman, B. E. (1976) Oral administration of insulin by encapsulation within liposomes. *FEBS Lett.* **62** 60–63.

Patel, H. M. and Ryman, B. E. (1977a) Orally administered liposomally entrapped insulin. *Biochem. Soc. Trans.* **5** 1739–1741.

Patel, H. M. and Ryman, B. E. (1977b) The gastrointestinal absorption of liposomally entrapped insulin in normal rats. *Biochem. Soc. Trans.* **5** 1054–1055.

Patel, H. M., Harding, N. G. L., Logue, F., Kesson, C., MacCuish, A. C., MacKenzie, J. C., Ryman, B. E. and Scobie, I. (1978) Intrajejunal absorption of liposomally entrapped insulin in normal man. *Biochem. Soc. Trans.* **6** 784–785.

Patel, H. M., Stevenson, R. W., Parson, J. A. and Ryman, B. E. (1982) Use of liposomes to aid intestinal absorption of entrapped insulin in normal and diabetic dogs. *Biochim. Biophys. Acta* **716** 188–193.

Patel, H. M., Tuzel, N. S. and Stevenson, R. W. (1985) Intracellular digestion of saturated and unsaturated phospholipid liposomes by mucosal cells. Possible mechanism of transport of liposomally entrapped macromolecules across the isolated vascularly perfused rabbit ileum. *Biochim. Biophys. Acta* **839** 40–49.

Pontefract, R. D. and Cunningham, H. M. (1973) Penetration of asbestos through the digestive tract of rats. *Nature (London)* **243** 352–353.

Richards, M. H. and Gardner, C. R. (1978) Effects of bile salts on the structural integrity of liposomes. *Biochim. Biophys. Acta* **543** 508–522.

Rowland, R. N. and Woodley, J. F. (1980) The stability of liposomes *in-vitro* to pH, bile salts and pancreatic lipase. *Biochim. Biophys. Acta* **620** 400–409.

Rowland, R. N. and Woodley, J. F. (1981a) The uptake of distearoyl-phosphatidylcholine/cholesterol liposomes by rat intestinal sacs *in-vitro*. *Biochim. Biophys. Acta* **673** 217–223.

Rowland, R. N. and Woodley, J. F. (1981b) Uptake of free and liposome-entrapped insulin by rat intestinal sacs *in-vitro*. *Biosci. Rep.* **1** 345–352.

Rowland, R. N. and Woodley, J. F. (1981c) Uptake of free and liposome-entrapped ^{125}I-labelled PVP by rat intestinal sac *in-vitro*: evidence for endocytosis. *Biosci. Rep.* **1** 399–406.

Rustum, Y. M., Dave, C., Mayhew, E. and Papahadjopoulous, D. (1979) Role and route of administration in the antitumor activity of liposome-entrapped 1-β-D-arabinofuranosylcytosine against mouse L 1210 leukemia. *Cancer Res.* **39** 1390–1395.

Sanders, E. and Ashworth, C. T. (1961) A study of particulate intestinal absorption and hepatocellular uptake. *Exp. Cell Res.* **22** 137–145.

Schwinke, D. L., Ganesan, M. G. and Weiner, N. D. (1984a) *In-situ* jejunal uptake from liposomal systems. *Int. J. Pharm.* **20** 119–127.

Schwinke, D. L., Ganesan, M. G. and Wiener, N. D. (1984b) Effect of entrapped markers on the *in-situ* jejunal uptake from liposomal systems. *Pharm. Res.* **1** 256–259.

Seiden, A. and Lichtenberg, D. (1979) Transport of liposomes components in rat everted intestinal loop. *J. Pharm. Pharmacol.* **31** 414–415.

Seifert, J., Sass, W. and Dreyer, H. P. (1983) Mucosal permeation of macromolecules and particles. In: Skadhauge, E. and Heintze, K. (eds) *Intestinal Absorption and Secretion*. Falk Symposium 36, Kluwer, Dordrecht, pp. 505–513.

Sessa, G. and Weissman, G. (1970) Incorporation of lysozyme into liposomes. *J. Biol. Chem.* **13** 3295–3301.

Shenfield, G. M. and Hill, J. C. (1982) Infrequent response by diabetic rats to insulin-liposomes. *Clin. Pharmacol. Physiol.* **9** 355–361.

Soehngen, E. C., Godin-Ostro, E., Fielder, F. G., Ginsberg, R. S., Slusher, M. A. and Weiner, A. L. (1988) Encapsulation of indomethacin in liposomes provides protection against both gastric and intestinal ulceration when orally administered to rats. *Arthr. Rheum.* **31** 414–422.

Tomlinson, E. (1987) Theory and practice of site-specific drug delivery. *Adv. Drug Deliv. Rev.* **1** 87–198.

Tragl, K. H., Pohl, A. and Kinast, H. (1979) Oral administration of insulin by means of liposomes in animal experiment. *Wien. Klin. Wochenschr.* **91** 448–451.

Ueno, M., Horikoshi, I., Takahashi, K. and Sakuragawa, N. (1982a) Studies on oral administration of concentrated factor IX preparation. *Yakugaku Zasshi* **102** 202–206.

Ueno, M., Nakasaki, T., Horikoshi, I. and Sakuragawa, N. (1982b) Oral administration of liposomally-entrapped heparin to beagle dog. *Chem. Pharm. Bull.* **30** 2245–2247.

Volkheimer, G. (1977) Persorption of particles: physiology and pharmacology. *Adv. Pharmacol. Ther.* **14** 163–187.

Volkheimer, G. and Schulz, F. H. (1968) The phenomena of persorption. *Digestion* **1** 213–218.

Weiner, M. L. (1988) Intestinal transport of some macromolecules in food. *Food Chem. Toxicol.* **26** 867–880.

Weiner, N. and Chiang, C. M. (1988) gastrointestinal uptake of liposomes. In: Gregoriadis, G. (ed.) *Liposomes as Drug Carriers.* Wiley, Chichester, pp. 599–607.

Weiner, N., Martin, F. and Riaz, M. (1989) Liposomes as a drug delivery system. *Drug Dev. Ind. Pharm.* **15** 1523–1554.

Weingarten, C., Moufti, A., Desjeux, J. P., Luong, T. T., Durand, G., Devissaguet, J. P. and Puisieux, F. (1981) Oral ingestion of insulin liposomes: effects of the administration route. *Life Sci.* **28** 2747–2752.

Weingarten, C., Moufti, A., Delattre, J., Puisieux, F. and Couvreur, P. (1985) Protection of insulin from enzymatic degradation by its association to liposomes. *Int. J. Pharm.* **26** 251–257.

Wells, C. L., Maddaus, M. A. and Simmons, R. L. (1988a) Proposed mechanisms for the translocation of intestinal bacteria. *Rev. Infect. Dis.* **10** 958–979.

Wells, C. L., Maddaus, M. A., Erlandsen, S. L. and Simmons, R. L. (1988b) Evidence for the phagocytic transport of intestinal particles in dogs and rats. *Infect. Immunol.* **56** 278–282.

Whitmore, D. A. and Wheeler, K. P. (1979) The fate of liposomes in the rat small intestine. *Biochem. Soc. Trans.* **7** 929–931.

7

Intestinal bioadhesive drug delivery systems

C.-M. Lehr, J. A. Bouwstra, A. G. de Boer, J. C. Verhoef, D. D. Breimer and H. E. Junginger

INTRODUCTION

Bioadhesive drug delivery systems (BDDSs) for oral application are aimed at interacting with the mucous lining of the gastrointestinal (GI) tract. This may allow both the GI transit to these systems to be controlled and the contact with the absorbing biological membrane to be intensified. The first mechanism can be used either to keep controlled-release dosage forms for a prolonged period of time within the body or to fix the system in a specific area of the GI tract, where a given drug might be preferably absorbed or induce local therapeutic effects. Therapeutic advantages of these systems, however, are only indirect consequences of their bioadhesive properties. In contrast, bioadhesion may also be suited to improve drug absorption itself by direct interaction with the intestinal mucosa at the site of adhesion–absorption.

The primary aim of these investigations was to assess whether the principle of bioadhesion can be used to improve the oral bioavailability of peptide drugs. Previous research on oral bioadhesive drug delivery systems was aimed at controlling (delaying) their GI transit and hence was only dealing with indirect bioadhesion effects (Ch'ng *et al.*, 1985; Longer *et al.*, 1985). For this approach, it might be advantageous to make the system adhere in the stomach, where it acts as a permanent reservoir for the drug being delivered. For the direct bioadhesion approach, however, premature gastroadhesion has to be prevented by appropriate technological measures (e.g. enteric coating) until the system has reached the small intestines. Improvement of intestinal peptide absorption due to bioadhesion may be caused by various mechanisms (Fig. 1):

- decrease in diffusion path from the BDDS to the absorbing biological membrane;
- increase in local drug concentration at the site of adhesion–absorption;
- immediate absorption from the BDDS without previous dilution and possible degradation in the luminal fluids;
- penetration enhancers and/or enzyme inhibitors can be brought closer to their site of action in a well-defined area.

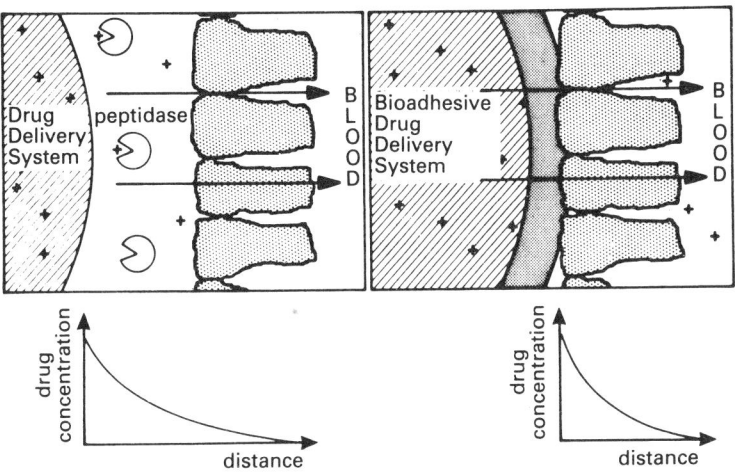

Fig. 1. Drug absorption from a bioadhesive and non-adhesive drug delivery system.

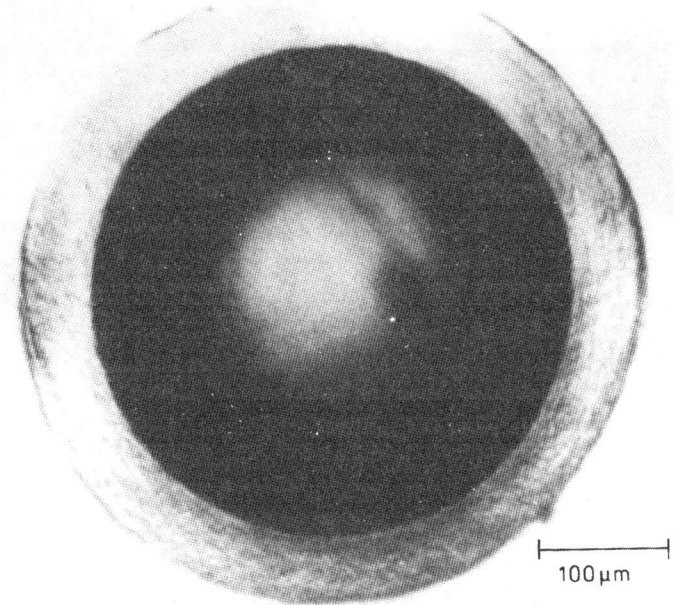

Fig. 2. Photomicrograph of a PHEMA microsphere coated with mucoadhesive polymer in a swollen state.

PHARMACEUTICAL–TECHNOLOGICAL ASPECTS

To study the effect of bioadhesion on intestinal peptide absorption, a suitable delivery system had to be developed first. In view of the available experience in preparing and characterizing hydrogels, a multiple-unit hydrogel matrix system has been designed. It is based on microspheres of poly(2-hydroxyethyl methacrylate) (PHEMA) to be coated with a mucoadhesive polymer (Fig. 2; Lehr et al., 1989). The peptide drug chosen as a model for these investigations was 9-desglycinamide-8-arginine vasopressin (DGAVP) which is metabolically relatively stable and was available in large amounts. The intact peptide could be measured in plasma by a highly sensitive radioimmunoassay (van Bree et al., 1988). With respect to the intended further investigations, it was important that drug release from the PHEMA system was not controlled by and hence was independent of the presence of the mucoadhesive coating (Fig. 3).

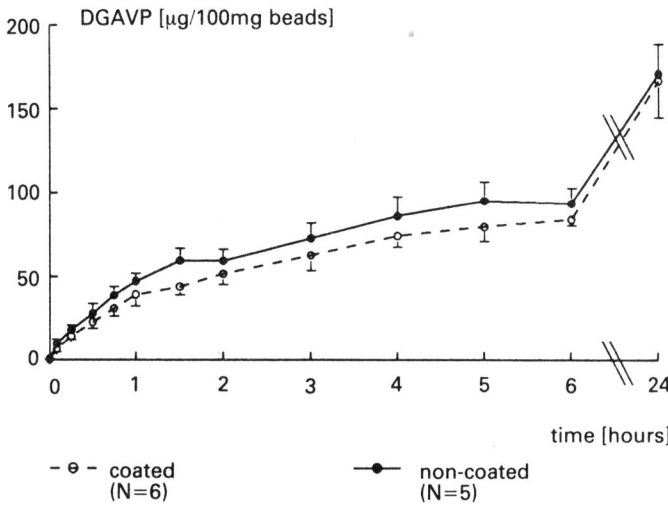

Fig. 3. Release of DGAVP from PHEMA microspheres in saline at 37°C with (o , $N = 6$) and without (• , $N = 5$) mucoadhesive Polycarbophil coating (USP paddle method, mean ± SD, $n = 3$).

BIOADHESION AND THE GI TRANSIT OF DRUG DELIVERY SYSTEMS

For peptide delivery, a delayed GI transit would be a minor aspect rather than the major mechanism of a possible increased absorption caused by bioadhesion. Nonetheless, a delay in (gastro)intestinal transit is suitable for verifying the bioadhesive properties of such a drug delivery system *in vivo* and hence this was studied first.

The intestinal transit of microspheres coated with different mucoadhesive polymers was studied in a chronically isolated intestinal loop model in the rat (Poelma and Tukker, 1987). Differences in mucoadhesive properties between polymers appeared to exist (Fig. 4; Lehr et al., 1990), but the results suggested that physiological rather than technological factors were limiting. The rat *in situ* loop was well suited to the study of some of those physiological factors under controlled conditions and permitted the turnover time of the intestinal mucus gel layer to be estimated to be in the order of some very few hours only (Lehr et al., (1991). Artificially increasing mucus output in this model simultaneously shortened the transit time of both mucoadhesive and non-adhesive particles (Fig. 5). The concept of mucoadhesion in controlling GI transit of drug delivery systems turned out to be ultimately limited by the relatively rapid mucus turnover. No difference in small intestinal transit was found after intraduodenal administration to rats between microspheres with and without mucoadhesive coating.

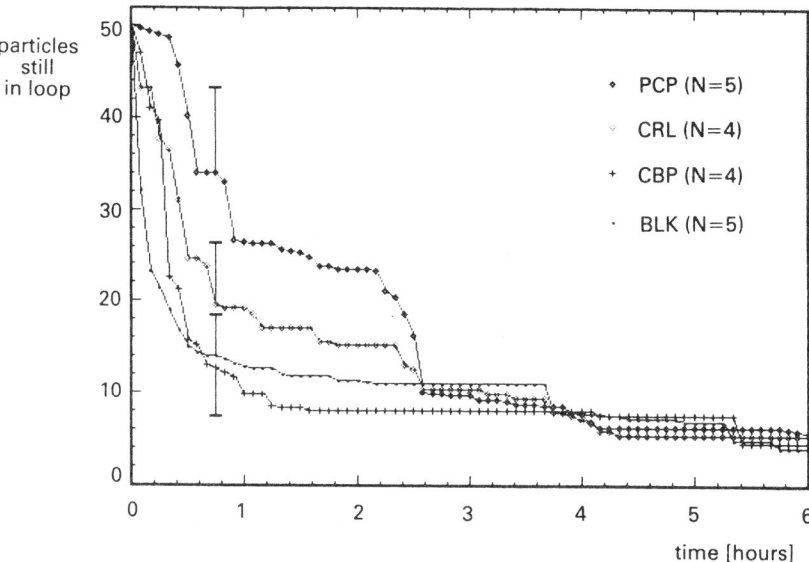

Fig. 4. Residence curves of PHEMA microspheres in the *in situ* perfused intestinal loop (mean ± SEM): PCP, Polycarbophil; CBP, Carbomer; CRL, blend of Carbomer + Eudragit® RL 100; BLK; non-coated.

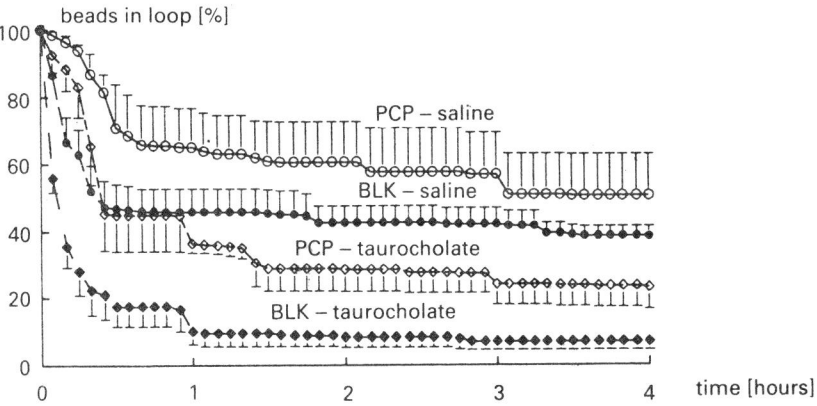

Fig. 5. Effect of stimulated mucus output by 10 mM sodium taurocholate on intestinal transit of microspheres (mean ± SEM, $n = 4$): PCP, Polycarbophil; BLK, non-coated.

BIOADHESION AND ORAL PEPTIDE DELIVERY

The results of some pilot experiments with isolated perfused rat intestinal tissue *in vitro* roughly supported the initial working hypothesis (Junginger *et al.*, 1990).

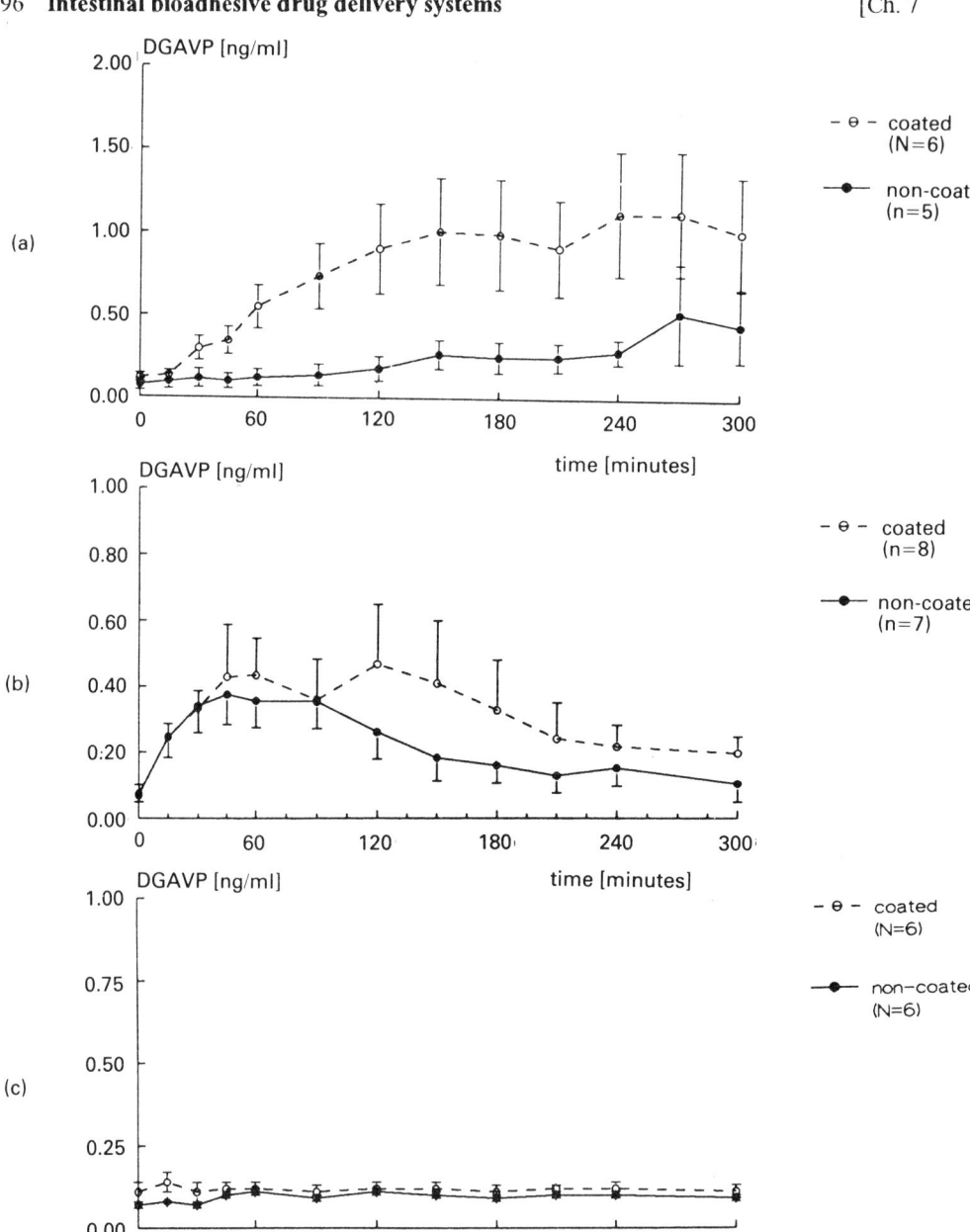

Fig. 6. Absorption of DGAVP from microspheres loaded with 100 mg of drug (a) *in vitro* (coated, $N = 6$; non-coated, $N = 5$), (b) *in situ* (coated, $N = 8$; non-coated, $N = 7$) and (c) in vivo (coated, $N = 6$; non-coated, $N = 6$) (mean ± SEM, $n = 5$–8): ○, coated; ●, non-coated.

The subsequent attempts to verify these findings *in vivo*, however, were at first disappointing, because the observed effect appeared to vanish with increasing physiological complexity of the test model (*in vitro – in situ – in vivo,* Fig. 6). However, as additional experiments revealed, the mucoadhesive polymer polycarbophil was virtually able to improve the intestinal absorption of DGAVP in all three models provided

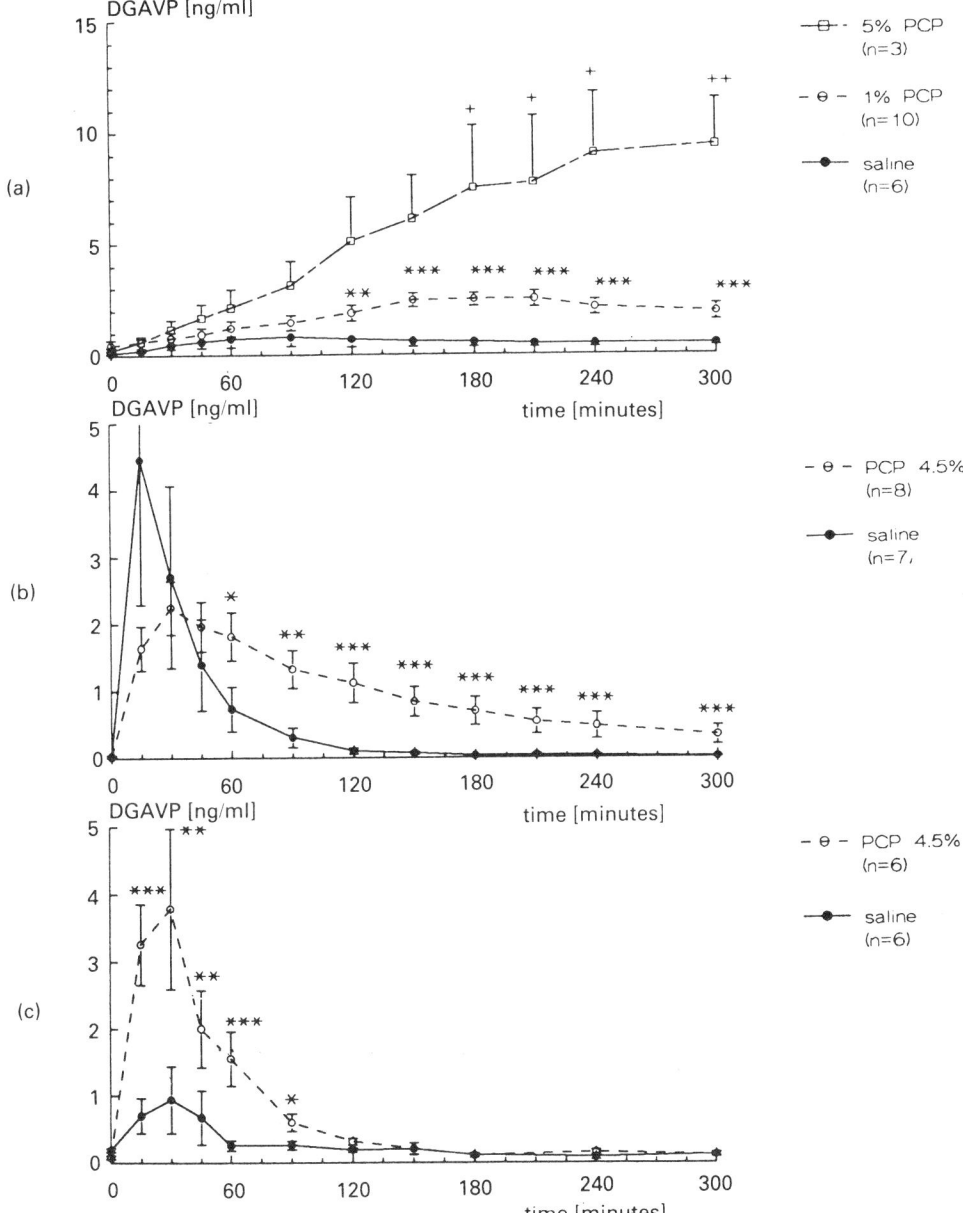

Fig. 7. Absorption of DGAVP from Polycarbophil (PCP) suspensions vs saline (mean ± SEM, n = 6–8): (a) *in vitro* (dose, 10 μg; □, 5% PCP (n = 3); ○, 1% PCP (n = 10); ●, saline (n = 6)); (b) *in situ* (dose, 100 μg; ○, 4.5% PCP (n = 8); ●, saline (n = 7)); (c) *in vivo* (dose, 500 mg; ○, 4.5% PCP (n = 6); ●, saline (n = 6)). * $P < 0,1$, ** $P < 0.05$, *** $P < 0,01$ compared with saline.

that the drug was delivered rapidly (Fig. 7). In addition to being only mucoadhesive, poly(acrylic acid) appeared to possess intrinsic penetration enhancing effects, in particular inhibiting the enzymatic degradation of the drug by mucosal peptidases. Oral delivery of peptide drugs using poly(acrylic acid) appears to be possible.

SPECIFIC ADHESION

Whereas the long-time realization of bioadhesion by means of non-specific mucoadhesion turned out to be limited *in vivo*, the possible advantages of bioadhesion in general were still considered to be valid. A new concept for achieving the intended fixation of drug delivery systems consists of the application of specific, receptor-mediated interactions between suitable macromolecules (e.g. lectins) and the epithelial cell surface. Tomato lectin was chosen as first candidate for safety reasons and in view of some promising effects reported by others (Naisbett and Woodley, 1990). As a proof of principle, it could be demonstrated that tomato lectin can be used to render bioadhesive properties to potential drug delivery systems in the form of fluorescently labelled microspheres (Figs 8 and 9). An enterocyte radio binding assay (ERBA), developed for that purpose, permitted the study of lectin binding in a quantitative way. The same affinity was found to fixed pig enterocytes and to monolayers of human Caco2 cells. Lectin adhesion is preferred in a neutral rather than in an acidic environment but could

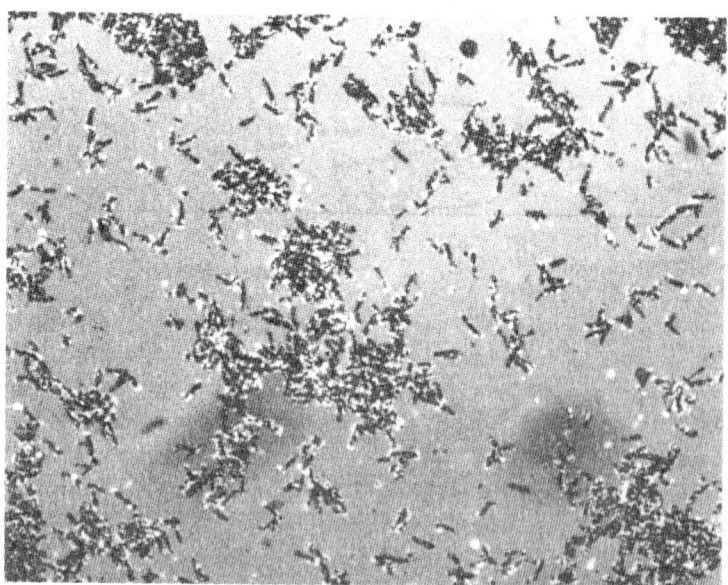

Fig. 8. Fluorescently labelled polystyrene microspheres (1 µm, Polysciences) coated with tomato lectin adhere to isolated fixed pig enterocytes.

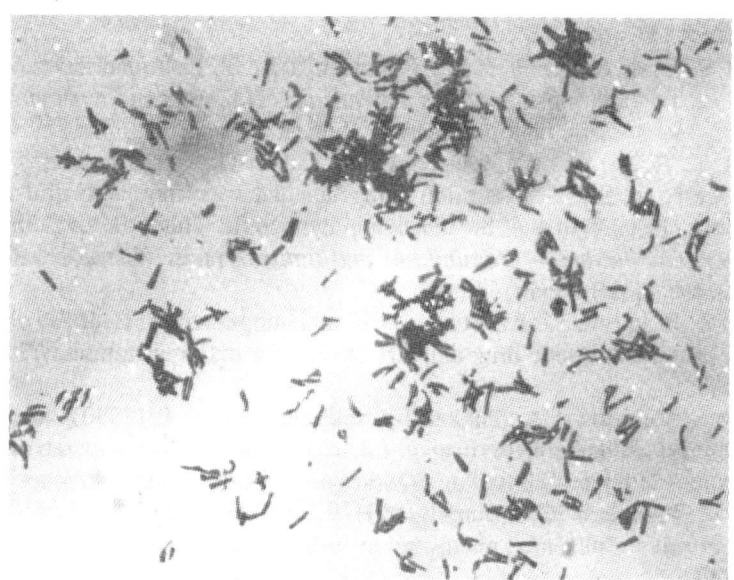

Fig. 9. The same microspheres as in Fig. 8 coated with bovine serum albumin do not adhere.

be specifically inhibited by mucus glycoproteins. To evaluate the practical significance of this cross-reactivity *in vivo* will be the subject of future studies.

In comparison with the former approach based on mucoadhesive polymers, the concept of specific adhesion has set a new stage for bioadhesion in drug delivery. Essentially, adhesion via specific mechanisms implicates the principal possibility of adherence with high selectivity on a cellular level. Moreover, specific binding needs not be restricted to simple adhesion but might permit the triggering of activated cellular drug absorption in future (Pusztai, 1989).

CONCLUSIONS

Achieving long-term bioadhesion by means of non-specific mucoadhesive polymers was found to be substantially limited by the rapid turnover of the intestinal mucus gel layer. Nonetheless, the mucoadhesive polymer polycarbophil led to an improved intestinal absorption of the peptide drug DGAVP *in vivo*. Probably other mechanisms, such as penetration enhancement and enzyme inhibition, are involved. as well as bioadhesion. Future research on bioadhesive drug delivery systems should focus on a new approach to the application specifically binding molecular structures.

REFERENCES

van Bree, J. B. M. M., de Boer, A. G., Danhof, M., Verhoef, J. C., van Wimersma Greidanus, T. B. and Breimer, D. D. (1988) Radioimunoassay of desglycinamide–

arginine vasopressin and its application in a pharmacokinetic study in the rat. *Peptides* **9** 555–559.

Ch'ng, H. S., Park, H., Kelly, P. and Robinson, J. R. (1985) Bioadhesive polymers as platforms for oral controlled drug delivery. II. Synthesis and evaluation of some swelling, water insoluble bioadhesive polymers. *J. Pharm. Sci.* **74** 399–405.

Junginger, H. E., Lehr, C.-M., Bouwstra, J. A., Tukker, J. J., and Verhoef, J. C. (1990) Site specific intestinal absorption using bioadhesives: improved oral delivery of peptide drugs by means of bioadhesive polymers. In: Gurny, R. and Junginger, H. E. (eds) *Bioadhesion — Possibilities and Future Trends*. Wissenschaftliche Verlagsgesellschaft, Stuttgart, 117 pp.

Lehr, C.-M., Bouwstra, J. A., Tukker, J. J. and Junginger, H. E. (1989) Design and testing of a bioadhesive drug delivery system for oral application. *STP Pharma* **5** 857–862.

Lehr, C.-M., Bouwstra, J. A., Tukker, J. J. and Junginger, H. E. (1990) Intestinal transit of bioadhesive microspheres in an *in situ* loop in the rat — a comparative study with copolymers and blends based on poly(acrylic acid). *J. Control. Release* **13** 51–62.

Lehr, C.-M., Poelma, F. G. J., Junginger, H. E. and Tukker, J. J. (1991) An estimate of turnover time of intestinal mucus gel layer in the rat *in situ* loop. *Int. J. Pharm.* **70** 235–240.

Lehr, C.-M., Bouwstra, J. A., Kok, W., Noach, A. B. J., de Boer, A. G. and Junginger, H. E. (1992a) Bioadhesion by means of specifically binding tomato lectin. *Pharm. Res.*, **4** 547–553.

Lehr, C.-M., Bouwstra, J. A., Kok, W., de Boer, A. G., Tukker, J. J., Verhoef, J.C., Breimer, D. D. and Junginger, H. E. (1992b) Effects of the mucoadhesive polymer polycarbophil on the intestinal absorption of a peptide drug, *J. Pharm. Pharmacol.* **44** 402–407.

Longer, M. A., Ch'ng, H. S. and Robinson, J. R. (1985) Bioadhesive polymers as platforms for oral controlled drug delivery. III. Oral delivery of chlorothiazide using a bioadhesive polymer. *J. Pharm. Sci.* **74** 406–411.

Naisbett, B. and Woodley, J. F. (1990) Binding of tomato lectin to the intestinal mucosa — potential for oral drug delivery. *Biochem. Soc. Trans.* **18** 879–880.

Poelma, F. G. J. and Tukker, J. J. (1987) Evaluation of a chronically isolated internal loop in the rat for the study of drug absorption kinetics. *J. Pharm. Sci.* **76** 433–436.

Pusztai, A. (1989) Transport of proteins through the membranes of the adult gastrointestinal tract — a potential for drug delivery? *Adv. Drug Deliv. Rev.* **3** 215–228.

8

Pellets and multi-unit dosage forms: state of the art

Jasper G. Fokkens

INTRODUCTION

In the last ten years the use of multi-unit dosage forms has become more popular. The main reasons can be found in some advantages over unit dose systems, e.g.

- a limited risk of dose dumping, and
- small particles can be mixed with food, which is done in practice to ease drug intake in the elderly.

In order to produce multi-unit dosage forms several techniques can be used:

- spray drying;
- wet granulation, followed by sieving and drying;
- one-step granulation in a fluidized bed;
- built-up granulation on core material;
- extrusion, followed by spheronization.

The last two techniques mentioned are becoming more popular in pharmaceutical industries, with the major role for extrusion–spheronization. Usually particles with a diameter of around 1 mm are produced, which then are coated (taste coating, enteric coating, controlled release coating). In this chapter critical factors in built-up granulation and extrusion–spheronization will be mentioned. Finally, some attention will be given to *in vivo* behaviour.

BUILT-UP GRANULATION

Built-up granulation is a technique in which drug-containing material is sprayed on or bound to core material. Hence, the starting material is always important with regard to binding properties, shape, particle size and particle size distribution. By spraying a solution or suspension, containing binder, drug and/or other excipients, on core material such as sugar spheres, it is possible to produce particles with diameters of a few hundred micrometres up to millimetres. It is possible to spray several drug-containing layers alternatively with non-drug-containing layers. This is illustrated in Fig. 1. In this way it is possible to regulate (at least *in vitro*) accurately the release of drug in time.

Built-up granulation is usually carried out in a rotor–granulator. A schematic drawing of a Freund rotor–granulator is presented in Fig. 2.

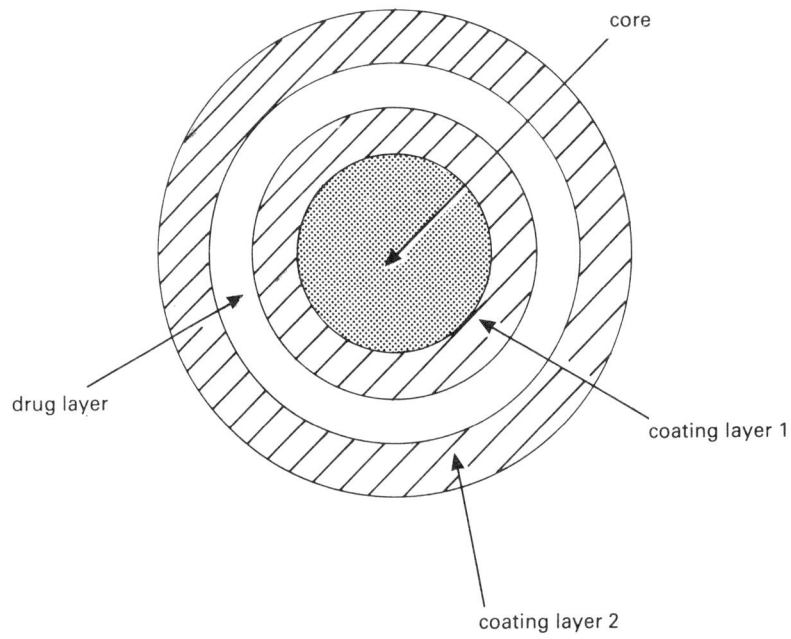

Fig. 1.

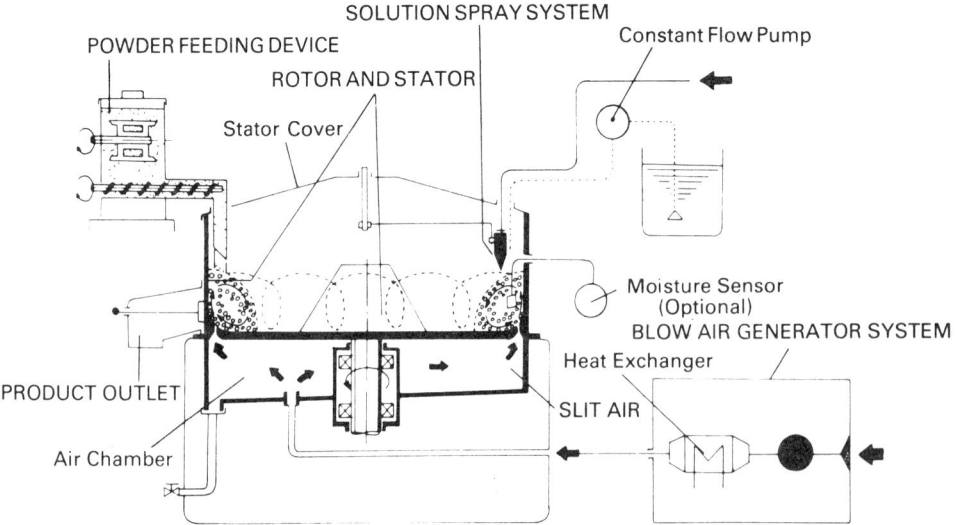

Fig. 2. Schematic diagram of the CF Granulator. (Adapted from technical brochures, Vector Corporation, Marion, IA.)

Firstly the core material is put on the rotating plate. This core material can have 'any' shape and particle size. However, mostly the starting materials are sugar spheres or sugar crystals or crystalline drug material. Because of the building of one or more layers, one can always end up with spherical particles, reflecting the particle size distribution of the starting material. Apart from the spraying of solution or suspension on the core material it is also possible to add dry powder on the wetted cores.

The main advantages of built-up granulation are as follows:

- It is flexible with regard to release of the drug; by playing around with drug and excipients many different release profiles can be obtained.
- The process is very reproducible.
- The end product is in general spherical and the particle size distribution reflects that of the starting material.

The disadvantages are:

- The process is a batch-process and therefore time consuming.
- The process is laborious (intensive monitoring is required; e.g. the distance between the spray nozzle and product must be adjusted constantly, because of the increase in mass).

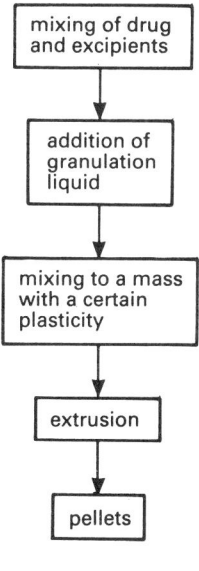

Scheme 1.

EXTRUSION AND SPHERONIZATION

Extrusion

Extrusion is the process of pressing a mass through an opening. Because of the compression the mass density is increased and pellets are formed. A simplified scheme represents the important steps in the extrusion process (Scheme 1). In Fig. 3 some types of extruders are shown. The pressure building on the mass depends on the type of extruder (Rowe, 1986). However, before a mixture can be extruded, a number of other factors have to be taken into account:

(a) physical–chemical properties of excipients;
(b) amount and composition of the granulation liquid;
(c) mixing process;
(d) plasticity of mass before extrusion.

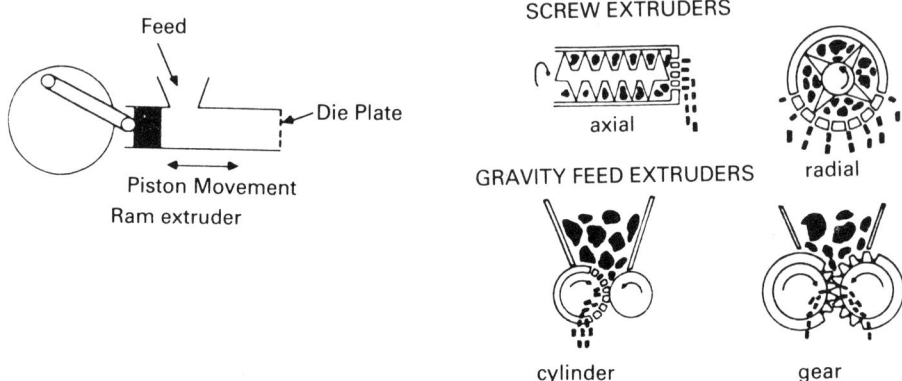

Fig. 3.

Excipients

The mass to be extruded (and spheronized) must possess a certain plasticity. Therefore, most of the time it is necessary to add excipients which can bind water to a certain

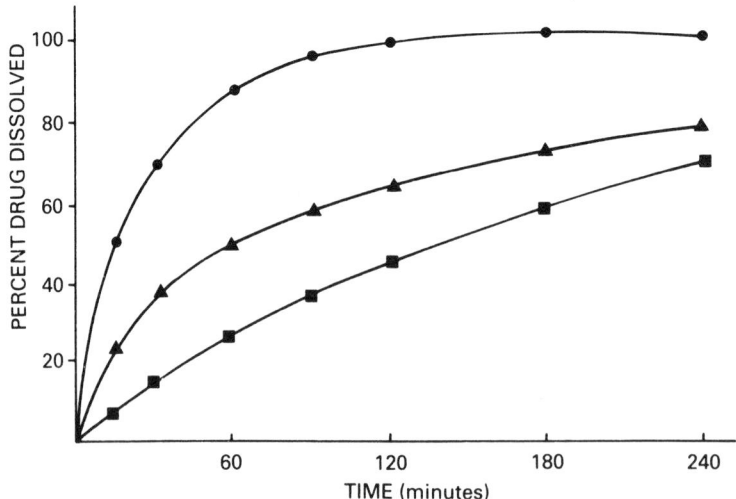

Fig. 4. Dissolution profiles for pellets containing 50% theophylline in different Avicel MCC types: ●, Avicel PH-101; ▲, Avicel RC-581; ■, Avicel CL-611.

extent. The most well-known and widely used excipients are the microcrystalline celluloses. Depending on the type of microcrystalline cellulose, one has different binding properties which may result in different drug release profiles. Some examples are shown in Figs 4 and 5. The main difference between the Avicel PH-101 and RC-581 and CL-611 is that the latter two contain carboxymethylcellulose which has excellent binding properties. This results in a slower drug release. However, it is noted that an increase in theophylline affects the internal binding in the granules and hence the release profile (O'Connor and Schwartz, 1989).

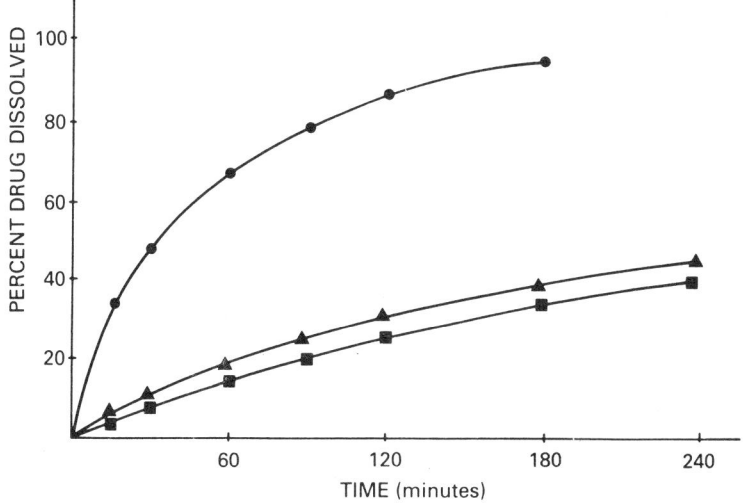

Fig. 5. Dissolution profiles for pellets containing 10% theophylline in different Avicel MCC types: ●, Avicel PH-101; ▲, Avicel RC-581; ■, Avicel CL-611.

Amount and composition of the granulation liquid

The amount of granulation liquid is related to the plasticity of the mass as is shown in Fig. 6. (The plasticity was measured using a method similar to that described by Alleva and Schwartz, 1986).

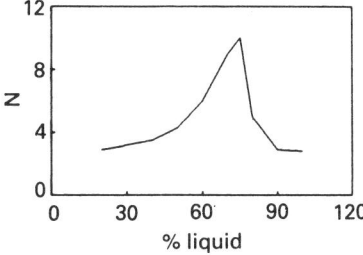

Fig. 6. Plasticity curve (Collette high shear mixer) for 1:1 isopropanol:water.

Mixing of theophylline with Avicel RC-581 (1:1) in a Collette high shear mixer with isopropanol:water (1:1) results in a curve with maximal plasticity after addition of 75% liquid (per cent by dry weight) (Fig. 7). Changing the granulation liquid from isopropanol:water to ethanol:water (1:1 and 1:9 respectively) results in a shift of the plasticity curve. Hence, more liquid is needed to obtain a high plasticity. Furthermore, it is noticed that the shape of the curve also changes, indicating a different bonding force in the granulate.

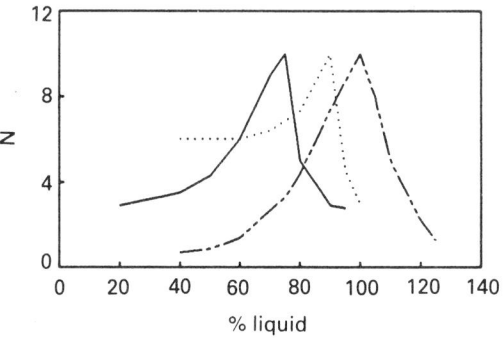

Fig. 7. Plasticity curves (Collette high shear mixer) for 1:1 isopropanol:water (———), 1:1 ethanol:water (- - - - -) and 1:9 ethanol:water (—— - -).

Mixing process
The distribution of liquid through a dry powder is determined, among other factors, by the type of mixer used. In Fig. 8 the plasticity curves are shown for a screw mixer (Nauta) and a planet mixer (Peerless). The mixing process was identical in both mixers with regard to load, time and rotational speed. From these curves and from the curves shown in Fig. 7 it is concluded that the mixing process has a relatively large influence on plasticity.

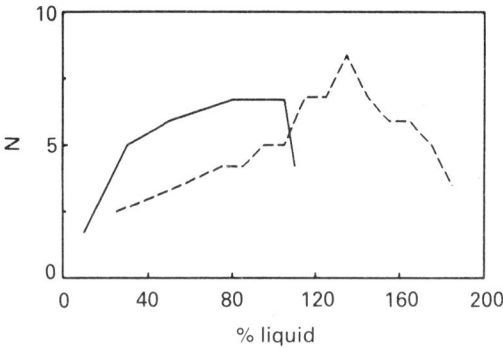

Fig. 8. Plasticity curves for 1:1.5 ethanol:water in a Nauta screw mixer (———) and a Peerless planet mixer (- - - - -).

Plasticity of mass before extrusion

In Fig. 9 the plasticity curve is shown of a mixture of 10% theophylline and 90% Avicel RC-581 with water as granulation liquid (Elbers *et al.*, 1991). Between 100% and 140% liquid addition a decrease in plasticity is found, which is followed by an increase. It turned out that pellets containing between 140% and 180% water could be spheronized, whereas pellets from the granulate with a lower water content could not be spheronized.

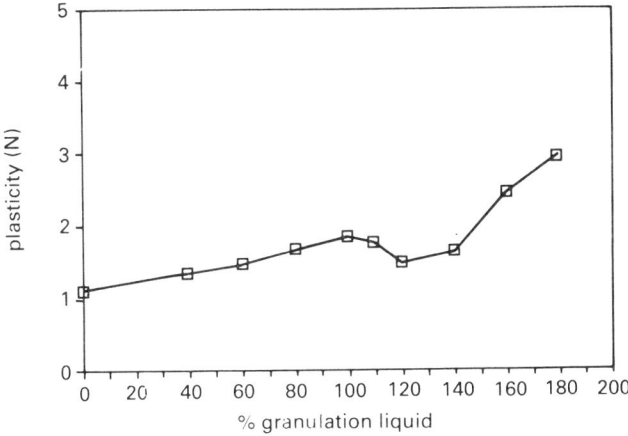

Fig. 9. Plasticity curve for a mixture of 10% theophylline and 90% Avicel RC-581 with water as the granulation liquid.

The extrusion of the above-mentioned masses was carried out in a Schlter extruder. A schematic drawing of the screen with the collar is shown in Fig. 10. The mass is pressed through the holes in the screen and the pellets formed can be cut by a knife. The diameter of the pellets depends on the diameter of the holes and can vary between 400 and more than 2000 μm. Normally pellets are produced with a diameter of 0.8, 1.0 or 1.2 mm.

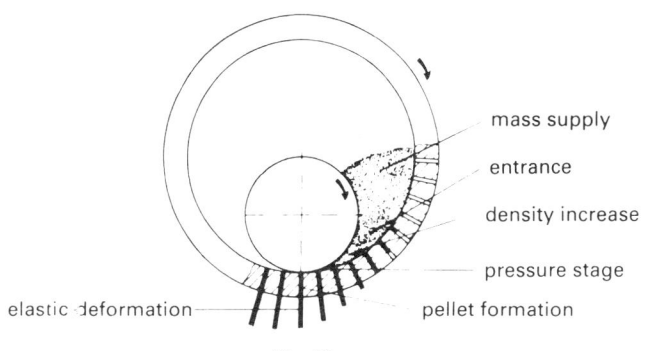

Fig. 10.

SPHERONIZATION

The pellets are broken (ideally in pieces just as long as their diameter) on the rotating plate of a spheronizer. This plate has a special structure (see Fig. 11) for this purpose. Because of the centrifugal force the particles are transported to the wall of the spheronizer where they roll one over another, while running with the speed of the plate. During this process the cylindrical particles are spheronized, following various stages as depicted in Fig. 12 (Chapman *et al.*, 1988).

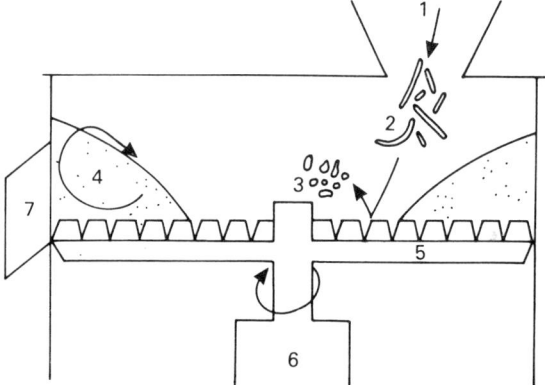

Fig. 11. Schematic drawing of spheronizer (Marumerizer): 1, feed inlet; 2, extrudate; 3, breakage into short rods; 4, rope-shaped bed; 5, friction plate; 6, drive unit; 7, product outlet.

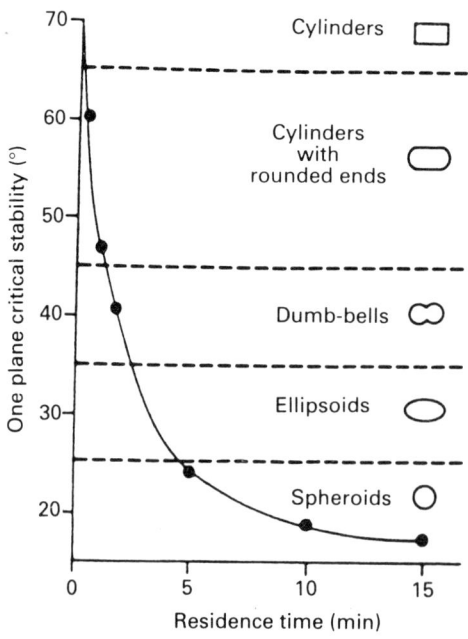

Fig. 12.

As can be seen, eventually spheroids are formed after a dwell time which can vary between a few and 15–20 min. (The one-plane critical stability is the angle indicating when a particle placed on a plate, which is lifted, starts to move.)

Important factors in the spheronization process are

- liquid content,
- peripheral velocity of the spheronizer plate, and
- dwell time.

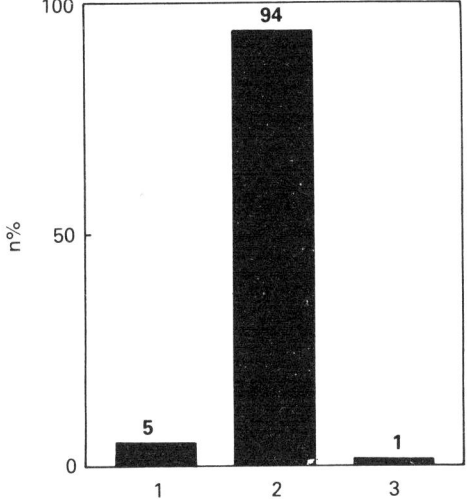

Fig. 13. Influence of a peripheral velocity of 400 rpm on the particle size distribution of pellets (extruded through a 1 mm screen; 50% theophylline–50% Avicel RC-581; ethanol:water = 1.0:1.5 (90% dry); 7 min; the number % of particles in each size range is shown): column 1, 500–710 μm; column 2, 710–1000 μm; column 3, >1000 μm.

An illustration of the influence of peripheral velocity on the particle size distribution of pellets (extruded through a 1 mm screen) is shown in Fig. 13 and Fig. 14. These figures also illustrate that it is possible to obtain a relatively narrow particle size distribution.

Summarizing, it can be stated that the extrusion–spheronization process has the following advantages:

- in general a wide range of drug concentrations can be handled;
- the end product consists of spheres;
- the spheres have a relatively high density;
- the particle size can be chosen by using the relevant screen;
- the particle size distribution is narrow.

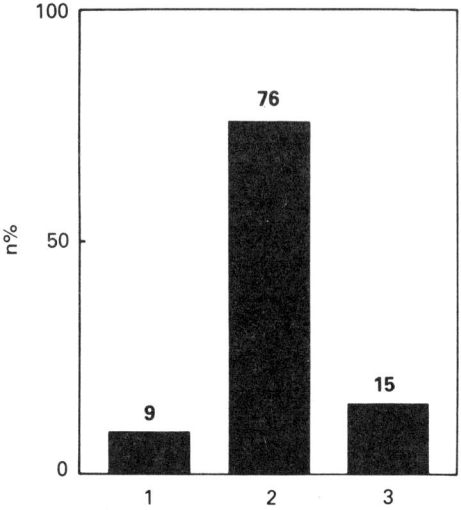

Fig. 14. Influence of a peripheral velocity of 500 rpm on the particle size distribution of pellets (extruded through a 1 mm screen; 50% theophylline–50% Avicel RC-581; ethanol:water = 1.0:1.5 (90% dry); 7 min; the number % of particles in each size range is shown): column 1, 500–710 µm; column 2, 710–1000 µm; column 3, >1000 µm.

IN VIVO VICISSITUDES

It is well known that small particles (diameter ≤2 mm) can freely pass the pylorus. Hence, the gastric retention time of these particles is relatively short compared with, for example, the retention time of tablets (e.g. see Bechgaard, 1982; Davis *et al.*, 1984). In Fig. 15 the *in vivo* transit time of pellets through the gastrointestinal tract is presented (as percentage activity of labelled material in time) (Christensen *et al.*, 1985).

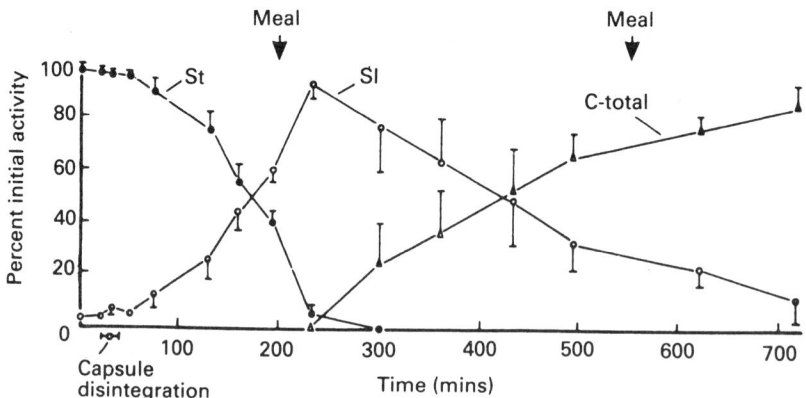

Fig. 15. *In vivo* transit time of pellets.

After disintegration of the capsule, the particles pass the stomach (ST) within 3 h. Most of the particles are transported through the small intestine (SI) in about 3.5 h, whereafter they enter the colon (C) (Davis, 1985). It is known that food influences the transit times, which is illustrated in Fig. 16 (Davis, 1985). There is a significant retention in gastric transit time after taking a heavy breakfast (HB) in comparison with a light breakfast (LB). As can be seen from the figures the transit through the small intestine is rather constant and independent of food. Furthermore, it was found that this transit time is also independent of dosage form: 3.5 ± 0.5 h.

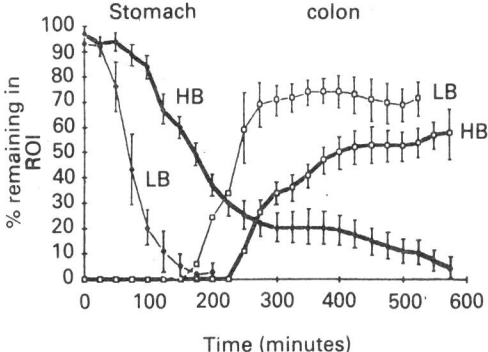

Fig. 16. Effect of food on transit time (mean values ± SD for gastric emptying and arrival in the colon): HB, heavy breakfast; LB, light breakfast.

Transit times for multiple unit dose systems are given in Table 1. From these values it is clear that non-dissolving particles reach the colon after a few hours. In recent years drug uptake from the colon has been studied for a number of drugs. Some examples of drugs absorbed from the colon are shown in Table 2 (Bieck, 1987).

Table 1. Transit times for multiple unit dose sytems

Stomach	30 min–5 h, depending on meal
Small intestine	3.5 h 0.5 h
Large intestine	~20 h

Table 2. Drugs absorbed from the colon: some examples

Clioquinol
Digoxin
Diclofenac
Glibenclamide
Metoprolol
Oxprenolol
Theophylline

Apart from the extra opportunity offered for these drugs (with regard to controlled release formulations, e.g. theophylline preparations releasing the drug over 24 h), a number of companies and institutes are still working on formulations which release the drug only in the colon. This way of drug targeting (mainly used for treatment of ulcerative colitis or Crohn's disease with 5-ASA- or 5-ASA-like compounds) is done mainly by coating granules with a pH-sensitive polymer. This coating material should dissolve only at pH values of about 7.5, whereafter the drug is released. Other groups are working on pH-sensitive hydrogels and coating material with aza bonds (to be cleaved by micro-organisms) (e.g. see Rubinstein, 1990; Tozer, 1990; Dong and Hoffman, 1991; Klokkers-Bethke and Fischer, 1991).

ACKNOWLEDGEMENTS

The author thanks Mr J. Elbers for determining the plasticity curves and for carrying out the extrusion and spheronization experiments.

REFERENCES

Alleva, D. S. and Schwartz, J. B. (1986) *Drug Dev. Ind. Pharm.* **12** 471–487.
Bechgaard, H. (1982) *Acta Pharm. Technol.* **28** 149–157.
Bieck, P. R. (1987) *Acta Pharm. Technol.* **33** 109–114.
Chapman, S. R. *et al.* (1988) *J. Pharm. Pharmacol.* **40** 503–505.
Christensen, F. N. *et al.* (1985) *J. Pharm. Pharmacol.* **37** 91–95.
Davis, S. S. (1985) *J. Control. Release* **2** 27–38.
Davis, S. S. *et al.* (1984) *Int. J. Pharm.* **21** 167–177.
Dong, L. and Hoffman, A. S. (1991) *J. Control. Release* **15** 141–152.
Elbers, J. E. *et al.* (1991) *Drug Dev. Ind. Pharm.* **12** 501–517.
Klokkers-Bethke, K. and Fischer, W. (1991) *J. Control. Release* **15** 105–112.
O'Connor, R. E. and Schwartz, J. B. (1989) In: Ghebre-Sellarsie, I. (ed.) *Pharmaceutical Pelletization Technology.* Dekker, New York, Chap. 9.
Rowe, R. C. (1986) *Proc. 25th Int. Colloq. Ind. Pharm., Gent, 1986.* pp. 1–17.
Rubinstein, A. (1990) *Biopharm. Drug Disp.* **11** 465–475.
Tozer, T. N. (1990) *Proc. Int. Symp. Control. Release Bioact. Mater.* **17** 126–127.

9

Oral uptake of microparticles across the gastrointestinal mucosa

Alexander T. Florence and Praful U. Jani

INTRODUCTION

Research over the past 30 years suggests that there is need to revise current views on the barriers to drug absorption offered by the gastrointestinal epithelium. Overcoming barriers to macromolecular and colloidal carrier uptake, and an understanding of the mechanisms of uptake and transport, should allow us to harness the potential of the oral route more effectively. There has been, for some time, evidence (Sanders and Ashworth, 1961) of the transepithelial passage of small particles across the gastrointestinal wall. The process termed 'persorption' suggested by Volkheimer (1969, 1975) to allow the passage of particles up to 100 µm in diameter, which subsequently reach the portal venous blood and the thoracic lymph (of dogs), has been a subject of considerable controversy, with the consequence that until recently there have been few attempts to use the potential of oral administration of microparticulate carriers for the systemic delivery of drugs in intact carriers. Here some of the evidence for particulate uptake by the gut-associated lymphoid tissue and the potential for drug delivery and for oral immunisation (Mestecky and McGhee, 1989) by this mechanism is discussed.

Vesicular systems and microspheres have been administered almost exclusively by the parenteral route. The oral use of microencapsulated systems has concentrated, until recently, on slow release to provide controlled absorption and gastrointestinal protection or site direction through enteric coating of granules. Various mechanisms of drug transport from micelles or emulsion droplets have been proposed, there having been some suggestion of the possibility of uptake of intact micelles and droplets *via* the fat absorption pathways resulting in enhanced uptake to the lymphatics (Hashida *et al.*, 1979). Surfactant-based systems such as emulsions might allow enhanced penetration of drugs through the induction of increased membrane permeability (Attwood and Florence, 1983).

There seems now to be the possibility of taking advantage of the specialized uptake of submicron particulate carriers, although it has been said that 'transport of intact carriers across the GI tract is restricted to exceptional and unusual circumstances'

(O'Mullane et al., 1987). Certainly in some pathological conditions, such as Crohn's disease, the normal permeability of the gut (to small molecules at least) is increased (Glaison et al., 1989). However, there are data in the literature, dating back as far as 1922, that suggest that the gastrointestinal mucosa does allow particulate absorption at least under some circumstances. Le Fevre and his colleagues (1978, 1989) have made extensive studies of the uptake and translocation of polystyrene latices, and recently we (Jani et al., 1989, 1990) have obtained unequivocal evidence of the absorption of intact polystyrene latex particles in the 50 nm to 1 µm size range. Particles from animals fed orally for up to 10 days were taken up *via* Peyer's patches, then transported by the mesentery lymph vessels towards the lymph nodes. This suggests the need to re-examine the possibilities of particulate oral delivery, as well as the potential toxicity of ingested particulates such as titanium dioxide and other insoluble materials found in pharmaceuticals (Florence et al., 1990).

Macromolecular uptake and particulate uptake
It is known that the neonatal mammalian small intestine has the capacity to ingest macromolecules by a process of endocytosis principally by the Peyer's patches in the gut, which comprise membraneous epithelial (M) cells overlying lymphoid follicles (Bye et al., 1984; Owen and Jones, 1974). The number of Peyer's patches changes with age and is maximal at puberty. Viral and bacterial particles can penetrate the mucosal barrier by way of the Peyer's patches which endocytose and transport macromolecules and microorganisms into the associated lymphoid tissues (Walker and Owen, 1990; Grutzkau et al., 1990). It seems not unreasonable that, if bacterial particles can be transported from the lumen via M-cells, then, so too, might some synthetic particles of appropriate size and surface character. Such absorbable particles, loaded with drug, could be used as carriers of labile drug molecules, such as proteins or other poorly absorbed materials. Questions to be addressed include what surface characteristics of the particles aid or indeed prevent uptake? What is the extent in terms of the dose of administered particles? Is there site-specific uptake? What is the ultimate fate of administered particles?

Bacterial transport
The manner in which bacterial and viral particles are absorbed in the gut may be instructive in the design of carrier systems. Recently there has been renewed interest in the role of failure of the intestinal barrier in the development of systemic infection. Deitch (1990) states that, based on current knowledge, bacteria do not translocate from the normal gut because of the presence of an intact epithelial barrier, normal host immune defences and an intestinal flora which prevents bacterial overgrowth. However, bacteria (such as *Vibro cholerae* and *Campylobacter jejuni*) (Owen et al., 1986; Walker et al., 1988) and viruses have been found not only to be associated with the Peyer's patches but to translate across the epithelial barrier via the M-cells. Walker and Owen (1990), in discussing M-cell uptake and transport of virulent organisms, point out the marked differences in adherence capacity of different organisms, a feature that might be utilized in the design of systems with specific affinities for Peyer's patches. Newton et al. (1989) have incorporated the cholera toxin epitope into *Salmonella*

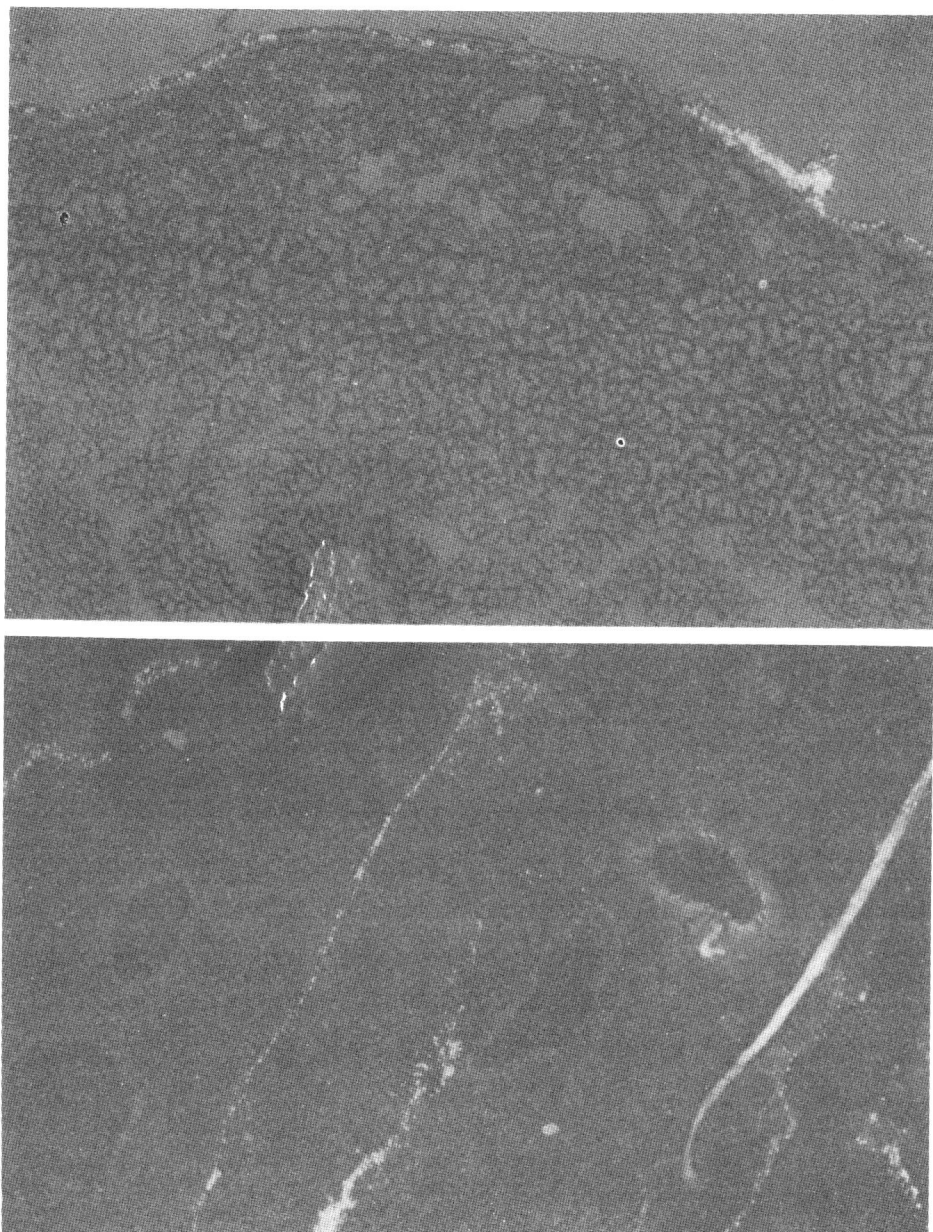

Fig. 1. (a) Photomicrograph of a frozen section of a region of the rat gut showing a Peyer's patch. 500 nm fluorescent polystyrene beads can be seen at the serosal edge of the patch and a few particles can be seen transversing the patch. (b) Subsequent movement of the 500 nm fluorescent polystyrene within the mesenteric lymph vessels can be seen in this photomicrograph. Both slides were obtained after 10 days feeding by oral gavage of the latex at a dose of 12.5 (mg/kg)/day.

flagellin. Walker and Owen (1990) suggest that improved delivery systems will facilitate the use of lymphokines and immunomodulators, thereby giving the potential to enhance nonspecific resistance to enteric pathogens.

EVIDENCE OF MICRO- AND NANOPARTICULATE UPTAKE

We have conducted investigations to elucidate the extent of uptake and the particle size dependency of uptake of model (polystyrene) particles. The clear evidence of oral uptake of nondegradable particles (Fig. 1) obtained by feeding a suspension of latex particles to female Sprague–Dawley rats daily for 10 days suggests that the evidence of the absorption of liposomes and other carriers should be re-examined. Whether or not sufficient quantities of drug-loaded colloidal carriers can be taken up to elicit useful therapeutic responses reliably remains to be seen. Details of the experimental method are given in Jani *et al.* (1989, 1990). Location of the microspheres was observed microscopically using frozen histological sections and the quantity of polystyrene uptake measured by extraction of tissues and gel permeation chromatography of the extracts.

Fig. 2 suggests that total uptake ranges from about 33% (50 nm latex) to about 7% (1 μm latex) of the administered dose; the figure demonstrates the size dependency of uptake in all tissues examined. While these data and those which include gastrointestinal tissue (Figs 3 and 4) may be inflated because of the possible inclusion of *adsorbed* particles not penetrating the epithelial barrier, there is no doubt that particles found in

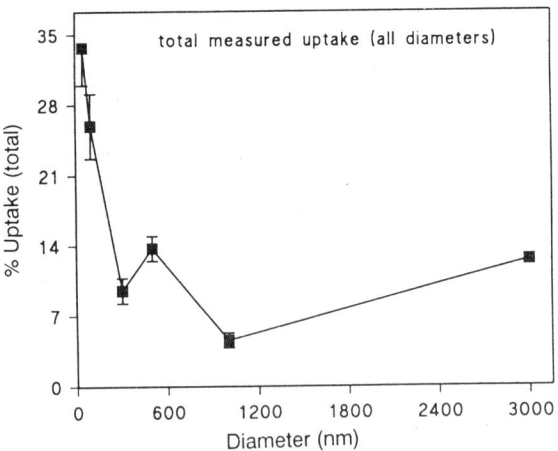

Fig. 2. The total uptake of polystyrene microspheres from the gastrointestinal tract of female Sprague–Dawley rats ($n = 3$) following oral administration for 10 days at a dose of 12,5 mg/kg as measured by extraction of polystyrene from the tissues mentioned in the text, the data being plotted as a function of the particle size of the latex. (Reproduced from Jani *et al.* (1990).)

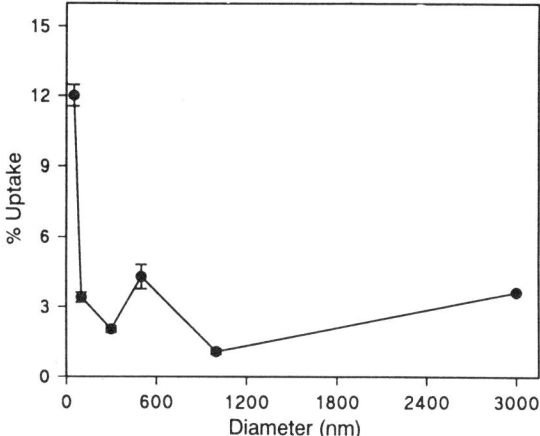

Fig. 3. The uptake of orally administered polystyrene latex by the small intestine as analysed by gel permeation chromatography, as a function of particle diameter. Histological evidence showed that the microspheres are present mainly in the Peyer's patches and the mesentery network of the small intestine. (Reproduced from Jani et al. (1990)).

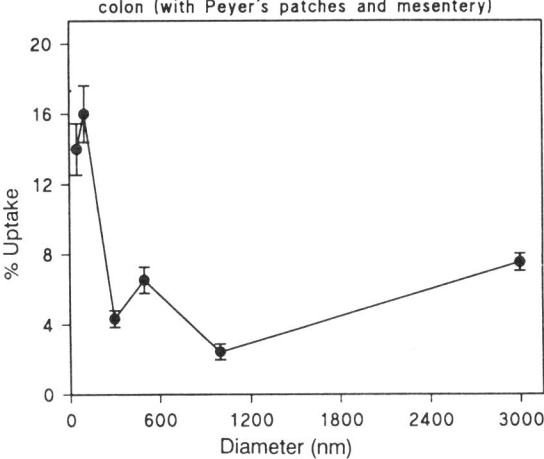

Fig. 4. Uptake of orally administered polystyrene latex particles by the colon, as a function of latex size. Histological evidence points to the accumulation of particles in the lymphoid aggregates present in the colon. (Reproduced from Jani et al. (1990)).

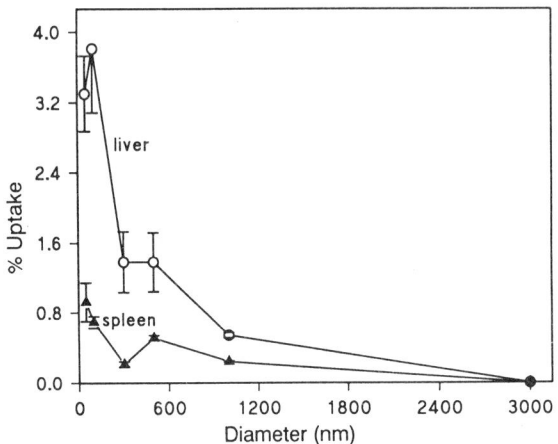

Fig. 5. The concentration of orally administered polystyrene latex in the liver and spleen as a percentage of administered dose plotted as a function of particle size. The particles are present mainly in the macrophage cells of the liver and the granular follicles of the spleen. (Reproduced from Jani et al. (1990).)

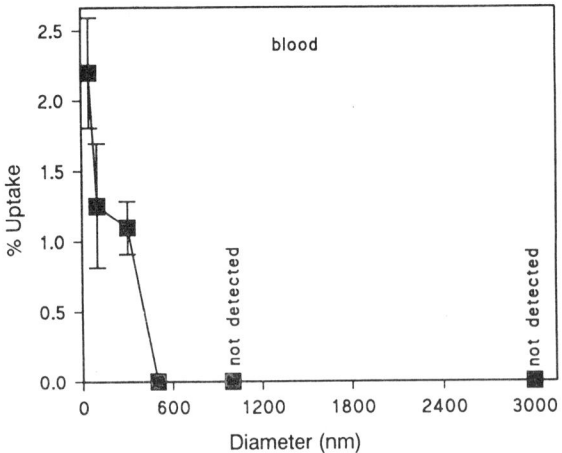

Fig. 6. The presence of polystyrene latex particles of varying size in the blood. No evidence of polystyrene was found in blood after administration of particles in the size range 500 nm to 3 μm; the limit of detection of 6.25×10^{-5}% (w/v) does not allow a conclusion that there are no particles in the blood, but the probability is reduced at these larger diameters. (Reproduced from Jani et al. (1990).)

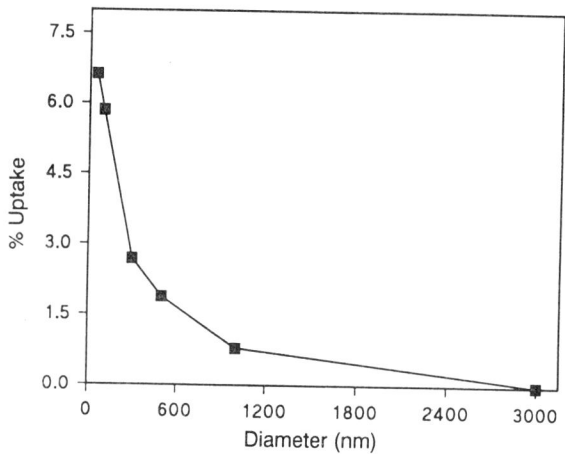

Fig. 7. The cumulative uptake of polystyrene, orally administered to female Sprague–Dawley rats for 10 days at a dose of 12.5 mg/kg, as a function of particle diameter in the liver, spleen, blood, bone marrow and kidney. In the case of particles of 500 nm and 1 μm these data refer only to liver and spleen as no microspheres were detected in blood, bone marrow and kidney. For the 300 nm latex the data refer to liver, spleen and blood. (Reproduced from Jani et al. (1990).)

tissues physically separate from the gut lumen are conclusive proof of transport. The results show the presence in such organs (Figs 5 and 6) of polystyrene particles in the size range 50 nm–1 μm, although the largest particles studied, which are 3 μm particles (Fig. 7), appear to be confined to the Peyer's patches.

Although 3 μm latex beads were not detected either in the systemic circulation or in the liver and the spleen, the histological evidence indicated that these particles were absorbed, immobile within the submucosal layer of the thicker mucosa and the Peyer's patches. The smaller beads are quickly translocated into the serosal layer and thence into the systemic circulation. The apparently high uptake of the 3 μm particles may be explained in part by adsorption. However, adsorption of smaller particles is undoubtedly a prelude to absorption. Heart and lungs revealed no latex particles, and, except for the 50 nm particles, no polystyrene was detected in the kidney, while 100 nm latex particles seem to represent the upper limit for transport into the bone marrow.

Both the rate and size dependency of uptake of particles are of interest. Both have been illustrated recently by the work of Eldridge et al. (1989) from whose data, on biodegradable lactide–glycolide microparticles, Fig. 8 is taken. Our initial studies were

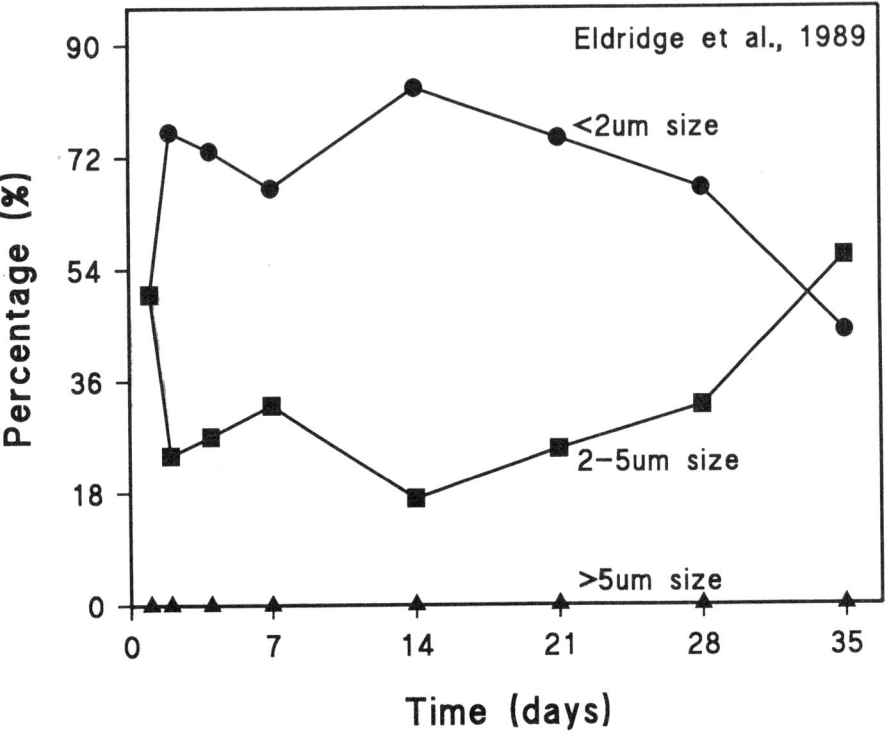

Fig. 8. Data showing the time scale and size dependence of migration, plotted from the figures presented by Eldridge et al. (1989). The figure shows the percentage of dye-labelled polylactide–glycolide particles of different sizes (<2 μm, 2–5 μm and >5 μm) moving with time in and through the mesenteric lymph nodes.

conducted by feeding the experimental animals daily for 10 days. However, single-dose studies (Jani et al., 1991) show that uptake is rapid. Table 1 illustrates our recent data on the size and time dependence of polystyrene latex uptake in rats after a single oral dose.

CHALLENGES OF THE ORAL ROUTE

The future use of particulate carriers by the oral route thus offers several challenges principally: in the design of carriers resistant to the ravages of the GI milieu but which are taken up effectively by the epithelial cells for transport to the systemic circulation, where this is required, or to induce cellular or humoral immunity (Mestecky and McGhee, 1989). Particles used with the intention of being absorbed via the Peyer's patches have to interact with these extremely small target zones. The role of mucosa in this process is not yet clear. The long residence time of latex particles such as found in the lumen of the small intestine of the mouse (Ebel, 1990), might be important in facilitating uptake. Another approach is through the design of selectively adhesive particles. Improved intestinal absorption of a peptide from bioadhesive microspheres

Table 1. Size and time dependence of latex uptake observed microscopically

Sizes of Latex	50 nm	500 nm	1 μm	50 nm	500 nm	1 μm	50 nm	500 nm	1 μm	50 nm	500 nm	1 μm	50 nm	500 nm	1 μm
Organs examined	6 h			12 h			18 h			24 h			36 h		
Payer's patches	+++	+	+	+++	+	+	++	+++	++	−	++	+	−	+	+
Mesentery lymph network and nodes	+++	++	−	+++	+++	+	++	++	+	+	++	++	−	+	+
Liver	−	−	−	+	−	−	++	+	+	++	++	+	+	+	+
Spleen	−	−	−	−	−	−	+	+	−	++	+		+	+	+

−, no evidence of uptake or presence of the latex spheres; +, very little extent of uptake and presence of the latex spheres; ++, good extent of uptake and presence of the latex spheres; +++, significant extent of uptake and presence of the latex spheres.

of Carbopol-coated PHEMA microspheres has been demonstrated (Lehr et al., 1990). The real test of the approach is the measurement of a biological response following the administration of drug-laden microspheres (Damgé et al., 1988). Andrieu et al. (1989) administered indomethacin-containing polyisobutylcyano-acrylate nanocapsules in the size range 200–300 nm. Although indomethacin is normally absorbed from the gut, nanoencapsulation was claimed to accelerate the extravascular distribution of the drug, partly because of enhanced uptake of the colloidal carrier by the reticuloendothelial system. The results were attributed to an increase in the extent or duration of contact of the encapsulated drug with the gut wall or to absorption via paracellular pathways. This work is discussed in Chapters 6 and 7 of this volume.

Convincing data derive from the delivery of therapeutic agents, such as insulin, which are normally very poorly absorbed by the gut. Fed orally to diabetic rats, insulin encapsulated in 200 nm polycyacrylate nanospheres decreased fasting glycaemia by 50–60% by the second day (Damgé et al., 1988). Insulin absorbed at the surface of the nanocapsules did not produce responses (Couvreur et al., 1980). Aprahamian and colleagues (1987) used polyalkylcyanoacrylate nanocapsules loaded with Lipiodol, an iodized oil, as a tracer for X-ray microparticle analysis. When administered into the lumen of the jejunum, these nanocapsules increased absorption of the tracer, levels in the blood capillaries being fourfold higher than after intrajejunal administration of a Lipiodol emulsion.

UNWANTED ABSORPTION OF PARTICLES

It is clear that Peyer's patches and M-cells cannot distinguish between particulates unless there are specific biological–biophysical interactions between the particle and the membraneous epithelial cells. This leads naturally to the notion that many sub-micron particles administered in pharmaceuticals might be inadvertently taken up by this route. We have recently studied the uptake and distribution of titanium dioxide particles of 500 nm size (Florence et al., 1990) (Table 2). Further studies of this type are necessary to investigate the possible outcomes from such unwanted absorption and translocation. Perhaps we should be less sanguine about the impermeability of the gastrointestinal mucosa.

Table 2. Titanium dioxide (rutile) particles (500 nm diameter) in tissues

Peyer's patches	SI	MN	Colon	Liver	Spleen	Kidney	Heart	Lung
++	+	+++	++	++	+	0	0	+

0, no evidence of uptake and presence; +, very little extent of uptake and presence; ++, moderate extent of uptake and presence; +++, significant extent of uptake and presence.
SI, small intestine; MN, mesentery network and nodes.

CONCLUSIONS

We and others have shown that particulate uptake in the gastrointestinal tract takes place mainly at the Peyer's patches, which are rich in lymphatic supply and mononuclear phagocytic cells; particles absorbed in this way are translocated to the mesentery network especially to the mesentery nodes, if below 2–5 μm in diameter. The microspheres, within the size constraints discussed, while circulating in the lymph, eventually enter the liver and general circulation. The venous circulation would transfer the microspheres to the liver, the blood circulation of which transports them to the liver. It is pertinent that there is a direct lymphatic portal circulation connection from the mesometrial wall of the Peyer's patches and the mesentary network and the other parts of the gastrointestinal tract.

The possibility of taking advantage of the oral route for immunization has been addressed by several groups (O'Hagan *et al.*, 1989; Eldridge *et al.*, 1989, 1990) who have examined the role of the carrier particle on uptake and immunological response. It is further work on these lines that will lead to realizing the full potential of the oral route for both drug and vaccine delivery (O'Hagan, 1990). Particles in the 50 nm size range possibly offer the best compromise between extent of uptake and carrying or protective capacity for drug molecules, but there are still many hurdles to be overcome.

Sternson (1987) has pointed out that the effectiveness of this route will depend on (a) its efficiency and capacity (which is deemed to be low), (b) the delay in eliciting pharmacological response due to slow processing within lymphoid tissue and the slow movement of lymph itself, and (c) the loss of drug to lymphocytes or macrophages or their passage to mesenteric lymph nodes. These are some factors that must be considered in any evaluation of the route.

ACKNOWLEDGEMENTS

The experimental work discussed in this chapter on polystyrene latex particles and titanium dioxide uptake has been supported by Syntex Research Centre, Edinburgh, and by the Maplethorpe Fellowship programme of the University of London.

REFERENCES

Andrieu, V., Fessi, H., Dubrasquet, M., Devissaguet, J.-P., Puisieux, F. and Benita, S. (1989) Pharmacokinetic evaluation of indomethacin nanocapsules, *Drug Des. Deliv.* **4** 295–302.

Aprahamian, M., Michel, C., Humert, W., Devissaguet, J.-P. and Damgé, C. (1987) Transmucosal passage of polyalkyl cyanoacrylate nanocapsules as a new drug carrier in the small intestine. *Biol. Cell.* **61** 69–76.

Attwood, D. and Florence, A. T. (1983) *Surfactant Systems: Their Chemistry Pharmacy and Biology.* Chapman and Hall, London.

Bye, W. A., Allan, C. H. and Trier, J. S. (1984) Structure, distribution and origin of M-cells in Peyer's patches of mouse ileum. *Gastroenterology* **86** 789–801.

Couvreur, P., Lenaerts, V., Kante, B., Roland, M. and Speiser, P. (1980) Oral and parenteral administration of insulin associated to hydrolysable nanoparticles. *Acta Pharm. Technol.* **26** 220–221.

Damgé, C., Michel, C., Aprahamian, M. and Couvreur, P. (1988) New approach for oral administration of insulin with polycyanoacrylate nanocapsules as drug carrier. *Diabetes* 37 246–351.

Deitch, E. A. (1990) The role of intestinal barrier failure and bacterial translocation in the development of systemic infection and multiple organ failure. *Arch. Surg.* 125 403–404.

Ebel, J. P. (1990) A method for quantifying particle absorption from the small intestine of the mouse. *Pharm. Res.* 7 848–851.

Eldridge, J. H., Gilley, R. M., Staas, J. K., Moldoreanu, Z., Meulbroek, J. A. and Tice, T. R. (1989) Biodegradable microspheres: vaccine delivery system for oral immunization. In: Mestecky, J. and McGhee, J. R. (eds) *New Strategies for Oral Immunization.* Current Topics in Pharmacology and Immunology, No. 146, Springer, Berlin, pp. 59–66.

Eldridge, J. H., Hammond, C. J., Meulbroek, J. A., Staas, J. K., Gilley, R. M. and Tice, T. R. (1990) Controlled vaccine release in the gut-associated lymphoid tissues. Orally administered biodegradable microspheres target the Peyer's patches. *J. Control. Release* 11 205–214.

Florence, A. T., Jani, P. U. and McCarthy, D. (1990) Toothpaste and Crohn's disease. *Lancet* 336 1580–1581.

Glaison, G., Sjodahl-Leandersson, P. and Tagesson, C. (1989) Abnormal intestinal permeability pattern in colonic Crohn's disease. *Scand. J. Gastroenterol.* 24 571–576.

Grutzkau, A, Hanski, C., Hahn, H. and Riecken, E. O. (1990) Involvement of M-cells in the bacterial invasion of Peyer's patches: a common mechanism shared by *Yersinia enterocolitica* and other enteroinvasive bacteria, *Gut* 31 1011–1015.

Hashida, M., Muranishi, S., Sezaki, H., Tanigawa, N., Satomura, K. and Hikasa, Y. (1979) Increased lymphatic delivery of bleomycin by microsphere in oil emulsion and its effect on lymph node metastasis. *Int. J. Pharm.* 2 245–256.

Jani, P. U., Halbert, G. W., Langridge, J. and Florence, A. T. (1989) The uptake and translocation of latex nanospheres and microspheres after oral administration to rats. *J. Pharm. Pharmacol.* 41 809–812.

Jani, P. U., Halbert, G. W., Langridge, J. and Florence, A. T. (1990) Nanoparticle uptake by the rat gastrointestinal mucosa: quantitation and particle size dependency. *J. Pharm. Pharmacol.* 42 821–826.

Jani, P. U., Florence, A. T. and McCarthy, D. (1991) Polystyrene nanosphere and microsphere uptake and translocation via the GIT mucosa after a single oral dose. *J. Pharm. Pharmacol.* 43 29P.

Le Fevre, M. E., Vanderhoff, J. W., Laissue, J. A. and Joel, D. D. (1978) Accumulation of 2 mm latex particles in mouse Peyer's patches during chronic latex feeding. *Experientia* 34 120–122.

Le Fevre, M. E., Boccio, A. M. and Joel, D. D. (1989) Intestinal uptake of fluorescent microspheres in young and aged mice. *Proc. Soc. Exp. Biol. Med.* 190 23–27.

Lehr, C.-M., Bouwstra, J. A., de Boer, A. G., Tukker, J. J., Verhoef, J. C., Breimer, D D. and Junginger, H. E. (1990) Intestinal absorption of a peptide drug using a bioadhesive drug delivery system. In: Gurny, R. and Junginger, H. E. (eds) *Bioadhesion — Possibilities and Future Trends.* WVG, Stuttgart, pp. 177–190.

Mestecky, J. and McGhee, J. R (eds) (1989) *New Strategies for Oral Immunization.* Current Topics in Pharmacology and Immunology, No. 145, Springer, Berlin.

Newton, S. M. C., Jacob, C. O. and Stocker, B. A. D. (1989) Immune response to cholera toxin epitope inserted in *Salmonella* flagellin. *Science* **244** 70–72.

O'Hagan, D T. (1990) Intestinal translocation of particulates — implications for drug and antigen delivery. *Adv. Drug Deliv. Res.* **5** 265–285.

O'Hagan, D. T., Palin, K., Davis, S. S., Artursson, P. and Sjoholm, I. (1989) Microparticles as potentially orally immunological adjuvants. *Vaccine* **7** 421–424.

O'Mullane, J. E., Artursson, P. and Tomlinson, E. (1987) Biological approaches to the controlled delivery of drugs. *Ann. NY Acad. Sci.* **507** 117–128.

Owen, R. L. and Jones, A. L. (1974) Epithelial cell specialization with human Peyer's patches: an ultrastructural study of intestinal lymphoid filloids. *Gastroenterology,* **66** 189–203.

Owen, R. L., Pierce, N. F., Apple, R. T. and Cray, W. C. (1986) M cell transport of *Vibrio cholerae* from the intestinal lumen into Peyer's patches: a mechanism for antigen sampling and for microbial transepithelial migration. *J. Infect. Dis.* **153** 1108–1118.

Sanders, E. and Ashworth, C. T. (1961) A study of particulate intestinal absorption and hepatocellular uptake. Use of polysterene latex particles. *Exp. Cell Res.* **22** 137–145.

Sternson, L. A (1987) Obstacles to polypeptide delivery. *Ann. NY Acad. Sci.* **507** 19–21.

Volkheimer, G. (1975) Haematogenous dissemination of ingested polyacrylchloride particles, *Ann. NY Acad. Sci.* **246** 164–170.

Volkheimer, G. and Schultz, F. H. (1968) The phenomenon of persorption. *Digestion* **1** 213–218.

Volkheimer, G., Schultz, F. H., Lindenau, A. and Beitz, V. (1990) Resorption of metallic iron particles. *Gut* **10** 32–33.

Walker, R. I. and Owen, R. L. (1990) Intestinal barriers to bacteria and their toxins. *Annu. Rev. Med.,* **41** 393–400.

Walker, R. I., Schmauder-Chock, E. A., Parker, J. L. and Burr, D. (1988) Selective association and transport of *Campylobacter jejuni* through M-cells of rabbit Peyer's patches. *Can. J. Microbiol.* **34** 11142–11147.

Part III
Pulmonal route

10

Pulmonary surfactant: basic physiology and its use for replacement therapy

B. Lachmann and E. P. Eijking

INTRODUCTION

In 1929, von Neergaard wrote 'It may be possible that the surface tension of the alveoli is diminished by concentration of surface-active substances against other physiological solutions' (von Neergaard, 1929). He was referring to the existence of a surface film in the alveoli and his assumption was based on the following observations. Von Neergaard measured pressure–volume diagrams from human and animal lungs, first filling them with air and then with liquid. The surprising result was that the pressure necessary for filling the lung with liquid was only half the pressure necessary for filling the lung with air. His explanation of this remarkable difference was based on the assumption that in each alveolus there must be a barrier between air and fluid (such as in the wall of a soap bubble) with a tendency to diminish its size according to the law of Laplace. The amount of retraction pressure for the lung is larger than the retraction force of the elastic fibres. By filling the alveoli with liquid, the air–liquid barrier is replaced by a liquid-to-liquid barrier without any surface tension. The retraction pressure, measurable in the fluid-filled lung, is therefore equal to the retraction pressure of the elastic fibres. The same procedure for determining the influence of surface tension on the overall retraction of the lung was later reported by other scientists, and is now a well-established method.

Pattle (1955) showed that bubbles resulting from lung oedema, as well as bubbles squeezed from a lung cut, are very stable. Pattle assumed that the walls of these bubbles consist of surface-active materials and that their stability depended on the quantity and quality of the surfactant phospholipids. Clements (1957) was the first to investigate lung extracts in a Wilhelmy balance and demonstrated that these extracts had, in contrast to detergents or plasma, genuine hysteresis properties.

Avery and Mead (1959) were the first to call attention to the possibility that lungs of infants with respiratory distress syndrome (RDS) may have abnormal surface tension properties, due to a deficiency in lung surfactant.

BIOCHEMICAL COMPOSITION

Biochemical characterization has shown that surface-active phospholipids, proteins and mucopolysaccharides are the main constituents of the surfactant system of the lung. Generally, between 80% and 90% of surfactant lipid is phospholipid. The major representative (70% to 80%) of surfactant phospholipids is phosphatidylcholine (PC) and about 60% of the PC molecules contain two saturated acyl chains. This disaturated PC (DSPC) is largely dipalmitoylphosphatidylcholine (DPPC). Monoenoic PC molecules constitute most of the unsaturated PC in surfactant. In most adult mammalian species, phosphatidylglycerol (PG) is the second most abundant phospholipid class, accounting for up to 10% of total surfactant lipid. Surfactant contains, in addition, small proportions of phosphatidylinositol (PI), phosphatidylserine, phosphatidylethanolamine and sphingomyelin (for review see Van Golde et al., 1988).

Phospholipids are synthesized in the type II alveolar cells. They are stored in these cells as so-called lamellar bodies, before being released to the surface of the alveoli. The surfactant lipids spread as a monolayer or multilamellar layer at the air–liquid boundary. They reduce the net contractile force of the alveolar surface, thus preventing the airspaces from collapsing at low lung volumes.

To date, the functional importance of the other components of the surfactant system, including proteins and mucopolysaccharides, has not yet been fully explained. However, recently, it could be demonstrated that for optimal function of lipids the presence of a few small proteins is a prerequisite for optimal *in vivo* function of artificial surfactant and surfactant extracted from mammalian lungs (for details see Van Golde et al., 1988).

FUNCTION OF THE SURFACTANT SYSTEM
Mechanical stabilization of the lung

The integrity of the surfactant system of the lung is a prerequisite for normal breathing with the least possible effort. The surfactant system acts by decreasing surface tension of the interface between alveoli and air. This provides an explanation as to why we have to generate a 'negative' pressure of only 5–10 cmH_2O during each inspiration; in the absence of surfactant the surface tension at the air–liquid interface would be that of plasma and the pressure needed to maintain lung aeration would be 25–30 cmH_2O (depending on the radius of the alveoli). This is a well-known problem in patients with respiratory failure.

In alveoli with different radii an equal lowering of surface tension would not, however, produce stabilization of the alveolar system. It would instead, according to the law of Laplace, lead to the collapse of the smaller bubbles or alveoli, and to their emptying into the larger bubbles. Since alveoli *in vivo* do not exhibit such behaviour, one can conclude that the second remarkable quality of the alveolar lining layer is that it can change the surface tension in a manner related to the size of the alveoli. Meanwhile, there are also other explanations for this behaviour, but also these are not yet finally proved to be correct.

Surfactant as anti-oedema factor

Another function of the pulmonary surfactant system is stabilization of the fluid balance in the lung, and protection against lung oedema. The normal plasma oncotic pressure of 37 cmH$_2$O is opposed by the oncotic pressure of interstitial fluid proteins of 18 cmH$_2$O, the capillary hydrostatic pressure of 15 cmH$_2$O and by the surface tension conditioned suction of 4 cmH$_2$O (Fig. 1).

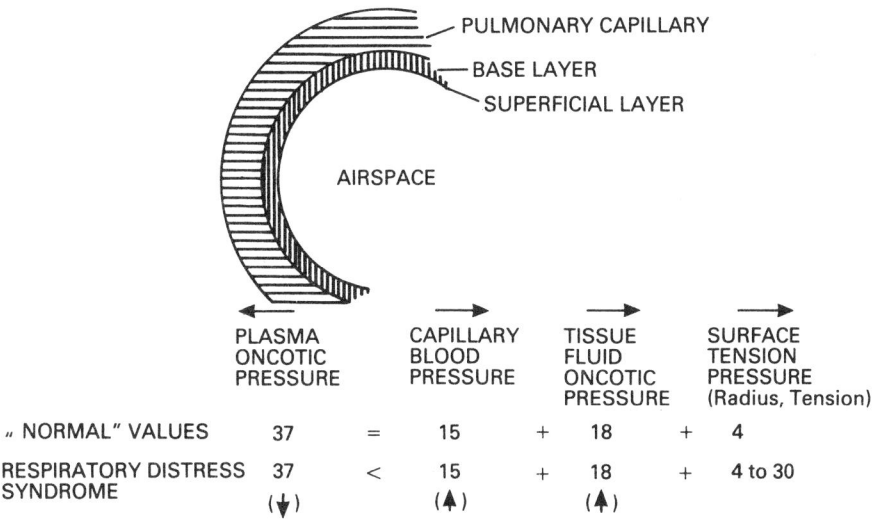

Fig. 1. Simplified schematic diagram representing the factors influencing the fluid balance in the lung.

In general, alveolar flooding will not occur as long as the suction force in the pulmonary interstitium exceeds the pressure gradient generated by surface tension in the alveolar air–liquid interface. Since this pressure gradient is inversely related to the radius of the alveolar curvature there is, for each combination of interstitial resorptive force and average surface tension, a critical value for surface tension and for alveolar radius, below which alveolar flooding occurs (Guyton *et al.*, 1984). From these facts it can also be concluded that established statements in the literature concerning the fluid exchange according to the law of Starling and the development of lung oedema have to be reconsidered, at least for those cases where the lung oedema appears to be due to a surfactant disturbance, because in this concept the surface tension is not included in the formula.

Surfactant and local defence mechanisms

Observations in patients have shown that, following a decrease in lung compliance (thus, surfactant deficiency), pneumonia will often develop, despite the application of high doses of antibiotics. Therefore, it is possible that the surfactant system is also involved in local defence mechanisms of the lung. It has been demonstrated that alveolar phagocytic macrophages ingest bacteria (or destroy them intracellularly) only in the presence of sufficient surface-active material (Huber *et al.*, 1976; Jarstrand, 1984). In this context surfactant seems to reduce the surface forces of bacterial membranes and it is also an energy-rich substrate which supports the macrophages' high rate of metabolism. Recently we have demonstrated that the pulmonary surfactant system may also be involved in protecting the lung against its own mediators (e.g. angiotensin II) and in protecting the cardiocirculatory system against mediators produced by the lung (Hein et al., 1987).

Surfactant and airways stabilization

As early as 1970, Macklem et al. (1970) called attention to the significance of bronchial surfactant for the stabilization of the peripheral airways and hinted that lack of stabilization may cause airway obstruction or collapse of the small bronchi with air trapping. Just recently this could be proved in our laboratory in an animal model where the bronchial surfactant was almost selectively destroyed (Lachmann, 1985). It was demonstrated that the pressure needed to open up the collapsed bronchi is about 20 cmH$_2$O.

In addition to its role in mechanical stabilization, bronchial surfactant also has a transporting function for mucus and inhaled particles. This has been proven, *in vitro*, in a study showing that particles on a surface film move in one direction only if the surface film is compressed and dilatated, comparable with the compression and expansion during expiration and inspiration (Lachmann, 1985). Furthermore, bronchial surfactant also acts as an antiglue factor preventing the development of large adhesive forces between mucus particles, as well as between mucus and the bronchial wall (Fig. 2) (Reifenrath, 1983).

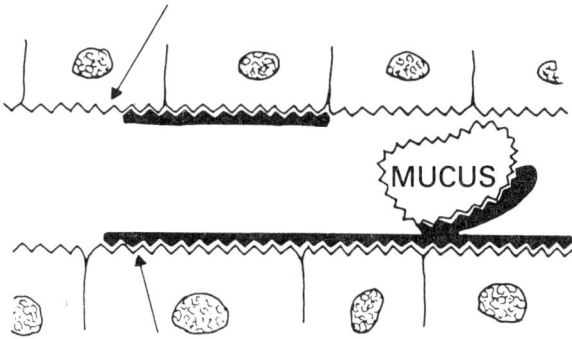

Fig. 2. Schematic diagram demonstrating the interaction between mucus and airways. Note that there will be non-adhesive forces only if the mucus particle and the airways are covered with surfactant (thick solid line).

A further possible function of bronchial surfactant, which to date has scarcely been discussed, is its masking of receptors on smooth muscle with respect to substances which induce contraction and could lead to airway obstruction. We have recently demonstrated that lining the airway with surfactant in ovalbumin-sensitized guinea pigs prevented significant bronchial obstruction during antigen challenge in these animals.

This means that the bronchial surfactant could also be involved in asthma (Lachmann and Becher, 1986). This is further supported by the fact that the most effective bronchodilatory drugs (corticoids and betamimetics) lead to a release of surfactant.

FUNCTIONAL CHANGES DUE TO A 'DISTURBED' SURFACTANT SYSTEM

When considering the main physiological functions of the alveobronchial surfactant system it can easily be understood that alteration in its functional integrity will lead to

- decreased lung distensibility and thus to increased work of breathing and increased oxygen demand by the respiratory muscles,
- atelectasis,
- transudation of plasma into the interstitium and into the alveoli with decreased diffusion for oxygen and CO_2,
- inactivation of the surfactant by plasma and specific surfactant inhibitors,
- hypoxaemia,
- metabolic acidosis secondary to increased production of organic acids under anaerobic conditions,
- enlargement of functional right-to-left shunt due to perfusion of non-ventilated alveoli (the von Euler–Liljestrand reflex does not 'work' in surfactant-deficient alveoli), and
- decreased production of surfactant as a result of hypoxaemia, acidosis and hypoperfusion.

This will finally lead to a vicious circle and the lung will fail as a gas exchange organ (Fig. 3) (Lachmann; 1988).

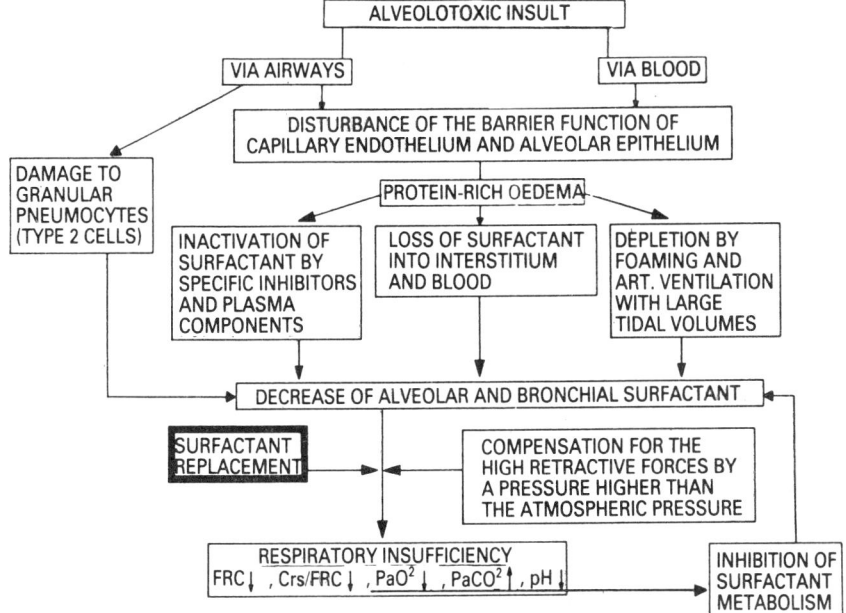

Fig. 3. Pathogenesis of ARDS with special reference to the surfactant system, including suggestions to compensate for a damaged surfactant system.

SURFACTANT REPLACEMENT THERAPY

Three decades of active research have resulted in the probability that surfactant treatment of surfactant deficiency states will soon be generally possible.

Exogenous surfactant therapy offers great promise for reducing the severity, morbidity and early mortality attributable to RDS. The RDS remains the primary cause of neonatal mortality; it is responsible for approximately one neonatal death per 1000 live births and it contributes to the number of infants with chronic pulmonary sequelae and neurodevelopmental handicaps, emphasizing the need to make efficacious therapies available.

Soon after the identification of dipalmitoylphosphatidylcholine (DPPC) as the principal surface-active component of surfactant and the recognition in 1959 that saline extracts from the lungs of infants who died of RDS had abnormal surface properties (Avery and Mead, 1959), aerosols of DPPC were used to treat RDS with little beneficial effect (Chu et al., 1967; Robillard et al., 1964). However, during the 1970s, Enhorning and Robertson and colleagues (Enhorning and Robertson, 1972) developed a sound experimental basis for the concept that RDS could be treated with exogenously administered surfactant. The idea was first successfully tested in infants by Fujiwara and coworkers (1980) and, subsequently, experimental and clinical investigations have increased exponentially (Tables 1 and 2).

The terminology used to describe various surfactants in the experimental and clinical literature is inconsistent; there are four general categories of surfactants that are being evaluated for clinical use.

Natural surfactant is the surfactant that can be removed from fresh alveolar washes or from amniotic fluid by simple centrifugation and/or filtration procedures designed to recover the large surface-active aggregates of surfactant (Hallman et al., 1983; Jobe and Ikegami, 1984). Such natural surfactant contains more protein than the more highly purified surfactant, but it can be recovered in the large amounts necessary for treatment protocols. Surfactants prepared after lipid extraction procedures is specifically excluded from this category since the native surfactant aggregates are disrupted.

Modified natural surfactants are made from homologous or heterologous lungs or alveolar lavage of various species. Such surfactants are prepared by extraction of lipids followed by selective addition and/or removal of compounds, sterilization and suspension procedures designed to restore the desired surface properties (Egan et al., 1983; Fujiwara, 1984; Taeusch et al., 1986). The final surfactant may contain as much as 1% lipophilic surfactant-specific proteins (Whitsett et al., 1986). Modified natural surfactants are designed to reproduce or improve upon the characteristics of natural surfactant, to decrease protein contamination and to ensure sterility.

Artificial surfactants are those surfactants made from a mixture of synthetic compounds that may or may not be normal components of natural surfactant. The most studied artificial surfactant is a mixture of dipalmitoylphosphatidylcholine (DPPC) and phosphatidylglycerol (PG) made from egg phosphatidylcholine (Morley et al., 1981). While both phospholipids are present in natural surfactant, the proportions differ and the acyl groups of the PG are different from those found in the PG of natural surfactant. Another artificial surfactant contains compounds foreign to natural surfactant such as hexadecanol and tyloxapol.

Table 1. Prophylactic surfactant treatment

Type of surfactant	Source	Number of patients	Number of controls	Treatment criteria	Outcome
Surfactant TA (supplemented bovine homogenate)	Soll et al. (1988)	79	81	Birth weight 750–1250 g, intubated 4–37 min after birth	$FiO_2\downarrow$, chest X-photo improved, patients who weighed 750–999 g responded better
Bovine lung lavage extract	Enhorning et al. (1985)	39	33	<30 wk gestation	Incidence of death ↓, incidence of IVH ↓ incidence of air leaks decreased
CLSE	Shapiro et al. (1985)	16	16	25–29 wk gestation	Severity of RDS decreased transiently
	Wood et al. (1987)	25	35 (saline) 20 (air)	25–29 wk gestation	Incidence of RDS ↓, chest X-photos show decreased severity of RDS in treated group
	Kendig et al. (1988)	34	31	25–29 wk gestation	Severity of RDS ↓, incidence of air leaks decreased

Table 1 cont.

Type of surfactant	Source	Number of patients	Number of controls	Treatment criteria	Outcome
	Shennan et al. (1988)	39 (phase 1) 29 (phase 2)	33 27	<30 wk gestation <30 wk gestation	(See Enhorning et al. 1985); both phases, incidence and severity of RDS decreased, PIE ↓, FiO_2 ↓, a/A PO_2 ↑, incidence of BPD ↓, phase 2: no decrease in IVH and mortality
Infasurf (CLSE)	Kwong et al. (1985)	16 14	17 13	30–33 wk gestation 24–28 wk gestation	No effect Severity of RDS was decreased at 48 h, FiO_2 decreased, ventilatory support was decreased
	Kwong and Egan (1988)	315	0	23–29 wk gestation	Incidence of death ↓
	Egan and Kwong (1988)	1437 (262 were treated too late)	0	≤32 wk gestation	Severity of RDS was higher in patients who were treated too late, mortality ↓ compared with earlier studies

Table 1 cont.

Type of surfactant	Source	Number of patients	Number of controls	Treatment criteria	Outcome
	Shapiro et al. (1988)	78 (prophylaxis) 81 (rescue)	0	24–29 wk gestation, RDS: $FiO_2 > 0.4$, MAP ≥ 7 cm H_2O, X-photo showing RDS	Both groups: identical mortality, no difference in incidence of complications
	Bloom et al. (1987a)	43 (Infasurf) 13 (HAF)	30	24–31 wk gestation	Incidence of death ↓, incidence of PIE ↓, FiO_2 ↓
	Bloom (1988)	30 (Infasurf) 10 (HAF)	30	24–31 wk gestation	Mortality ↓, BPD ↓, PIE ↓, incidence of pneumothorax ↓: FiO_2, CLSE < HAF; MAP, CLSE < HAF; a/A PO_2, CLSE > HAF
HAF	Merritt et al. (1986)	31	29	24–29 wk gestation, L/S ratio ≤ 2.0	Incidence of death ↓, incidence of BPD ↓, incidence of air leaks decreased

Table 1 cont.

Type of surfactant	Source	Number of patients	Number of controls	Treatment criteria	Outcome
	Merritt et al. (1988b)	23 (prophylaxis) 23 (rescue)	0	24–29 wk gestation, 23 twin pairs: one half → prophylaxis, the other half → rescue	<6 h after treatment, blood gas values better in prophylaxis group; >6 h, MAP ↓ and FiO$_2$ ↓ in rescue group
Synthetic phospholipids (ALEC)	Morley et al. (1981)	22	33	≤34 wk gestation	Incidence of death ↓
	Wilkinson et al. (1982)[a]	16	16	≤32 wk gestation	No effect
	Milner et al. (1984)[a]	10	6	≤34 wk gestation	No effect
	Morley et al. (1985)[a]	243	220	25–34 wk gestation	Incidence of death ↓ before 30 wk
	Morley et al. (1987)	159	149	25–29 wk gestation	Mortality ↓, incidence of IVH ↓, hours of ventilation ↓

Table 1 cont.

Type of surfactant	Source	Number of patients	Number of controls	Treatment criteria	Outcome
	Morley (1988)	163	164	23–34 wk gestation	Before 30 wk gestation: incidence of death ↓, IVH ↓, dependence on O_2 therapy ↓
Exosurf (synthetic surfactant)	Phibbs (1988)	29 (prophylaxis)	32	≤34 wk gestation, 700–1350 g birth weight	No effect on survival, FiO_2 ↓ and PIP ↓ during first 72 h
		45 (rescue)	40	≥650 g birth weight, RDS: FiO_2 ≥0.4, MAP ≥7 cm H_2O, X-photo showing RDS	Treated group shows higher survival, FiO_2 ↓ during first 48 h
DPPC + HDL	Halliday et al. (1984)	49	51	25–33 wk gestation	No effect

[a]Cited in Merritt and Hallman (1988a).

Explanation of abbreviations used: a/A PO_2, arterial–alveolar PO_2 ratio; BPD, bronchopulmonary dysplasia; CLSE, calf lung surfactant extract; HAF, human amniotic fluid; HMD, hyaline membrane disease; IVH, intraventricular haemorrhage; MAP, mean airway pressure; PDA, patent ductus arteriosus; PIE, pulmonary interstitial emphysema; PIP, positive inspiratory pressure; ↑, increase; ↓, decrease.

Table 2. Rescue surfactant treatment

Type of surfactant	Source	Number of patients	Number of controls	Treatment criteria	Outcome
Surfactant TA (supplemented bovine homogenate)	Fujiwara et al. (1980)	10	0	RDS	PaO_2 ↑, $PaCO_2$ ↓, a/A PO_2 ↑, 9 patients had PDA
	Fujiwara (1981)	19	0	RDS	PaO_2/FiO_2 ↑, FiO_2 ↓, incidence of PDA ↑
	Fujiwara et al. (1984)[a]	20	10	RDS	a/A PO_2 ↑, MAP ↓, chest X-photos improved
	Fujiwara (1984)	37	5	RDS	a/A PO_2 ↑, FiO_2 ↓, chest X-photos improved, incidence of PDA ↑
	Fujiwara et al. (1987)	91	Yes	RDS	Early improvement, IVH ↓, BPD ↓, incidence of death ↓, pneumothorax ↓
	Raju et al. (1987)	17	13	Birth weight 751–1750 g, MAP >8 cm H_2O, a/A PO_2 ≤ 0.24, age ≤ 6 h, HMD	a/A PO_2 ↑, FiO_2 ↓, incidence of PDA ↓, BPD ↓, air leaks ↓

Table 2. cont.

Type of surfactant	Source	Number of patients	Number of controls	Treatment criteria	Outcome
	Gitlin et al. (1987)	18	23	Birth weight ≥1000 g, FiO$_2$ ≥0.4, age <8 h	a/A PO$_2$ ↑, MAP ↓, time on ventilator ↓, number of days with FiO$_2$ ≥0.4 ↓
	Fujiwara et al. (1988)	96	0	Birth weight 520–2400 g, MAP >7 cm H$_2$O, FiO$_2$ > 0.4, RDS	'Pure RDS': sustained improvement 'RDS + PDA': at first improvement, secondly relapse, after treatment of PDA: recovery
	Horbar et al. (1988b)	38	46	Birth weight 750–1750 g, RDS	a/A PO$_2$ ↑, MAP ↓, incidence of IVH ↑
	Horbar et al. (1988a)	78	81	Birth weight 750–1750 g	FiO$_2$ ↓, MAP ↓, a/A PO$_2$ ↑, incidence of ventilatory support >48 h decreased

Table 2. cont.

Type of surfactant	Source	Number of patients	Number of controls	Treatment criteria	Outcome
	Konishi et al. (1988b)	206	0	23–39 wk gestation, birth weight 600–3401 g, MAP >7 cm H_2O, FiO_2 > 0.4, RDS	Group I (good response): mortality, 10%; FiO_2 ↓, MAP ↓, a/A PO_2 ↑ Group II (poor response): mortality, 22%; no increase in a/A PO_2
	Konishi et al. (1988a)	23 (high dose) 23 (low dose)	0	Birth weight 1000–1499 g, RDS	Both groups, a/A PO_2 ↑; high dose: prolonged effect of treatment, lower incidence of IVH and BPD, lower number of patients treated with O_2 for 30 days
	Charon et al. (1989)	29	23	Birth weight 750–1750 g, age <8 h, RDS	(See Gitlin et al., 1987); in the lasting response group the a/A PO_2 ratio improved >48 h

Table 2. *cont.*

Type of surfactant	Source	Number of patients	Number of controls	Treatment criteria	Outcome
Bovine lung lavage extract	Smyth *et al.* (1981)	3	0	Severe RDS	PaO_2 ↑, FiO_2 ↓, chest X-photo improved
	Smyth *et al.* (1983)	6	0	Severe HMD	a/A PO_2 ↑ (24 h effect)
	Shennan *et al.* (1988)	22 (1 dose) 17 (≥1 dose) (phase 3)	20	30–36 wk gestation, RDS	Prolonged improvement of gas exchange in group receiving ≥1 dose, no significant difference in mortality and morbidity between treated groups and control group
Bovine surfactant (SF-RI 1)	Gortner *et al.* (1988)	15 (high dose) 19 (low dose)	0	24–31 wk gestation, birth weight 430–1500 g, RDS, $FiO_2 > 0.5$	High dose survival ↑; both groups, FiO_2 ↓, MAP ↓, a/A PO_2 ↑

Table 2. cont.

Type of surfactant	Source	Number of patients	Number of controls	Treatment criteria	Outcome
CLSE	Davis et al. (1988)	35	0	RDS, $FiO_2 \geq 0.4$	Improvement of gas exchange, improvement of lung mechanics only during spontaneous breathing
Bovine or porcine surfactant	Mortensson et al. (1987)	10	0	27–32 wk gestation, birth weight 795–1680 g, RDS	Chest X-photo: improvement of aeration, distension of bronchioli, right-left shunt ↓
	Noack et al. (1987)	10	0	Same patient group as Mortensson et al. (1987)	a/A PO_2 ↑, see Mortensson et al. (1987)
Porcine surfactant	Svenningsen et al. (1987)	4	4	Birth weight 700–1400 g, FiO_2 >0.6, RDS	Transcutaneous O_2 ↑; chest X-photo: improved aeration
	McCord et al. (1988b)	12	8	RDS, $FiO_2 > 0.6$	Incidence of IVH ↓ and pneumothorax ↓

Table 2. cont.

Type of surfactant	Source	Number of patients	Number of controls	Treatment criteria	Outcome
	McCord et al. (1988a)	14	15	Birth weight < 2000 g, RDS, FiO_2 > 0.6	a/A PO_2 ↑, incidence of IVH ↓ and pneumothorax ↓
Porcine CK	Kobayashi et al. (1981)[a]	1	0	RDS	PaO_2/FiO_2 ↑, $PaCO_2$ ↓, chest X-photo improved
	Ohta et al. (1981)[a]	1	0	RDS	'Improvement'
	Nohara et al. (1983)[a]	6	0	RDS	PaO_2 ↑ in 4 patients, chest X-photos improved
Curosurf (porcine surfactant)	Berggren et al. (1984)[a]	4	0	Severe RDS	PaO_2 ↑, $PaCO_2$ ↓, incidence of air leaks decreased
	Robertson et al. (1988)	77	69	Severe RDS, birth weight 700–2000 g	Incidence of death ↓, BPD↓
	Robertson (1988)	55	0	Severe RDS, birth weight 700–2000 g	Same outcome

Table 2. cont.

Type of surfactant	Source	Number of patients	Number of controls	Treatment criteria	Outcome
	Speer et al. (1988)	14	20	Severe RDS	Oxygenation ↑, gas exchange ↑, duration of PIP and FiO_2 >0.4 was decreased in treated group, mortality ↓, pneumothorax ↓, PDA ↑, no difference in BPD and IVH
HAF	Hallman et al. (1982)	3	0	RDS	PaO_2 ↑, FiO_2 ↓, MAP ↓
	Hallman et al. (1983)[a]	6	6	<29 wk gestation, age <10 h, L/S ratio ≤2.0	PaO_2 ↑, $PaCO_2$ ↓, chest X-photos improved
	Hallman et al. (1983)	5	5	Mean birth weight 974 ± 61 g, RDS	PaO_2 ↑, $PaCO_2$ ↓, pH ↑, chest X-photo improved, severity of RDS decreased

Table 2. cont.

Type of surfactant	Source	Number of patients	Number of controls	Treatment criteria	Outcome
	Merritt et al. (1983)	4	3	Preterm infants with severe RDS	$PaO_2 \uparrow$, $PaCO_2 \downarrow$, $FiO_2 \downarrow$, MAP $\downarrow$, chest X-photo improved
	Hallman et al. (1985)	25	28	Birth weight <1500 g, age <10 h, severe RDS, L/S ratio ≤2.0	Incidence of death $\downarrow$, BPD $\downarrow$, incidence of air leaks $\downarrow$, numbers of infants who required $FiO_2 >$ 0.3 at 30 days was decreased
	Heldt et al. (1988)	49	?	25–29 wk gestation, birth weight 450–1580 g, RDS	Maturity of ductus arteriosus parallels the maturity of the lung and is independent of surfactant therapy
	Lang et al. (1988)	10	14	25–32 wk gestation, severe RDS; mean treatment time, 5.6 h	$PaO_2 \uparrow$, $FiO_2 \downarrow$, MAP $\downarrow$, a/A $PO_2 \uparrow$
Synthetic phospholipids (ALEC)	Milner et al. (1983)[a]	10	0	RDS	No effect

Table 2. cont.

Type of surfactant	Source	Number of patients	Number of controls	Treatment criteria	Outcome
	Weintraub et al. (1985)[a]	22	0	RDS, FiO_2 >0.6, PIP ≥20 cm H_2O	$PaCO_2$ ↓, PIP ↓, 8 patients died
	Wilkinson et al. (1985)[a]	12	0	≤32 wk gestation, RDS	No effect, L/S ratio in tracheal fluid ↑
	Wilkinson et al. (1985)	16 (trial I) 12 (trial II)	16 12	≤32 wk gestation, L/S ratio immature, RDS	No significant difference in ventilator pressures or O_2 therapy used, nor in mortality and morbidity <2 years
Liposomal phospholipids (artificial surfactant)	Obladen et al. (1988)	10	0	<30 wk gestation, birth weight <1500 g, RDS	a/A PO_2 ↑, FiO_2 ↓, lung compliance ↑, 3 patients died
Artificial improved surfactant (DPPC, etc.)	Friedman and Doody (1982)	3	0	RDS	Chest X-photos improved in 2 patients before clinical improvement
Synthetic L-α-lecithin	Robillard et al. (1964)	11	0	RDS	Cyanosis ↓, retraction score ↓
Dipalmitoyl L-α-lecithin	Chu et al. (1967)	27	21	RDS	No beneficial effect

[a]Cited in Merritt and Hallman (1988a).

Explanation of abbreviations used: a/A PO_2, arterial–alveolar PO_2 ratio; BPD, bronchopulmonary dysplasia; CLSE, calf lung surfactant extract; HAF, human amniotic fluid; HMD, hyaline membrane disease; IVH, intraventricular haemorrhage; MAP, mean airway pressure; PDA, patent ductus arteriosus; PIE, pulmonary interstitial emphysema; PIP, positive inspiratory pressure; ↑, increase; ↓, decrease.

Synthetic natural surfactants are just beginning to be a possibility. With the recent isolation and characterization of the surfactant proteins, synthetic natural surfactants are being tested. In the near future, such surfactants will be reconstructed *in vitro* from surfactant-specific proteins synthesized using molecular biological techniques and from mixtures of lipids and phospholipids.

CONCLUSIONS

Initial reports suggest that surfactant treatments will simplify care sufficiently that hospital stay and thus cost of care will be decreased (Enhorning *et al.*, 1985). Many practical aspects of the treatment of infants with surfactant have not been evaluated. The dose, the best method of administration and the benefits from repetitive doses are not well defined. While a number of surfactants have been evaluated clinically, they are 'home made' and were not well standardized. Different surfactants have not been compared directly in clinical trails. The surfactant with the best clinical response may not be a surfactant that can be easily standardized and prepared in bulk as a pharmaceutical. Practical considerations of formulation and licensure will probably in part dictate which surfactants will ultimately be available for clinical use.

Surfactant therapy should be beneficial not only to those infants in need of supplemental surfactant, but also indirectly to infants who suffer secondarily to surfactant deficiency. Other uses of surfactant are now being considered. Experimental models of lung injury in adult animals such as saline lavage (Berggren *et al.*, 1986; Kobayashi *et al.*, 1984), oxygen injury (Matalon *et al.*, 1987), viral and bacterial pneumonia, oxygen free radicals, anti-lung serum and pulmonary oedema (Lachmann *et al.*, 1983, 1987a,b; Lachmann and Bergmann, 1987), together with first clinical trails (Lachmann, 1988) suggest that there is a role for surfactant in the treatment of adult respiratory distress syndrome (ARDS). Surfactant treatments will become a major advance in the care of preterm infants with severe RDS and may ultimately prove useful in other lung disease.

ACKNOWLEDGEMENT

This study was financially supported by a grant from the Dutch Foundation for Medical Research (SFMO).

REFERENCES

Avery, M. E. and Mead, J. (1959) Surface properties in relation to atelectasis and hyaline membrane disease. *Am. J. Dis. Child.* 97 517.

Berggren, P., Lachmann, B., Curstedt, T. *et al.* (1986) Gas exchange and lung morphology after surfactant replacement in experimental adult respiratory distress syndrome induced by repeated lung lavage. *Acta Anaesthesiol. Scand.* 30 321–328.

Bloom, B. T. (1988) Human surfactant and calf lung surfactant extract: moderation of respiratory distress in preterm infants by a single prophylactic dose in a randomized and controlled clinical trial. In: Lachmann, B. (ed.) *Surfactant Replacement Therapy* in *Neonatal and Adult Respiratory Distress Syndrome*. Springer, Berlin, pp. 150–157.

Charon, A., Taeusch, T., Fitzgibbon, C. *et al.* (1989) Factors associated with surfactant treatment in infants with severe respiratory distress syndrome. *Pediatrics* **83** 348–354.

Chu, J., Clements, J. A., Cotton, E. K. *et al.* (1967) Neonatal pulmonary ischemia. *Pediatrics* **40** 709–782.

Clements, J. A. (1957) Surface tension of lung extracts. *Proc. Soc. Exp. Biol. Med.* **95** 170–172.

Davis, J. M., Veness-Meehan, K., Notter, R. H. *et al.* (1988) Changes in pulmonary mechanics after the administration of surfactant to infants with respiratory distress syndrome. *N. Engl. J. Med.* **319** 476–479.

Egan, E. A. and Kwong, M. S. (1988) Clinical results of a multicenter open trial of Infasurf. In: *Ross Laboratories Special Conference: Hot Topics '88 in Neonatology,* pp. 86–96.

Egan, E. A., Notter, R. H., Kwong, M. S. and Shapiro, D. L. (1983) Natural and artificial lung surfactant replacement therapy in premature lambs. *J. Appl. Physiol.* **55** 875–883.

Enhorning, G. and Robertson, B. (1972) Lung expansion in the premature rabbit fetus after tracheal deposition of surfactant. *Pediatrics* **50** 58–66.

Enhorning, G., Shennan, A., Possmayer, F. *et al.* (1985) Prevention of neonatal respiratory distress syndrome by tracheal instillation of surfactant: a randomized clinical trial. *Pediatrics* **76** 145–153.

Friedman, Z. V. I. and Doody, M. (1982) Artificial surfactant: a therapeutic trial in infants with hyaline membrane disease. *Pediatr. Res.* **16** 287A.

Fujiwara, T. (1981) Tracheal instillation of artificial surfactant for the treatment of hyaline membrane disease. In: *Newer Management of Hyaline Membrane Disease. Ann. Nestlé* **48** 24–29.

Fujiwara, T. (1984) Surfactant replacement in neonatal RDS. In: Robertson, B., Van Golde, L. M. G. and Batenburg, J. J. (eds) Pulmonary surfactant Elsevier, Amsterdam, pp. 479–503.

Fujiwara, T., Chida, S., Watabe, Y. *et al.* (1980) Artificial surfactant therapy in hyaline-membrane disease. *Lancet* **1** 55–59.

Fujiwara, T., Konishi, M., Nanby, H. *et al.* (1987) Surfactant supplementation treatment of neonatal respiratory distress syndrome. *Shonika Rinsho* **40** 549–568.

Fujiwara, T., Konishi, M., Chida, S. *et al.* (1988) Factors affecting the response to a postnatal single dose of a reconstituted bovine surfactant (Surfactant TA). In: Lachmann, B. (ed.) *Surfactant Replacement Therapy in Neonatal and Adult Respiratory Distress Syndrome*. Springer, Berlin, pp. 91–107.

Gitlin, J. D., Soll, R. F., Parad, R. B. *et al.* (1987) Randomized controlled trial of exogenous surfactant for the treatment of hyaline membrane disease. *Pediatrics* **79** 31–37.

Gortner, L., Pohlandt, F., Bartmann, P. *et al.* (1988) Surfactant replacement with SF-RI 1 in premature infants with respiratory distress syndrome: a clinical pilot study. In:

Lachmann, B. (ed.) *Surfactant Replacement Therapy in Neonatal and Adult Respiratory Distress Syndrome.* Springer, Berlin, p. 133.
Guyton, A. C., Moffatt, D. S. and Adair, T. A. (1984) Role of alveolar surface tension in transepithelial movement of fluids. In: Robertson, B., van Golde, L. M. G. and Batenburg, J. J. (eds) *Pulmonary Surfactant.* Elsevier, Amsterdam, pp. 171–185.
Halliday, H. L., Reid, M. McMeban, C. *et al.* (1984) Controlled trial of artificial surfactant to prevent respiratory distress syndrome. *Lancet* 1 476–478.
Hallman, M., Schneider, H., Merritt, T. A. *et al.* (1982) Human surfactant substitution. *Pediatr. Res.* 16 691A.
Hallman, M., Merritt, T. A., Schneider, H. *et al.* (1983) Isolation of human surfactant from amniotic fluid and a pilot study of its efficacy in respiratory distress syndrome. *Pediatrics* 71 473–482.
Hallman, M., Merritt, T. A., Jarvenpaa, A. L. *et al.* (1985) Exogenous surfactant for treatment of severe respiratory distress syndrome: a randomized prospective clinical trial. *J. Pediatr.* 106 963–969.
Hein, T., Lachmann, B., Armbruster, S., Smit, J. M., Voelkel, N. and Erdmann, W. (1987) Pulmonary surfactant inhibits the cardiovascular effects of platelet activating factor (PAF), 5-hydroxytryptamine (5-HT) and angiotensin II. *Am. Rev. Resp. Dis.* 135 A506.
Heldt, G. P., Pesonen, E., Merritt, T. A. *et al.* (1988) Dynamic lung compliance, closure of the patent ductus arteriosus and surfactant therapy. *Pediatr. Res.* 23 510A.
Horbar, J. D., Sutherland, J., Philip, A. G. S. *et al.* (1988a) Multicenter trial of single dose surfactant-TA for treatment of respiratory distress syndrome. *Pediatr. Res.* 23 410A.
Horbar, J. D., Linderkamp, O., Schachinger, H. *et al.* (1988b) European trial of single dose surfactant-TA for treatment of respiratory distress syndrome. *Pediatr. Res.* 23 510A.
Huber, G., Mullane, J. and LaForce, F. M. (1976) The role of alveolar lining material in antibacterial defenses of the lung. *Bull. Eur. Physiopathol. Resp.* 12 178–179.
Jarstrand, C. (1984) Role of surfactant in the pulmonary defence system. In: Robertson, B., van Golde, L. M. G. and Batenburg, J. J. (eds) *Pulmonary Surfactant.* Elsevier, Amsterdam, pp. 187–201.
Jobe, A. and Ikegami, M. (1984) The prematurely delivered lamb as a model for studies of neonatal adaptation. In: Nathanielsz, P. W. (ed) *Animal Models in Fetal Medicine.* Perinatology Press, Ithaca, NY, pp. 1–30.
Kendig, J. W., Notter, R. H., Cox, C. *et al.* (1988) Surfactant replacement at birth: final analysis of a clinical trial and comparisons with similar trials. *Pediatrics* 82 756–762.
Kobayashi, T., Kataoka, H., Ueda, T. *et al.* (1984) Effects of surfactant supplement and end-expiratory pressure in lung-lavaged rabbits. *J. Appl. Physiol.* 57 995–1001.
Konishi, M., Fujiwara, T., Naito, T. *et al.* (1988a) Surfactant replacement therapy in neonatal respiratory distress syndrome: a multicentre, randomized clinical trial: comparison of high- versus low-dose of surfactant TA. *Eur. J. Pediatr.* 147 20–25.
Konishi, M., Fujiwara, T., Chida, S. *et al.*(1988b) Response to a single dose of exogenous surfactant: a multicenter study. In: *Ross Laboratories Special Conference: Hot Topics '88 in Neonatology,* pp. 48–61.

Kwong, M. S. and Egan, E. A. (1988) Routine use of Infasurf (calf lung surfactant extract) at birth for prematures ≤ 32 wks gestation. *Pediatr. Res.* **23** 415A.

Kwong, M. S., Egan, E. A., Notter, R. H. *et al.* (1985) Double-blind clinical trial of calf lung surfactant extract for the prevention of hyaline membrane disease in extremely premature infants. *Pediatrics* **76** 585-592.

Lachmann, B. (1985) Possible function of bronchial surfactant. *Eur. J. Respir. Dis.* **67** 49-61.

Lachmann, B. (1988) Surfactant replacement in acute respiratory failure: animal studies and first clinical trials. In: Lachmann, B, (ed.) *Surfactant Replacement Therapy in Neonatal and Adult Respiratory Distress Syndrome*. Springer, Berlin, pp. 212-223.

Lachmann, B. and Becher, G. (1986) Protective effect of lung surfactant on allergic bronchial constriction in guinea pigs. *Am. Rev. Respir. Dis.* **133** A118.

Lachmann, B. and Bergmann, K. C. (1987) Surfactant replacement improves thorax-lung compliance and survival rate in mice with influenza infection. *Am. Rev. Respir. Dis.* **135** A6.

Lachmann, B., Fujiwara, T., Chida, S. *et al.* (1983) Surfactant replacement therapy in the experimental adult respiratory distress syndrome (ARDS). In: Cosmi, E. V. and Scarpelli, E. M. (eds) *Pulmonary Surfactant Systems*. Elsevier, Amsterdam, pp. 231-235.

Lachmann, B., Saugstad, O. D. and Erdmann, W. (1987a) Effect of surfactant replacement on respiratory failure induced by free oxygen radicals. In: Schlag, G. and Redl, H. (eds) *Congress Report 1st Vienna Shock Forum*. Alan Liss, New York, pp. 305-313.

Lachmann, B., Hallman, M. and Bergmann, K. C. (1987b) Respiratory failure following anti-lung serum: study on mechanisms associated with surfactant system damage. *Exp. Lung Res.* **12** 163-180.

Lang, M. J., Rhodes, P. G., Reddy, S. *et al.* (1988) Limitation of the effective use of human surfactant in established respiratory distress syndrome. *Pediatr. Res.* **23** 513A.

Macklem, P. T., Proctor, D. F. and Hogg, J. C. (1970) The stability of peripheral airways. *Resp. Physiol.* **8** 191-203.

Matalon, S., Holm, B. A. and Notter, R. H. (1987) Mitigation of pulmonary hyperoxic injury by administration of exogenous surfactant. *J. Appl. Physiol.* **62** 756-761.

McCord, F. B., Curstedt, T., Halliday, H. L. *et al.* (1988a) Surfactant treatment and incidence of intraventricular haemorrhage in severe respiratory distress syndrome. *Arch. Dis. Child.* **63** 10-16.

McCord, F. B., Halliday, H. L., McClure, G. *et al.* (1988b) Changes in pulmonary and cerebral blood flow after surfactant treatment for severe respiratory distress syndrome. In: Lachmann, B. (ed.) *Surfactant Replacement Therapy in Neonatal and Adult Respiratory Distress Syndrome*. Springer, Berlin, pp. 195-200.

Merritt, T. A. and Hallman, M. (1988a) Surfactant replacement: a new era with many challenges for neonatal medicine. *Am. J. Dis. Child.* **142** 1333-1339.

Merritt, T. A. and Hallman, M. (1988b) Human surfactant treatment of respiratory distress syndrome: recent experiences in prophylactic versus rescue treatment and an analysis of the role of SP-A in surfactant function. In: *Ross Laboratories Special Conference: Hot Topics '88 in Neonatology,* pp. 82–85.

Merritt, T. A., Cochrane, C. G., Hallman, M. *et al.* (1983) Reduction of lung injury by human surfactant treatment in respiratory distress syndrome. *Chest* **5** 27S–31S.

Merritt, T. A., Hallman, M., Holcomb, K. *et al.* (1986) Human surfactant treatment of severe respiratory distress syndrome: pulmonary effluent indicators of lung inflammation. *J. Pediatr.* **108** 741–748.

Morley, C. J. (1988) Artificial surfactant: prophylaxis for respiratory distress syndrome. In: Lachmann, B. (ed.) *Surfactant Replacement Therapy in Neonatal and Adult Respiratory Distress Syndrome.* Springer, Berlin, pp. 158–167.

Morley, C. J., Miller, N., Bangham, A. D. *et al.* (1981) Dry artificial surfactant and its effect on very premature babies. *Lancet* **1** 64–68.

Morley, C. J., Lloyd, D., Duffty, P. *et al.*(ten centre study group) (1987) Ten centre trial of artificial surfactant (artificial lung expanding compound) in very premature babies. *Br. Med. J.* **294** 991–996.

Mortensson, W., Noack, G., Curstedt, T. *et al.* (1987) Radiologic observations in severe neonatal respiratory distress syndrome treated with the isolated phospholipid fraction of natural surfactant. *Acta Radiol.* **28** 389–394.

Noack, G., Berggren, P., Curstedt, T. *et al.* (1987) Severe neonatal respiratory distress syndrome treated with the isolated phospholipid fraction of natural surfactant. *Acta Paediatr. Scand.* **76** 697–705.

Obladen, M., Stevens, P. and Kattner, E. (1988) Rapid response of oxygenation, slow response of compliance after liposomal phospholipid substitution in respiratory distress syndrome. In: Lachmann, B. (ed.) *Surfactant Replacement Therapy in Neonatal and Adult Respiratory Distress Syndrome.* Springer, Berlin, pp. 168–180.

Pattle, R. E. (1955) Properties, function, and origin of the alveolar lining layer. *Nature (London)* **175** 1125–1126.

Phibbs, R. H. (1988) A preliminary report of initial trial of Exosurf, a synthetic surfactant for the prevention and early treatment of hyaline membrane disease. In: *Ross Laboratories Special Conference: Hot Topics '88 in Neonatology,* pp. 202–208.

Raju, T. N. K., Vidyasagar, D., Bhat, R. *et al.* (1987) Double-blind controlled trial of single-dose treatment with bovine surfactant in severe hyaline membrane disease. *Lancet* **1** 651–656.

Reifenrath, R. (1983) Surfactant action in bronchial mucus. In: Scarpelli, E. M. (ed.) *Pulmonary Surfactant System.* Elsevier, Amsterdam, pp. 339–347.

Robertson, B. (1988) The Curosurf experience in Europe. In: *Ross Laboratories Special Conference: Hot Topics '88 in Neonatology,* pp. 62–72.

Robertson, B. *et al.* (Collaborative European Multicenter Group) (1988) Surfactant replacement therapy for severe neonatal respiratory distress syndrome: an international randomized clinical trial. *Pediatrics* **82** 683–691.

Robillard, E., Alarie, Y., Dagenais-Perusse, P. *et al.* (1964) Microaerosol administration of β-γ-dipalmitoyl-L-α-lecithin in the respiratory distress syndrome: a preliminary report. *Can. Med. Assoc. J.* **90** 55–57.

Shapiro, D. L., Notter, R. H., Morin III, F. C. *et al.*(1985) Double-blind, randomized trial of a calf lung surfactant extract administered at birth to very premature infants for prevention of respiratory distress syndrome. *Pediatrics* **76** 593–599.

Shapiro, D. L., Kendig, J. W., Notter, R. H. *et al.* (1988) A multicenter randomized trial of pre-ventilatory versus post-ventilatory administration of surfactant (calf lung surfactant extract). In: *Ross Laboratories Special Conference: Hot Topics '88 in Neonatology*, pp. 105–108.

Shennan, A. T., Dunn, M. S. and Possmayer, F. (1988) CLSE experience in Canada. In: *Ross Laboratories Special Conference: Hot Topics '88 in Neonatology*, pp. 116–142.

Smyth, J. A., Metcalfe, I. L., Duffty, P. *et al.* (1981) Surfactant therapy in hyaline membrane disease. *Pediatr. Res.* **15** 681A.

Smyth, J. A., Metcalfe, I. L., Duffty, P. *et al.* (1983) Hyaline membrane disease treated with bovine surfactant. *Pediatrics* **71** 913–917.

Soll, R. F., Hoekstra, R., Fangman, J. *et al.* (1988) Multicenter trial of single dose surfactant TA for prevention of respiratory distress syndrome. *Pediatr. Res.* **23** 425A.

Speer, C. P., Harms, K., Muller, U. *et al.* (1988) Treatment of severe respiratory distress syndrome in the premature infant with natural surfactant. *Monatsschr. Kinderheilkd.* **136** 65–70.

Svenningsen, S., Robertson, B., Andreason, B. *et al.* (1987) Endotracheal administration of surfactant in very low birth weight infants with respiratory distress syndrome. *Crit. Care Med.* **15** 918–922.

Taeusch, W. H., Keough, K. M. W. and Williams, M. (1986) Characterization of bovine surfactant for infants with respiratory distress syndrome. *Pediatrics* **77** 572–581.

Van Golde, L. M. G., Batenburg, J. J. and Robertson, B. (1988) The pulmonary surfactant system. Biochemical aspects and functional significance. *Physiol. Rev.* **68** 374–455.

Von Neergaard, K. (1929) Neue Auffassungen über einen Grundbegriff der Atemmechanik. *Z. Ges. Exp. Med.* **66** 373–394.

Whitsett, J. A., Ohning, B. L., Ross, G. *et al.* (1986) Hydrophobic surfactant-associated protein in whole lung surfactant and its importance for biophysical activity in lung surfactant extracts used for replacement therapy. *Pediatr. Res.* **20** 460–467.

Wilkinson, A., Jenkins, P. A. and Jeffrey, J. A. (1985) Two controlled trials of dry artificial surfactant: early effects and later outcome in babies with surfactant deficiency. *Lancet* **2** 287–291.

Wood, B. P., Sinkin, R. A., Kendig, J. W. *et al.* (1987) Exogenous lung surfactant: effect on radiographic appearance in premature infants. *Radiology* **165** 11–13.

11

Molecular aspects of lung surfactant proteins and their use as pulmonal carriers

Klaus P. Schäfer

LUNG SURFACTANT — A FUNCTIONAL DESCRIPTION

Introduction

Lung surfactant is essential for all lung-breathing animals. It prevents collapse or overexpansion of the lungs by an adequate reduction of surface tension of the aqueous layer lining the alveoli. This process must be fast (in the range of seconds or less) and dynamically adjustable. Reduction of surface tension is achieved through a monomolecular film of phospholipids which covers the aqueous surface. The dynamics of film formation, however, depends on three surfactant-associated proteins, SP-A, SP-B and SP-C. During biosynthesis in alveolar type II pneumocytes, secretion and extra- as well as intracellular metabolism, these proteins cooperate with phospholipids to form various superstructures. Besides reduction of surface tension, the three proteins are known to or are supposed to cooperate with other molecules and a range of cells to mediate a host of different functions, including defense mechanisms against intruding bacteria or viruses (van Iwaarden et al., 1990; Manz-Keinke et al., 1992). The lack of surfactant quickly becomes life threatening as can be witnessed regarding the infant respiratory distress syndrome (Gortner et al., 1990; Lang et al., 1990) which is the major cause of death for prematurely born babies. A similar situation is found in adult patients suffering from the respiratory distress syndrome or shock lung (Richman et al., 1989) (for details see Chapter 10).

Formation and structures of natural lung surfactant

All components of lung surfactant (Table 1) are produced by alveolar type II pneumocytes. It forms inside these cells in the shape of lamellar bodies which are expelled into the aqueous lining phase towards the alveolar space (see Fig. 1). The lamellae in these structures are made up of stacks of phospholipid bilayers but incorporate also lung surfactant proteins (Schmitz and Müller, 1991).

Outside the cell, lamellar bodies unfold into a three-dimensional network of so-called tubular myelin (Beckmann and Dierichs, 1984). One can see tubular myelin as an intermediate form during hydration of the closely packed phospholipids. Tubular myelin subsequently dissolves by liberating the phospholipids which, under the influence of the hydrophobic surfactant proteins, spread rapidly on the air–water interface to form a monomolecular film.

Table 1. Phospholipid composition of natural surfactant

Component		H^a	D^a	R^a
(1)	Phosphatidylcholine	73.07	74	76.3
	Saturated	38.03	33	47.2
	Unsaturated	35.04	41	29.1
(2)	Phosphatidylserine	3.3	2	NI
(3)	Phosphatidylinositol	2.7	3	8.4^b
(4)	Phosphatidylinositol	12.4	10	5.1
	Saturated	ND	4.4	ND
	Unsaturated	ND	5.6	ND
(5)	Phosphatidylethanolamine	2.6	4	5.0
(6)	Sphingomyelin	3.7	5	—
(7)	Lysophosphatidylcholine	0.4	ND	—
(8)	Phosphatidic acid	ND	ND	ND
(9)	Diphosphatidylglycerol	ND	ND	3.7
(10)	Other components	1.9	1.3	0.9

Values are given as percentage of total mass. Surfactant-associated proteins are present in surfactant preparations usually between 1% and 5% of total mass. SP-A can only be found if no extraction by organic solvents was used during preparation. ND, not determined; NI, no information given.
[a]H, human (Hallman et al., 1982); D, dog (Pfleger and Thomas, 1971); R, rabbit (Baritussio et al., 1981).
[b]Sum of components (2), (3), (6) ad (7).

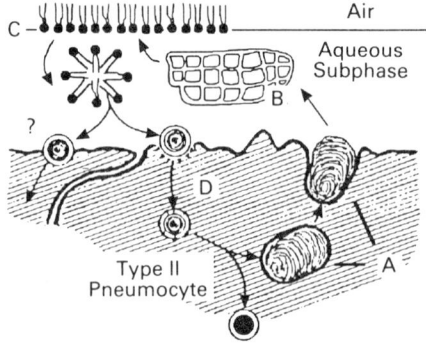

A Lamellar Bodies
B Tubular Myelin
C Surfactant Monolayer
D Recycling

Fig. 1. Biosynthesis and structural components of lung surfactant.

Physicochemistry of lung surfactant

The liquid layer lining the alveolar space of any healthy individual is covered completely by phospholipids. Their main function is to lower and adjust the surface tension of the aqueous surface in order to minimize the labour of breathing and to prevent a collapse of the alveoli upon exhalation. The reduction in surface tension is achieved by a monomolecular film of phospholipids covering the air–water interface. When this film is compressed during exhalation, part of the phospholipids are forced out from the interface and are sequestered to the aqueous subphase. Upon inhalation the surface film is expanded again and the phospholipids have to quickly move from the subphase to the free space in the interface to avoid any drastic increase in surface tension caused by an uncovered water surface. It turns out that the kinetics of spreading of phospholipids alone into the air–water interface is much too slow. However, the hydrophobic surfactant-associated proteins accelerate the spreading kinetics of the phospholipids sufficiently to ensure a properly covered surface at all times and under all conditions of breathing (see Fig. 2).

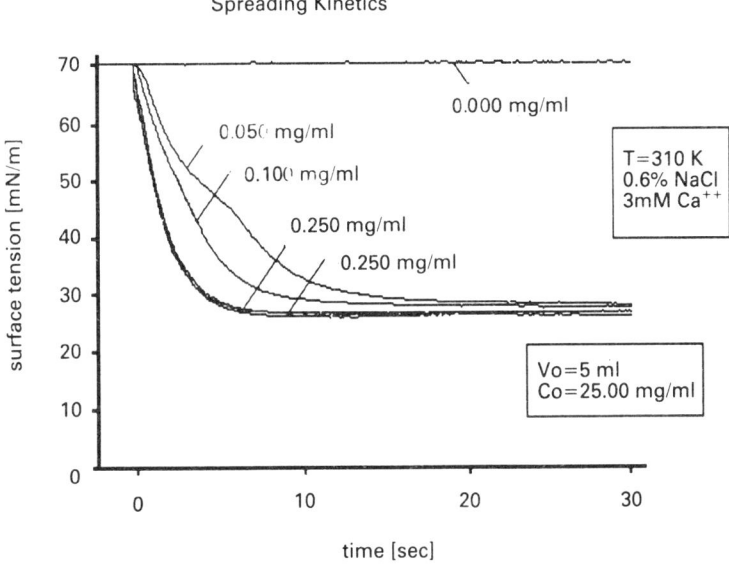

Fig 2. Spreading kinetics of a recombinant surfactant in a Wilhelmy balance.

Other proteins complement the above-mentioned hydrophobic species, creating a network of biochemical and metabolic feedback circles and thus maintaining the balance of the lung surfactant system.

It is this property of rapid spreading on an aqueous surface and the ability to readjust the surface film within fractions of a second which has caught the attention of people interested in drug delivery systems. Could the surfactant system be exploited as a carrier for drugs into the alveolar compartment and possibly even through the cellular barrier into the bloodstream?

On the one hand, this route of application would avoid burdening the whole organism with a drug which is intended to act in the lung. If we think, for example, of administering antibiotics to the lung to fight an infection of the airways, the dose could probably be lowered considerably since the antibiotics will reach their target without detour.

On the other hand, using the pulmonary route may even be attractive for the administration of 'classical' drugs such as insulin. In this case, there have already been successful attempts to use aerosolization and normal inhalation without the help of surfactant to get insulin across the pulmonary barrier into the system (Salzman et al., 1985). Of course, these attempts ran across other problems, such as dosing of the aerosolized drug and efficiency of its transcytotic transport. Nevertheless, the use of lung surfactant as a carrier for a variety of drugs remains an intriguing and yet to be explored possibility.

What types of surfactants are currently available and how can we assess their potential as drug carriers?

THE SURFACTANT SYSTEM

Available surfactant

An attempt to obtain a surfactant resembling as closely as possible the natural standard is represented by the use of lung lavage fluids or tissue extracts from animal lungs as well as extracts from human amniotic fluid. All of the surfactants obtained by these procedures contain the functionally essential components of surfactants, i.e. phospholipids and protein. The two small hydrophobic proteins SP-B and SP-C are present in about equal amounts together with a broad spectrum of phospholipids and other lipids (see Table 1). Except for amniotic extracts, the glycoprotein SP-A, however, is missing since the preparation procedure includes an extraction in organic media.

In vitro, such extracts exhibit excellent spreading properties in the Wilhelmy balance. In the pulsating bubble surfactometer they show egg-shaped hysteresis areas with surface tension reduction down to 19–20 dyn/cm (Fig. 3). In animal experiments, e.g. using immature rabbit foetuses (for details of the model see Chapter 10), lung mechanical parameters, e.g. compliance, as well as arterial oxygen pressure improve visibly and quickly. Various preparations have thus been used in clinical trials with highly satisfying results in the treatment of the infant respiratory distress syndrome (IRDS). Preventive and rescue studies have shown that a considerable reduction of infant mortality can be achieved.

Despite these advantages a number of reservations must be maintained against all these preparations.

- The composition of the mixtures is determined by the source of the material and the method of extraction, be it from bovine or porcine lung tissue, bovine lung lavage or human amniotic fluid. The complex mixture of the lipids in natural surfactants is well documented (Table 1). There are considerable differences among various phospholipids in different animal species, but also within the same species,

depending on age, health condition, and nutritional status of the animal. This can only partly be compensated by adjusting the level of some essential phospholipids up to a preset level. In addition, the method of extraction may alter the natural lipid composition.
- The lung surfactant proteins vary in their amino acid sequence among animal species and humans (see below for details). Differences in amino acid sequence in proteins used for therapy in humans are always a matter of concern because of potential immunological reactions in the treated patients. Although the immunogenic potential of the hydrophobic lung surfactant proteins seems to be low, one has to keep an eye on this problem. It may become even more serious if one considers use of surfactants in higher doses and over extended periods of time as may become necessary in the treatment of chronic diseases.
- Extracts of tissue or body fluids are prone to contamination by pathogens or toxins. All substances from 'natural' sources carry this risk which again increases with increasing time of application.

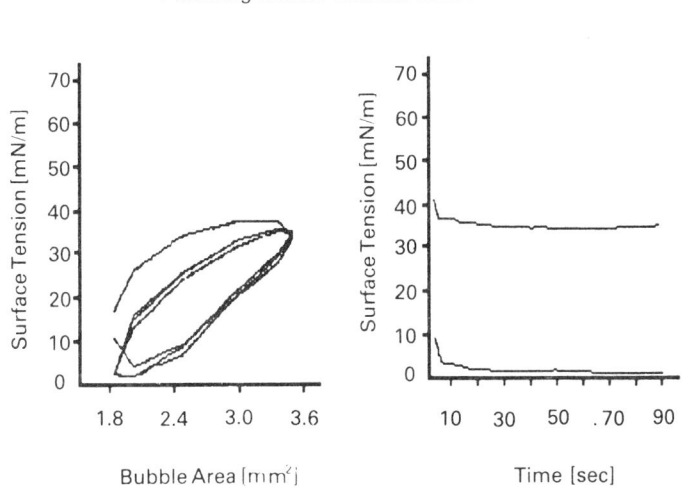

Fig. 3. Surface activity of a recombinant surfactant in the pulsating bubble surfactometer.

In an attempt to circumvent all of these problems, there have been approaches using protein-free, synthetic phospholipids alone (ALEC®) or phospholipids in combination with mild detergents (EXOSURF®) as completely artificial surfactants. Both types of preparations have been tested clinically as a substitution therapy in case of IRDS. EXOSURF® has, in the meantime, reached the market for this indication. However, there remain reservations against both products with regard to spreading efficiency (Hall *et al.*, 1991) when using phospholipids alone or problems with long-term use of detergents in humans. The body of available data indicates that omission of the hydrophobic protein component(s) strips the surfactant of its biologically active component. In return, this would certainly diminish is value as a carrier system.

'Recombinant' surfactant
Another approach for the design of an active surfactant to be used in respiratory distress syndrome therapy as well as in a carrier system could be the production of the hydrophobic surfactant protein(s) by means of recombinant DNA technology. Such a protein could be mixed with synthetic phospholipids in any desired composition and ratio. The activity of the surfactant can be tested by *in vitro* and *in vivo* models such as the Wilhelmy balance, the pulsating bubble surfactometer (Hallman *et al.*, 1985; Fuchimukai *et al.*, 1987), the premature rabbit foetus model (Grossmann *et al.*, 1984) or the lung lavage model (Lachmann, 1989).

It is possible to list some features of a recombinant surfactant.

- In a first approach, components should be selected from natural surfactants. Their concentration in the recombinant surfactant should not grossly vary from the limits set by nature. Successively, however, one could design variations from this standard to adjust the properties of the mixture to special requirements of the intended application. Hence, initially, phospholipid components are selected which are also found in natural surfactants but can be produced synthetically and subjected to a thorough analytical and quality control program.
- The phospholipids are combined with the recombinant proteins. Again, the proteins will be initially engineered in a way as to be structurally and functionally identical to their natural human counterparts. The cellular systems used for the production of the proteins should be selected so as to exclude any possibility for the presence of unwanted biological agents, i.e. viruses or toxins.

Surfactant by design
In a designed surfactant, phospholipids are chosen under the criterion of improving the efficacy of the complete surfactant with respect to

- velocity of spreading on aqueous surfaces as measured in a Wilhelmy balance,
- surface tension dynamics equalling that of natural surfactants as measured in a pulsating bubble surfactometer, and
- improving lung parameters (such as compliance, blood oxygen tension) as measured in the foetal rabbit model, the rat lung lavage model or other suitable animal models (see Chapter 10).

For practical reasons, a minimum set of natural phospholipids is selected.

Similar criteria applying to the protein component(s). Today, there are three *bona fide* surfactant proteins, namely SP-A, SP-B and SP-C, which are described in more detail below.

Biotechnology allows the maintenance of very high quality and safety standards in the production of proteins. However, it also solves the problem of sufficient supply of the proteins, which will be very hard to guarantee from natural sources. If expression of the desired protein in bacterial host cells or primitive eukaryotes, such as yeast or insect cells, is possible, the problem of contamination by animal viruses or other undesired substances which plague production in mammalian cell systems can be avoided. However, even when mammalian cells cannot be replaced, e.g. when a glycoprotein with the correct glycosylation pattern is required, there exist now a number of cell lines which have already been successfully used in the expression of therapeutic recombinant proteins (e.g. Chinese hamster ovary cells (CHO) for tissue-specific fibrinogen activator (tPA)).

In addition, the proteins can be produced, handled and purified in a way as to ascertain their structural identity with the natural human protein(s). This includes not only an identical amino acid sequence but also all aspects of secondary and tertiary structure as well as any post-translational modification. This provides safety with respect to the immunological potential of the protein. It should not be recognized as alien by the patient's immune system, and hence should be suitable even for extended periods of application and high dosage. Such extended periods of application will be common when application as a carrier is considered.

SURFACTANT AS CARRIER

The phospholipids

Any designed surfactant will have to use the natural standard as a basis for its composition. The phospholipid components of human lung lavage or amniotic fluid provide the basis for such mixtures.

Series of *in vivo* experiments using immature rabbits, lavaged dogs or rabbits and other animals have shown that a simple mixture of dipalmitoylphosphatidylcholine (DPPC) and dipalmitoylphosphatidylglycerol (DPPG) will not be sufficient to provide full efficacy in conjunction with surfactant proteins. It is mandatory that the phospholipids contain a certain percentage of unsaturated fatty acids, e.g. oleic acid, to lower the transition temperature of the lipid matrix and to provide the necessary flexibility during the dynamic changes between monolayer and subphase structures. From our experience with *in vitro* and *in vivo* experiments, it seems as if the distribution of the unsaturated fatty acid among the phospholipids is not of great importance and can be chosen, for example, according to the criterion of availability, quality or price of the phospholipid.

The proteins

Three major protein components are found in natural lung surfactants. They are designated as surfactant proteins A, B, and C, with decreasing molecular weights. Below a brief review is given for each protein.

SP-A

Lung surfactant protein SP-A is a glycoprotein of a molecular weight of 24 kDa, which on polyacrylamide gels forms a band at 29 kDa, when non-glycosylated, and shows a broad, diffuse band at 32–36 kDa when modified by carbohydrates. It was shown to have a highly complex structure by forming aggregates of 18 protein chains (Voss *et al.*, 1988). This protein is involved in the metabolic control of lung surfactant synthesis and recycling by alveolar type II pneumocytes, the natural producer cells of lung surfactant. It may also be involved in the clearance of complexes between inhibiting serum proteins and surfactant components via endocytosis in type II pneumocytes and/or macrophages (Wintergerst *et al.*, 1989). Lamellar bodies as well as tubular myelin have been shown to contain this protein. Monoclonal antibodies against this protein have been prepared and been used in the analysis of its location and traffic.

Its gene has been isolated and its interior structure elucidated by DNA sequencing. It is coded by a multigene family in the human genome (Fig. 4).

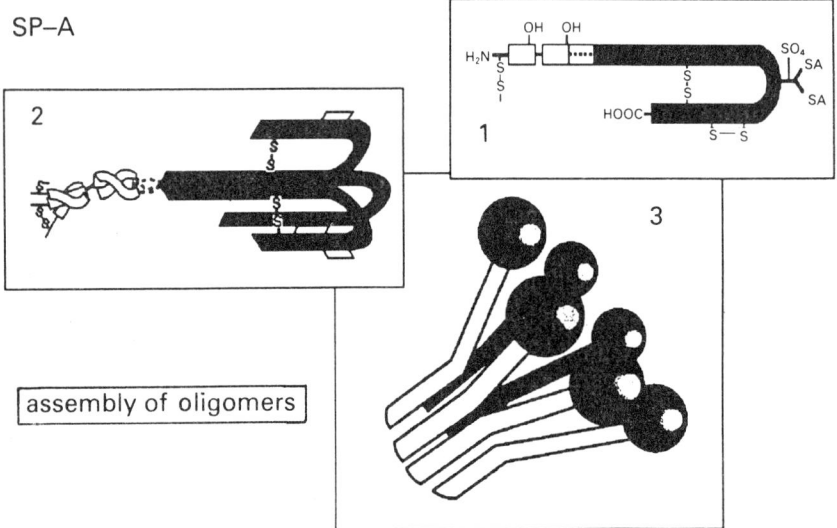

Fig. 4. Structure and assembly of SP-A protein : 1, monomeric protein chain (a type) ; (2) α3 complex (tulip) ; 3, hexameric complex.

Despite its multitude of functions and the fact that it is the major protein component in surfactant isolated from lung lavage by gentle methods excluding any extraction step by organic solvents, it does not seem to be necessary for the immediate enhancement of surface spreading of the phospholipids. It is assumed that it rather acts as a control protein as outlined above.

SP-B

Lung surfactant protein SP-B is a small hydrophobic protein of a molecular weight of 8.8 kDa. It has been shown *in vitro* to be required in the formation of tubular myelin from lamellar structures (Suzuki *et al.*, 1989). In its sequence is shows conserved regions with similarity to protease inhibitors (Emrie *et al.*, 1989). It has an extraordinarily high content in cysteine with 8 cysteines per 79 amino acids for human SP-B (~10% cys). Hence, it forms a couple of intramolecular disulphide bonds as well as in intermolecular disulphide bridge to form SP-B dimers. Otherwise it is unmodified. Its molecular structure has been partly determined for the porcine protein (Johansson *et al.*, 1991) and shows a serine protease kringle structure. Its primary sequence is characterized by a regular pattern of positively charged amino acids followed by a stretch of hydrophobic amino acids (Cochrane and Revak, 1991). In a mixture with phospholipids it improves the spreading characteristics of the lipids considerably though not to the same extent as SP-C.

The gene for this protein has also been isolated and sequenced together with a number of cDNA clones from a variety of species (Emrie et al., 1989) (Fig. 5).

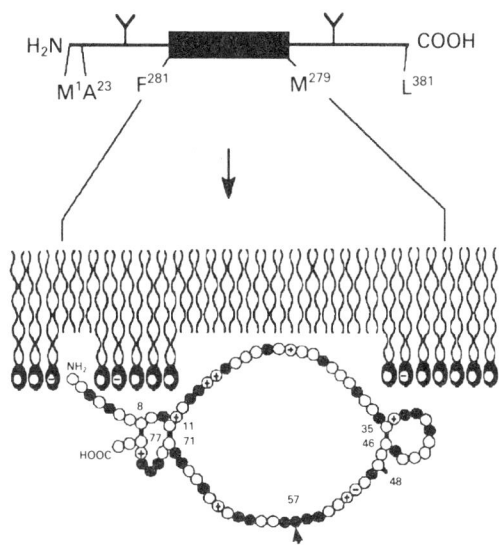

Fig. 5. Proposed structure and lipid matrix association of surfactant protein SP-B.

SP-C

Lung surfactant protein SP-C is the smallest and most hydrophobic of the lung surfactant proteins. In humans, it consists of a 1:1 mixture of a 35 (*N*-terminal phe) and a 34 (*N*-terminal gly) peptide species derived by limited proteolysis. It is the most important protein in terms of improving the spreading kinetics of phospholipids to the air/water interface. It is extremely hydrophobic ('... the most hydrophobic protein ever isolated' (J. Whitsett, Cincinnati)) and only soluble in organic solvents such as acidic chloroform–methanol mixtures. Its gene structure and sequence are also known for a couple of species (Fisher et al., 1989) and is highly conserved. Recently, it has been found that the SP-C protein is modified by fatty acid acylation (Curstedt et al., 1990; Voss et al., 1992). The two vicinal cysteine residues which are flanked on both sides by prolines form thioester bonds with palmitic acid. This modification further increases the hydrophobic nature of the SP-C protein. It has been shown that the C-terminal part of the protein forms a transmembrane α-helix which is inserted in the phospholipid matrix. The helix is oriented parallel to the acyl chains in the lipids (Vandenbusche et al., 1992) (Fig. 6).

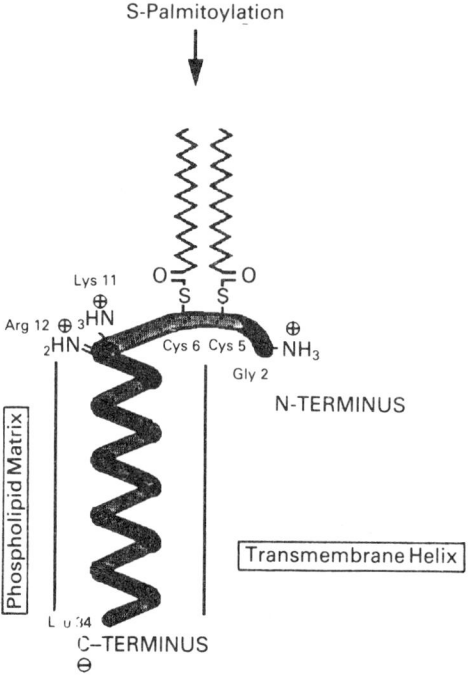

Fig. 6. Proposed structure of surfactant protein SP-C.

PROSPECTS AND SPECULATIONS

Of the three surfactant proteins described here, we have shown that recombinant, palmitoylated SP-C alone in conjunction with phospholipids forms a fully active surfactant (van Daal et al., 1992); (our unpublished results). It is equal to so-called 'natural' surfactants with respect to all parameters which can be determined by *in vitro* or *in vivo* methods. One can therefore predict that SP-C is an excellent candidate for any designed surfactant. What is needed now are experiments to show the ability of the surfactant system to carry drugs down the bronchial network to the alveolar space and to deliver it to the site of action. Up to now, we can only speculate that this approach will work, but the properties of the surfactant system make it a very attractive experimental target to look deeper into this matter.

REFERENCES

Baritussio, A. G., Magoon, M. W., Goerke, J. and Clements, J. A. (1981) Precursor-product relationship between rabbit type II cell lamellar bodies and alveolar surface-active material. Surfactant turnover time. *Biochim. Biophys. Acta* **666** 382–393.

Beckmann, H. J. and Dierichs, R. (1984) Extramembraneous particles and structural variations of tubular myelin figures in rat lung surfactant. *J. Ultrastruct. Res.* **86** 57–66.

Cochrane, C. G. and Revak, S. D. (1991) Pulmonary surfactant protein B (SP-B): structure–function relationships. *Science* **254** 566–568.
Curstedt, T., Johansson, J., Persson, P., Eklund, A., Robertson, B., Löwenadler, B. and Jörnvall, H. (1990) Hydrophobic surfactant-associated polypeptides: SP-C is a lipopeptide with two palmitoylated cysteine residues, whereas SP-B lacks covalently linked fatty acyl groups. *Proc. Natl. Acad. Sci. USA* **87** 2985–2989.
Emrie, P. A., Shannon, J. M., Mason, R. J. and Fisher, J. H. (1989) cDNA and deduced amino acid sequence for the rat hydrophobic pulmonary surfactant-associated protein, SP-B. *Biochim. Biophys. Acta* **994** 215–221.
Fisher, J. H., Shannon, J. M., Hofmann, T. and Mason, R. J. (1989) Nucleotide and deduced amino acid sequence of the hydrophobic surfactant protein SP-C from rat: expression in alveolar type II cells and homology with SP-C from other species. *Biochim. Biophys. Acta* **995** 225–230.
Fuchimukai, T., Fujiwara, T., Takahashi, A. and Enhorning, G. (1987) Artificial pulmonary surfactant inhibited by proteins. *J. Appl. Physiol.* **62** 429–437.
Gortner, L., Pohlandt, F., Bartmann, P. and Disse, B. (1990) Die Behandlung des Atemnotsyndroms (RDS) sehr kleiner Frühgeborener mit bovinem Surfactant. [Treatment of respiratory distress syndrome in very small premature infants with bovine surfactant.] *Monatsschr. Kinderheilkd.* **138** 8–12.
Grossmann, G., Larsson, I., Nilsson, R., Robertson, B., Rydhag, L. and Stenius, P. (1984) Lung expansion in premature newborn rabbits treated with emulsified synthetic surfactant; principles for experimental evaluation of synthetic substitutes for pulmonary surfactant. *Respiration* **45** 327–338.
Hall, S. B., Venkitaraman, A. R., Whitsett, J. A., Holm, B. A. and Notter, R. H. (1991) Importance of hydrophobic apoproteins as constituents of clinical exogenous surfactants. *Am. Rev. Respir. Dis.* **145** 24–30.
Hallman, M., Spragg, R., Harrell, J. H., Moser, K. M. and Gluck, L. (1982) Evidence of lung surfactant abnormality in respiratory failure. Study of broncho-alveolar lavage phospholipids, surface activity, phospholipase activity and plasma myoinositol. *J. Clin. Inv.* **70** 673–683.
Hallman, M., Enhorning, G. and Possmayer, F. (1985) Composition and surface activity of normal and phosphatidylglycerol-deficient lung surfactant. *Pediatr. Res.* **19** 286–292.
Johansson, J., Curstedt, T. and Jörnvall, H. (1991) Surfactant protein B: disulfide bridges, structural properties, and kringle similarities. *Biochemistry* **30** 6917–6921.
Lachmann, B. (1989) Animal models and clinical pilot studies of surfactant replacement in adult respiratory distress syndrome. *Eur. Respir. J. Suppl.* **2** 98s–103s.
Lang, M. J., Hall, R. T., Reddy, N. S., Kurth, C. G. and Merritt, T. A. (1990) A controlled trial of human surfactant replacement therapy for severe respiratory distress syndrome in very low birth weight infants. *J. Pediatr.* **116** 295–300.
Manz-Keinke, H., Plattner, H. and Schlepper-Schäfer, J. (1992) Lung surfactant protein A (SP-A) enhances serum-independent phagocytosis of bacteria by alveolar macrophages. *Eur. J. Cell Biol.* **57** 95–100.
Pfleger, R. C. and Thomas, H. G. (1971) Beagle dog pulmonary surfactant lipids. *Arch. Intern. Med.* **127** 863–872.

Richman, P. S., Spragg, R. G., Robertson, B., Merritt, T. A. and Curstedt, T. (1989) The adult respiratory distress syndrome: first trials with surfactant replacement. *Eur. Respir. J. Suppl.* **2** 109s–111s.

Salzman, R., Manson, J. E., Griffing, G. T., Kimmerle, R., Ruderman, N., McCall, A., Stoltz, E. I., Mullin, C., Small, D., Armstrong, J. (1985) Intranasal aerosolized insulin. Mixed-meal studies and long-term use in type I diabetes. *N. Engl. J. Med.* **312** 1078–1084.

Schmitz, G. and Müller, G. (1991) Structure and function of lamellar bodies, lipid–protein complexes involved in storage and secretion of cellular lipids. *J. Lipid Res.* **32** 1539–1570.

Suzuki, Y., Fujita, Y. and Kogishi, K. (1989) Reconstitution of tubular myelin from synthetic lipids and proteins associated with pig pulmonary surfactant. *Am. Rev. Respir. Dis.* **140** 75–81.

van Daal, G. J., Gommers, D., Bos, J. A. H., van Golde, P. H. M., van den Kamp, R. and Lachmann, B. (1991) Human recombinant surfactant is as effective as commercially available natural surfactants. *Eur. Respir. J. Suppl.* **14** 492s.

van Iwaarden, F., Welmers, B., Verhoef, J., Haagsman, H. P. and van Golde, P. L. M. (1990) Pulmonary surfactant protein A enhances the host-defense mechanism of rat alveolar macrophages. *Am. J. Respir. Cell Mol. Biol.* **2** 91–98.

Vandenbusche, G., Clercx, A., Curstedt, T., Johansson, J., Jörnvall, H. and Ruysschaert, J.-M. (1992) Structure and orientation of the surfactant-associated protein C in a lipid bilayer. *Eur. J. Biochem.* **203** 201–209.

Voss, T., Eistetter, H., Schäfer, K. P. and Engel, J. (1988) Macromolecular organization of natural and recombinant lung surfactant protein SP 28-36. Structural homology with the complement factor C1q. *J. Mol. Biol.* **201** 219–227.

Voss, T., Schäfer, K. P., Nielsen, P. F., Schäfer, A., Maier, C., Hannappel-Maaβen, J., Landis, B., Klemm, K. and Przybylski, M. (1992) Primary structure differences of human surfactant-associated proteins isolated from normal and proteinosis lung. *Biochim. Biophys. Acta* **1138** 261–267.

Wintergerst, E., Manz-Keinke, H., Plattner, H. and Schlepper-Schäfer, J. (1989) The interaction of a lung surfactant protein (SP-A) with macrophages is mannose dependent. *Eur. J. Cell Biol.* **50** 291–298.

Part IV
Dermal and transdermal routes

12

Skin penetration enhancers

Jonathan Hadgraft and Kenneth A. Walters

INTRODUCTION

In order to optimize topical or transdermal formulations it is often helpful to incorporate a skin penetration enhancer. This will aid the passage of drug both into and through the skin. The mechanisms by which enhancers act can only be appreciated by understanding the routes through which drugs diffuse in the skin. The mechanisms of skin penetration will be addressed. Examples of skin penetration enhancers will be described together with their proposed means of action. Various physicochemical techniques can be used to monitor the influence of enhancer on skin compounds and a number of these will be highlighted. It is often easier to analyse data obtained using more simple systems than something as heterogeneous as skin. Structured lipid bilayers in the form of liposomes have been used as an useful model of skin lipids and examples of their use will be provided.

MECHANISMS OF SKIN PENETRATION

Over the past couple of decades a large number of experiments have been conducted in order to identify the major routes of skin penetration. The major barrier to skin penetration resides, for most compounds, in the outer dead layer, the stratum corneum. A schematic representation is given in Fig. 1. Scheuplein (1967) suggested that at early times after drug application the appendageal route was dominant but little evidence to support substantial drug transfer through the appendages has been obtained. The major route therefore is either transcellular or intercellular (Fig. 1). Michaels *et al.* (1975) proposed an interesting model for the stratum corneum in which the structure was likened to a brick wall with the corneocytes being represented by the bricks and the intercellular channels by the mortar. Albery and Hadgraft (1979) used this model together with a kinetic model for skin penetration and demonstrated that the esters of nicotinic acid diffused predominantly through the intercellular space. At that time the nature of the constituents within the intercellular channels had not been identified. During the past decade considerable effort has been put into identifying the nature of the materials in the channels and it has been established that they contain a complex mixture of ceramides (50%), cholesterol (25%) free fatty acids (15%) cholesteryl sulphate (5%) and several minor constituents (Abraham and Downing, 1990). These lipids structure organize themselves into ordered bilayers and thus a molecule diffusing through the stratum corneum passes sequentially through a large number of bilayers. The rate-limiting step to drug transfer through the skin appears, therefore, to be the passage through the structured lipids that reside in the intercellular channels. A penetration enhancer may therefore be expected to act by interacting with the lipid bilayers. Its presence may affect the structure within the bilayer or it may influence the solubility characteristics.

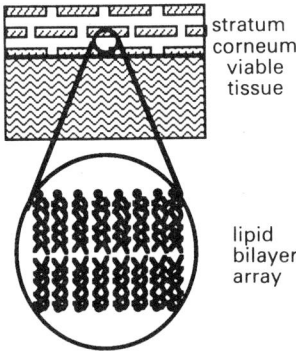

Fig. 1. A schematic representation of the skin

MOLECULAR STRUCTURE OF ENHANCERS

A large number of compounds have been examined and shown to modify the permeability characteristics of the skin (Walters, 1989). Because of their diverse nature, it is probable that they act by a variety of mechanisms. At a molecular level their shape will be important in determining their interaction with the lipid bilayer and it is instructive to use molecular graphics to examine their three-dimensional shape and charge distribution. Fig. 2 shows a graphics representation of four enhancers Azone® oleic acid, Transcutol® and N-methyl pyrrolidone (NMP). There are structural similarities between Azone and oleic acid in that they both possess head groups which are polar in nature and have long alkyl chains. It may be anticipated that the lactam functional group in Azone and the carboxyl group in oleic acid interact with the polar head group regions of the skin ceramides. The alkyl chains of the two compounds will then tend to reside in the less polar regions of the lipid bilayers. Their presence may therefore be expected to be one of imparting some disorder. On the other hand, Transcutol and NMP are smaller and would not be expected to be disruptive. They are good solvents and their presence in the skin may be expected to enhance drug solubility in the skin lipids. Such physicochemical properties as solubility parameters and related factors should provide information on their activity. However, this will have to be taken into consideration together with the solubility parameters of both the skin lipids and the diffusing drug.

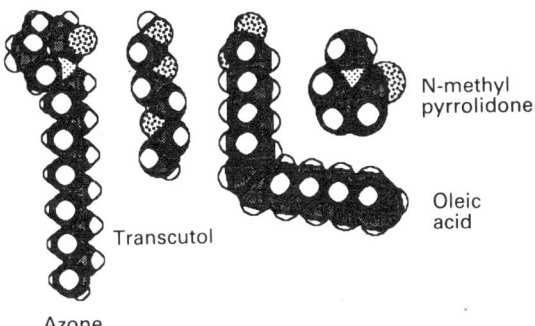

Fig. 2. Molecular graphics representations of the chemical structures of Azone, oleic acid, Transcutol and N-methyl pyrrolidone.

PHYSICOCHEMICAL TECHNIQUES TO PROBE PENETRATION ENHANCEMENT

A number of spectroscopic and other techniques have been used to monitor the influence of penetration enhancers on skin and structured lipids (such as dipalmitoyl-phosphatidyl choline (dppc) liposomes) thought to model the structured arrays in the skin. A summary of some of the techniques used is provided in Table 1.

Table 1. Some of the physicochemical techniques used to study skin or skin models

Technique	Skin		Model lipids
	In vitro	*In vivo*	
Fourier transform infrared	√	√	√
Differential scanning calorimetry	√		√
X-ray diffraction	√		√
Neutron scattering	√		√
Nuclear magnetic resonance	√		√
Electron spin resonance	√		√
Langmuir–Blodgett films			√
Fluorescence spectroscopy			√
Light scattering			√
Hot stage microscopy			√

Since many of the techniques require small samples of material to be placed inside sophisticated equipment most can only be applied to *in vitro* studies. The one spectroscopic method that can be used *in vivo* is reflectance Fourier transform infrared (FTIR). In the context of penetration enhancement this can provide information on how the enhancer modifies the disorder of the skin lipids and also the concentration distribution of the drug in the skin (Guy *et al.*, 1990). The former is achieved by monitoring the C–H asymmetric and symmetric stretching frequencies of the alkyl chains that occur at 2920 and 2850 cm^{-1}. The presence of oleic acid in the skin shifts the asymmetric peak to higher frequencies, indicating an increase in disorder of the alkyl chains. Recent work (Ongpipattanakul *et al.*, 1991) has indicated that oleic acid may act by creating regions of solid fluid phase separation and that enhanced permeation is a result of drug transfer at the interfacial defects. The concentration distribution of the drug in the stratum corneum can only be found if the penetrant has a discrete absorbance peak that does not overlap the peaks generated by the skin itself. The concentration can only be monitored invasively by tape stripping the site and relating the strips to the depth into the stratum corneum. Some penetration enhancers, particularly the ionic surfactants, can also alter the structure of the keratin in the skin. Beastall (1987) using FTIR, showed that *in vitro* keratin underwent a transformation after treatment with decylmethylsulphoxide whereas Azone had no effect on the keratin structure.

Differential scanning calorimetry (DSC) has been used to examine the phase transitions that occur as samples of stratum corneum are heated. Golden *et al.* (1987) have used the technique to examine the effect of skin penetration enhancers on the thermal transitions. They have demonstrated that there is a good correlation between penetration enhancement and the 'fluidization' or disordering of the skin lipids. In general there are three main transitions observed which occur near 65°C, 80°C and 95°C. Occasionally a fourth peak around 35°C is seen which has been attributed to changes within sebaceous lipids which are not relevant to the barrier function of the skin. Penetration enhancers which interact with the lipids usually have a marked effect on the peak at 65°C. Barry (1987) has shown that Azone can interact with the skin lipids in such a way as to remove the transitions at both 65°C and 80°C. Clearly DSC can be used to demonstrate interactions between penetration enhancers and skin lipids and there appears to be a correlation between the disruptive effect on the ordered lipids and enhancement activity.

From visualization techniques (Abraham and Downing, 1990) it has been suggested that the bilayer spacing changes between the corneocytes. There is some lipid that is bound to the corneocyte envelope and some more 'free' lipid. The higher temperature transition (85°C) is thought to be associated with the protein–lipid complex.

The fact that two distinct structures exist can be seen from small angle X-ray scattering (Bouwstra *et al.*, 1991). Bilayer repeat distances of 6.4 and 13.4 nm were found and theoretical calculations suggest that there are more than one bilayer present in a 13.4 nm unit cell. A change in the hydration state of the stratum corneum (from 6% to 60%) did not result in a swelling of the bilayers, implying that they have a robust nature.

Neutron scattering experiments on stratum corneum to probe the structure have been conducted by our group but the signal strength is small and the results inconclusive.

However, small angle neutron scattering on model bilayers (DPPC liposomes) shows that oleic acid incorporated into the lipid phase separates as suggested by the work of Ongpipattanakul et al. (1991).

The 'microviscosity' of the intercellular lipids can be probed by spectroscopic techniques such as electron spin resonance (ESR) and nuclear magnetic resonance (NMR). In the former Gay et al. (1989) used 5-doxylstearic acids in both DPPC liposomes and stratum corneum samples. The influence of various penetration enhancers on the order parameters monitored by the spin probe was measured. Materials such as oleic acid and decylmethyl sulphoxide (DecMSO) 'disorder' the lipid structure. Fig. 3 shows that the effect of DecMSO is concentration dependent, as is the non-ionic surfactant Brij36T. Oleic acid appears to have a saturable effect at the concentrations tested. The values of N-methyl pyrrolidone show a decrease in activity with increasing concentration. The precise reasons for this anomalous result are currently being investigated.

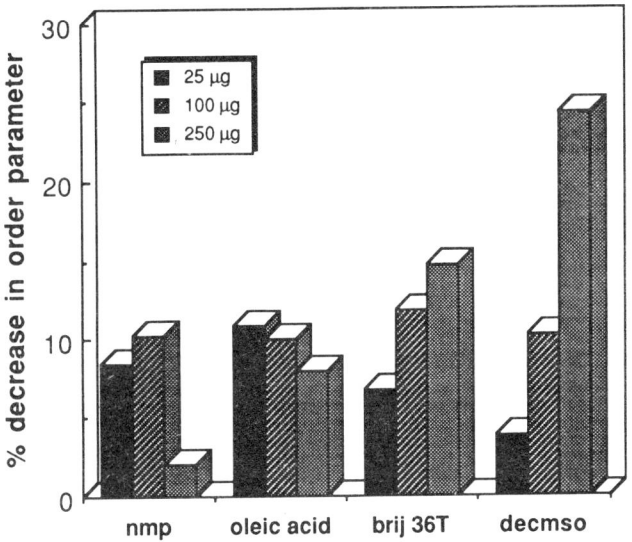

Fig. 3. The effect of the amount applied of various penetration enhancers on the order parameter of 5-doxyl stearic acid incorporated into samples of stratum corneum.

The wide variations in skin permeability and the associated enhancer effects can also be seen using ESR. Fig. 4 shows the results obtained for two subjects. There are marked differences and it is thought that the lipid composition of subject X is inherently more ordered and therefore the enhancer activity is more pronounced. It would be interesting to correlate skin lipid composition with skin permeability and enhancement activity.

NMR techniques can also be used to study molecular motion. The ^{19}F NMR spectrum of the propyl ester of flurbiprofen in stratum corneum was obtained using a pulsed NMR instrument (Jeol FX90Q). Typical spectra obtained are shown in Fig. 5. The 16% decrease in the line width in the stratum corneum sample treated with oleic acid is indicative that the drug is diffusing more rapidly.

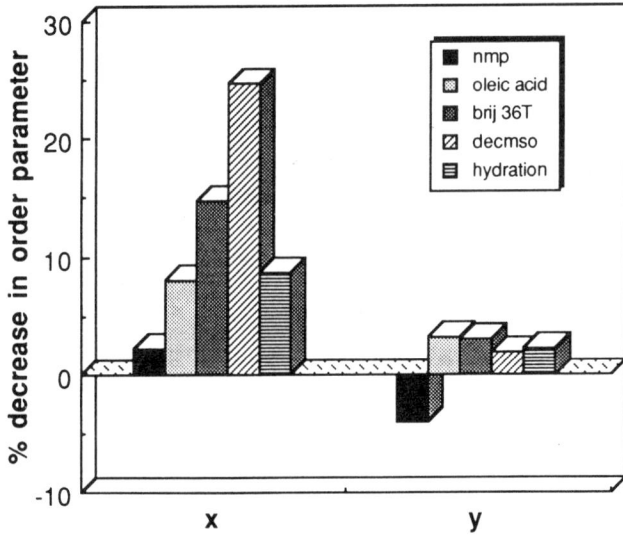

Fig. 4. The differential effects of penetration enhancers on stratum corneum samples obtained from two different subjects.

It is apparent from the above techniques that the enhancers are having a specific molecular action with the ordered lipids in the skin. Because of the complexity of the skin it is difficult to analyse the data in detail and often more information can be obtained considering a more simple model. Reference above has been made to the use of DPPC liposomes and these together with monolayer experiments have provided useful insight into the probable mechanism of action of enhancers.

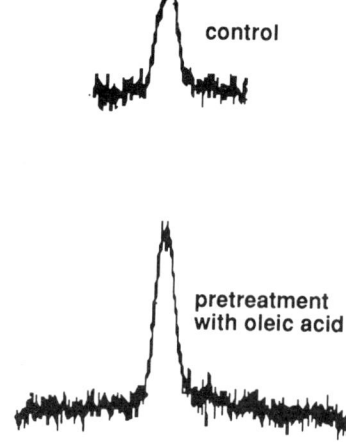

Fig. 5. The ^{19}F FT NMR spectrum of the propyl ester of flurbiprofen incorporated into the skin with and without pretreatment with oleic acid.

Azone is one of the interesting enhancers that has been examined in detail. Lewis and Hadgraft (1990) incorporated Azone into DPPC monolayers formed at an air–water interface and showed that the mean areas per molecule exhibited considerable expansion compared with the simple additivity rule (Fig. 6). Both Azone and oleic acid gradually reduced and finally abolished the liquid-expanded to liquid-condensed phase transition. The results indicated very clear differences in the two enhancers and the importance of the Azone head group conformation to its activity.

DPPC liposomes have also been used to investigate enhancer effects. Using a simple light scattering technique Beastall *et al.* (1988) showed that the presence of Azone lowered the phase transition temperature (T_c) of the DPPC. Recent work on a range of enhancers has indicated that there is a correlation between skin penetration enhancement and the ability of the enhancer to lower the T_c of DPPC liposomes (Williams, 1991). In addition to the light scattering work, Beastall *et al.* (1988) also monitored lipid disorder in DPPC liposomes using a fluorescent probe technique. Increase in Azone concentration increased lipid fluidity as determined by changes in pyrene fluorescence.

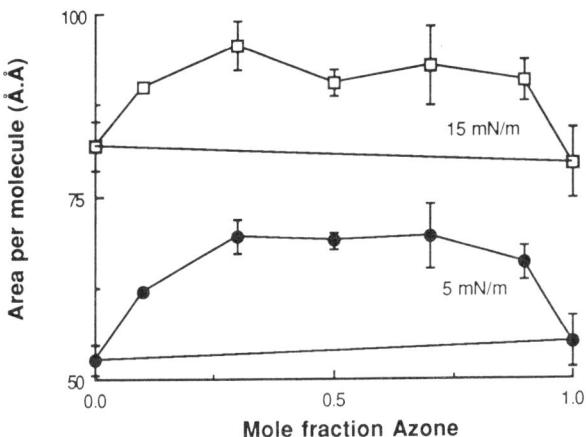

Fig. 6. The expansion that Azone induces in a DPPC monolayer.

It is interesting that Transcutol, a penetration enhancer which does not act by lipid disruption but rather by solubility effects, does not lower the T_c of DPPC liposomes (Watkinson *et al.*, 1990).

Lipids from the skin can be relatively easily extracted and thermal transitions examined by hot stage microscopy. Preliminary results (Walker and Hadgraft, 1991) tend to confirm the theory that oleic acid disrupts the intercellular lipid packing arrangement by the introduction of fluid-like channels at physiological temperature.

CONCLUSION

Penetration enhancers act in two major ways. Firstly they can disrupt the lipid ordering in the stratum corneum. Diffusion will be more rapid in the more 'fluid' environment.

Enhancement will be greater for less lipophilic penetrants where the rate-controlling step resides totally within the stratum corneum. Where the rate-controlling step is partitioning out of the stratum corneum enhancers which modify the solubility characteristics of the skin in a favourable manner are required. The way in which the enhancement should be vary as a function of the physicochemical properties of penetrant has been reviewed using mathematical modelling (Guy and Hadgraft, 1988). Whatever the enhancer it should have most of the characteristics described below:

(1) elicit no pharmacological action;
(2) be specific in its action;
(3) act immediately with predictable and reversible duration;
(4) be chemically and physically stable and compatible with all components of the formulation;
(5) be colourless, odourless and tasteless;
(6) be non-toxic, non-allergenic and non-irritant.

It is unlikely that any one enhancer will possess all of these and benefit-to-risk assessments need to be considered in any formulation strategy. It is likely that novel enhancers will be developed in the future which will have considerable utility in the formulation of topical and transdermal products. It is also possible that drugs which have been designed to act locally in the skin or to be absorbed transdermally will have functional attributes in their structure which provide self-enhancement.

REFERENCES

Abraham, W. and Downing, D. T. (1990) Factors affecting the formation, morphology and permeability of stratum corneum lipid bilayers *in vitro*. In: Scott, R. C., Guy, R. H. and Hadgraft, J. (eds) *Prediction of Percutaneous Penetration*. IBC Technical Services, London, pp. 110–122.

Albery, W. J. and Hadgraft, J. (1979) Percutaneous absorption: *in vivo* experiments, *J. Pharm. Pharmacol.* **31** 140–147.

Barry, B. W. (1987) Penetration enhancers. In: Shroot, B. and Schäfer, H. (eds) *Skin Pharmacokinetics*. Karger, Basel, pp. 121–137.

Beastall, J. C. (1987) The mechanism of action of Azone. *PhD Thesis*. The University of Nottingham.

Beastall, J. C., Hadgraft, J. and Washington, C. (1988) Mechanism of action of Azone as a percutaneous penetration enhancer: lipid bilayer fluidity and transition temperature effects. *Int. J. Pharm.* **43** 207–213.

Bouwstra, J. A., Gooris, G. S., van der Spek, J. A. and Bras, W. (1991) Structural investigations of human stratum corneum by small angle X-ray scattering. *J. Invest. Dermatol* **97** 1005–1012.

Gay, C. L., Murphy, T. M. Hadgraft, J., Kellaway, I. W., Evans, J. C. and Rowlands, C. C. (1989) An electron spin resonance study of skin penetration enhancers. *Int. J. Pharm.* **49** 39–45.

Golden, G. M., Mackie, J. E. and Potts, R. O. (1987) Role of stratum corneum lipid fluidity in transdermal flux *J. Pharm. Sci.* **76** 25–28.

Guy, R. H. and Hadgraft, J. (1988) Physicochemical aspects of percutaneous absorption and its enhancement. *Pharm. Res.* **5** 753–758.

Guy, R. H., Mak, V. H. W., Kai, T., Bommannan, D. and Potts, R. O. (1990) Percutaneous penetration enhancers, mode of action. In: Scott, R. C., Guy, R. H. and Hadgraft, J. (eds) *Prediction of Percutaneous Penetration.* IBC Technical Services, London, pp. 213–223.

Lewis, D. and Hadgraft, J. (1990) Mixed monolayers of dipalmitoylphosphatidylcholine with Azone or oleic acid at the air water interface. *Int. J. Pharm.* **65** 211–218.

Michaels, A. S., Chandrasekaran, S. K. and Shaw, J. E. (1975) Drug permeation through human skin: theory and *in vitro* experimental measurement. *AIChE J.* **21** 985–996.

Ongpipattanakul, B., Burnette, R. R., Potts, R. O. and Francoeur, M. L. (1991) Evidence that oleic acid exists in a separate phase within stratum corneum lipids. *Pharm. Res.* **8** 350–354.

Scheuplein, R. J. (1967) Mechanisms of percutaneous absorption II; transient diffusion and the relative importance of various routes of skin penetration. *J. Invest. Dermatol.* **45** 334–346.

Walker, M. and Hadgraft, J. (1991) Oleic acid — a membrane 'fluidiser' or fluid within the membrane. *Int. J. Pharm.* **71** R1–R4.

Walters, K. A (1989) Penetration enhancers and their use in transdermal therapeutic systems. In: Hadgraft, J. and Guy, R. H. (eds) *Transdermal Drug Delivery.* Dekker, New York, pp. 197–246.

Watkinson, A. C., Hadgraft, J. and Bye, A. (1990) Enhanced penetration of prostaglandin E2 through human skin *in vitro. J. Pharm. Pharmacol.* **42** 86P.

Williams, D. G. (1991) Mechanism of action of penetration enhancers. *PhD Thesis.* The University of Wales.

13

Skin cell cultures: reconstructed skin as a tool in the development of dermatological drugs and formulations

Paulette J. J. Wauben-Penris

INTRODUCTION

The object of research in skin pharmacology is to discover and develop effective drugs for the treatment of human skin diseases. For ethical and legal reasons, the evaluation of new drugs is not possible in man before they have been extensively tested for toxicity and efficacy. Therefore many animal tests have been developed to predict the effects of a substance in humans. However, animal tests are costly and time consuming, and are becoming more and more socially unacceptable. Furthermore, the animal skin is different from human skin in many respects, which results in very variable predictability.

As an alternative, *in vitro* tests using human skin have been developed. Excised human skin or isolated stratum corneum have been used extensively for the study of drug penetration and modulation by formulations (Franz, 1978). Also, explant cultures have been used (Prunieras *et al.*, 1976), but here tissue degradation will occur almost immediately after removal from the body, limiting the usefulness of this technique.

KERATINOCYTE CULTURES

Since the development of a method to culture human keratinocytes (Rheinwald and Green, 1975), epidermal cells grown in monolayers under conventional culture conditions have been used for testing the intrinsic toxicity and some of the pharmacological effects of substances (Reichert, 1986; Goldberg and Frazier, 1989; Ponec *et al.*, 1989). Chemically defined media have also been developed, which allow the omission of feeder cells and undefined components such as serum. This made it possible to test other types of substances, such as growth factors and peptides, and to analyse other features, such as cytokine production (Boyce *et al.*, 1990; Köck *et al.*, 1991; Luger and Schwartz, 1990; Barker *et al.*, 1991; see Fig. 1). Limited differentiation of keratinocytes

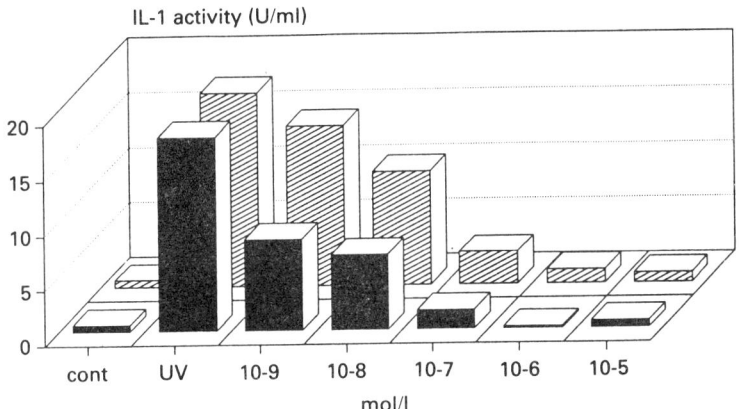

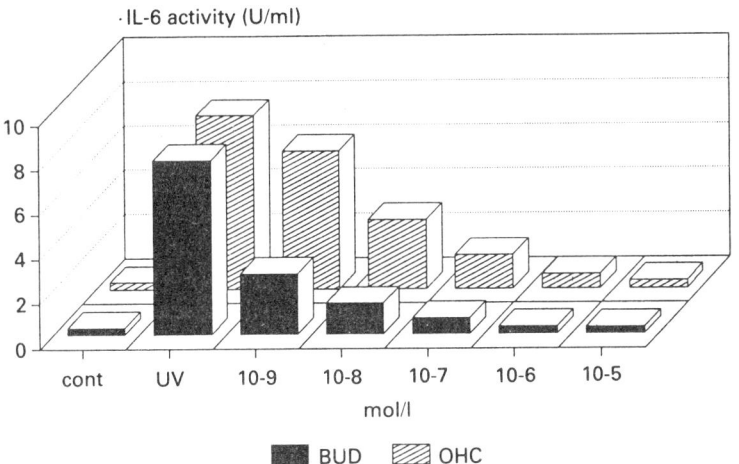

Fig. 1. Cytokine production by normal human keratinocytes: effects of corticosteroids. Normal human keratinocytes were stimulated with UV, and different concentrations of hydrocortisone (a weak corticosteroid) and budesonide (a potent corticosteroid) were added. Controls were included. Cytokine production was determined in the dialysed supernatants using bioassays. It can be seen that corticosteroids reduce stimulated IL-1 and IL-6 production in a dose- and potency-dependent way. (From Köck et al. (1991).)

can be induced by culturing them under physiological calcium conditions (Hennings et al., 1980), and by adherence to collagen, fibronectin or other extracellular matrix molecules (Hashimoto et al., 1990).

However, it turned out to be sometimes difficult to extrapolate the results obtained from keratinocytes cultured *in vitro* to the *in vivo* responses in diseased skin (Dubertret, 1990). *In vivo* cell–cell and cell–matrix interactions exist, which are responsible for both differentiation and some of the pharmacological responses.

DIFFERENTIATION

Differentiation of keratinocytes is a complex process involving the sequential expression and modification of specific differentiation products, resulting in defined morphological changes. Cell morphology changes drastically from the cuboidal basal cells to the large, flattened corneocytes. Among the earliest biochemical indicators of the onset of epidermal differentiation are the 'suprabasal' keratins K1 and K10 (Moll et al., 1982; Fuchs and Green, 1981; Boukamp et al., 1990). Other proteins, such as involucrin, a component of the cornified envelope (Rice and Green, 1979; Watt and Green, 1981), and filaggrin, a constituent of keratohyalin granules (Dale et al., 1978), are expressed at later stages, in more superficial cell layers. The formation of an organized stratum corneum with corneocytes and the strictly arranged intercellular lipids of unique composition is very important for the proper functioning of the skin (Potts, 1989).

When cultured under low calcium conditions, little or no differentiation of keratinocytes occurs. Under conventional submerged culture conditions, normal keratinocytes perform an incomplete program of differentiation as indicated by aberrant tissue architecture and the absence of certain ultrastructural features, such as keratohyalin granules, an electron-dense stratum corneum, and a structural basement membrane. Correspondingly filaggrin and the suprabasal keratins K1 and K10 are absent or only weakly expressed (Fuchs and Green, 1981; Bowden et al., 1987). Depletion of retinoids, regulators of epidermal proliferation and differentiation, triggers the expression of 'suprabasal' keratins and increases cornified envelope formation (Fuchs and Green, 1981). Other aspects of differentiation, such as regular stratification and morphological organization, have as yet not been achieved in conventional keratinocyte cultures.

DIFFERENTIATING KERATINOCYTE CULTURES

Therefore, attempts have been made to induce a complete program of keratinocyte differentiation *in vitro*, by culturing them at the air–liquid interface. Since the stratum corneum (SC) is the major permeability barrier in living skin, for drug testing it is important to develop a system where terminal differentiation elaborates a fully functional SC (Mak et al., 1991).

The first successful attempts to culture human epidermal cells on a dermal substrate were performed on dead pig dermis and were used in wound repair (Igel et al., 1974). Prunieras et al. (1979) combined human epidermal cells with human dead de-epidermized dermis DED. They developed a technique for removing the epidermis from the dermis, without removing the basement membrane, allowing a tight attachment between the growing epidermis and the DED. The culture then was lifted to the air–liquid interface. In this system differentiation occurs, which results in a morphology very similar to *in vivo* epidermis (Régnier *et al.*, 1988, 1990, Régnier and Darmon, 1989).

This system can be used for skin pharmacology, having two major advantages over classical submerged cultures: the degree of differentiation and barrier formation, and the exposure to air, which allows the testing of formulations.

Since the availability of human dermis forms a major problem, several alternative methods for *in vitro* reconstruction of human skin have been developed, in addition to the system using DED with intact basement membrane as a substrate for growing keratinocytes (Prunieras *et al.*, 1979):

- using collagen (Bell *et al.*, 1983) or collagen with glycosaminoglycans (Shahabeddin *et al.*, 1983) or chondroitin-6-sulphate (Boyce *et al.*, 1990) with living fibroblasts, forming a gel, on which keratinocytes can be grown;
- using completely non-cellular collagen-containing substrates (Boukamp *et al.*, 1990);
- using inert filters as a substrate (Bernstein *et al.*, 1986; Rosdy and Clauss, 1990);
- using hair follicles as the source for keratinocytes, inserting them in an upright position into collagen gels (Lénoir *et al.*, 1988);
- starting from a skin biopsy, allowing the keratinocytes to grow out over the substrate (Coulomb *et al.*, 1986);
- using the eye lens capsule as a substrate (Vermorken *et al.*, 1985);
- using animal DED as a substrate — we found that hairless rat and guinea pig dermis form a good substrate for differentiating human keratinocyte cultures (unpublished results);
- transplanting human keratinocytes to nude mice — this will increase the level of differentiation, but is not a complete *in vitro* model, and will not further be discussed.

These types of differentiating keratinocyte cultures have been used extensively (Bell *et al.*, 1983; Asselineau *et al.*, 1985; Boukamp *et al.*, 1990). However, the extent of maturation of keratinocytes was much more homogeneous on DED (Régnier *et al.*, 1988, Régnier and Darmon, 1989; Mak *et al.*, 1991; our unpublished observations). This system will now be discussed in more detail.

RECONSTRUCTED EPIDERMIS ON DED

A crucial point in this technique is the way the DED is prepared: by immersion of fresh human skin in phosphate buffer, until the epidermis can easily be peeled off (see Fig. 2). With this method the basal lamina remains intact with collagen IV, laminin and proteoglycans still present (Woodley *et al.*, 1982; Régnier *et al.*, 1990). Keratinocytes are isolated from newborn foreskins or from adult human skin. They are amplified according to the method of Rheinwald and Green (1975) and seeded on the dermis. After attachment, the cultures are lifted to the air–liquid interface (see Fig. 3).

After 3 days a stratified epidermis is observed. After 7 days bullous pemphigoid antiserum stains the basal cells and K1 and K10 keratins are expressed, and filaggrin

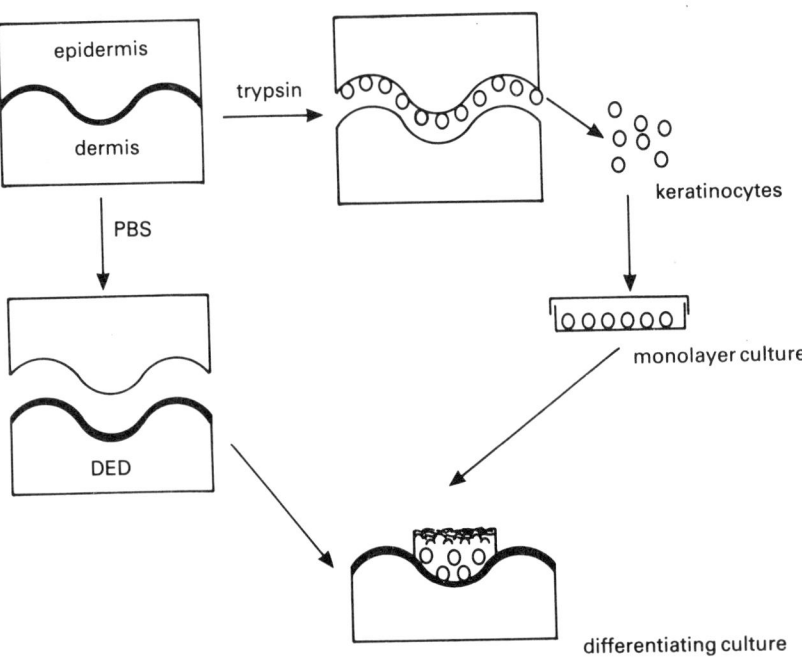

Fig. 2. Isolation of keratinocytes and preparation of DED from normal human skin. Keratinocytes are isolated using trypsin incubation (overnight at 4°C) and cultured in monolayers. DED is isolated using incubation in PBS, until epidermis can be peeled off. Basal lamina is still intact.

is present in the granular layer. At this time a compact stratum corneum is formed (Régnier et al., 1990). Hemidesmosomes, keratohyalin granules and intra- and extracellular membrane-coating granules (Régnier et al., 1990) and stratum corneum intercellular lipid bilayers (Madison et al., 1988; Ponec et al., 1988b; Boddé et al., 1990) are present. Protein (Asselineau et al., 1985; Kopan et al., 1987; Régnier et al., 1988, 1990; Boukamp et al., 1990) and lipid (Madison et al., 1988b; Ponec et al., 1988; Williams et al., 1988) profiles approach the in vivo situation. Substantial quantities of sphingolipids (Wertz and Downing, 1983), the critical constituents of the epidermal barrier (Elias, 1983) are generated. All classes of lipids are present, including acylceramide and lanosterol. However, the triglyceride content is generally higher and fatty acid content is lower than in normal epidermis (Ponec et al., 1988b). Ponec (1991) described that some of the abnormalities seen in differentiating cultures can be mimicked by culturing excised skin at the air–liquid interface.

Barrier function is present, but permeability to tritiated water was still 10 times higher than in excised normal human epidermis (Régnier et al., 1990). Penetration of nitroglycerin was 2 times lower, and of sucrose 100 times lower than through DED alone (Ponec et al., 1990). For both substances penetration is higher than through normal skin or stratum corneum. Recently Mak et al. (1991) reported increased barrier function to water by decreasing the relative humidity from almost 100% to 75%.

The reconstructed epidermis expresses many markers of hyperproliferation: involucrin (precursor of cornified envelope) and transglutaminase expression in spinous layers (Rice and Green, 1979; Dover and Watt, 1987; Régnier et al., 1988) as well as the hyperproliferation markers K6 and K16. Prolongation of the cultures leads to a gradual thinning of viable cell layers while a continuous sheet of SC is maintained. This suggests that under the in vitro conditions some signals controlling keratinocyte proliferation and differentiation, which should be tightly coordinated, are missing.

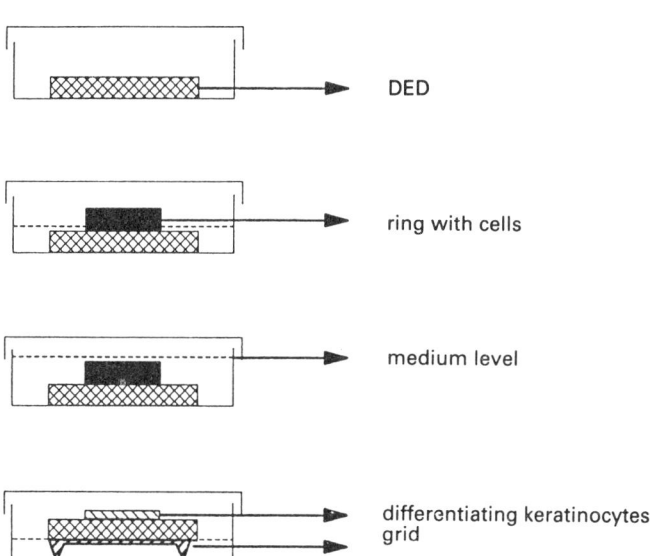

Fig. 3. Air-exposed keratinocyte cultures. DED is pre-incubated in medium. Keratinocytes are added, using a stainless steel ring. After attachment, the medium level is increased, to allow proper feeding of the cells. After 1 to 3 days the culture is placed on a stainless steel grid, and medium level is adapted to the level of the DED.

The higher penetration rates across reconstructed epidermis as compared with normal human skin could be explained either by deviations in lipid composition (Ponec et al., 1988b) or by local imperfections in intercorneocyte lipid depositions (Boddé et al., 1990). This could be a result of an essential fatty acid deficiency: the fatty acid profile of reconstructed epidermis (Madison et al., 1988; Ponec et al., 1988b) resembles that found in essential fatty acid deficient animals (Bowser et al., 1986; Burton, 1989; Ziboh, 1989). The epidermis of these animals is characterized by a hyperproliferation of basal cells which results in a thickening of the stratum granulosum and corneum and a marked increase in transepidermal water loss. However, in contrast to essential fatty acid deficient animals, supplementation of linoleic acid and arachidonic acid to reconstructed epidermis does not improve the barrier function (Ponec et al., 1990). This means that either essential fatty acids are not sufficiently incorporated into SC lipids or enzymes involved in epidermal lipogenesis are not optimally operative under the culture conditions used (Ponec et al., 1990).

Another explanation for the impaired barrier function could be local imperfections in the lipid structure as seen in freeze fracture EM (Boddé et al., 1990). As a result of such imperfections the lipid bilayer may be incomplete, providing shortcuts across the lipid bilayers.

LESIONAL KERATINOCYTE CULTURES

The system of reconstructing skin can also be used to culture keratinocytes from lesional skin, either on normal DED or on lesional DED. Attempts in this direction are promising: bullous skin can be mimicked *in vitro* by culturing lesional keratinocytes on normal DED (Hashimoto et al., 1990). Squamous cell carcinoma keratinocytes also show abnormal differentiation behaviour on DED (Ponec et al., 1988a). Attempts have been made to culture psoriatic skin *in vitro*, but results are varying. Since reconstructed skin of normal keratinocytes shows several features of hyperproliferative skin, it is as yet very difficult to interpret these results. *Pemphigus vulgaris* antibodies were reported to induce acantholysis in differentiating cultures of normal keratinocytes (Hunziker et al., 1989).

DRUG TESTING IN RECONSTRUCTED SKIN

One of the great advantages of reconstructed epidermis is that drugs can be tested mimicking both systemic and topical applications (see Fig. 4). Addition of retinoic acid (10^{-6} M) into the culture medium of differentiating keratinocyte cultures resulted after 7 days in disappearance of K1 and K10 keratins and filaggrins, while the SC became parakeratotic (Régnier et al., 1990). Application of a retinoic acid formulation on top of the cultures also resulted in total disappearance of K1 synthesis, and parakeratotic effects (Régnier et al., 1990).

Differentiating cultures in the absence of retinoic acid resulted in hyperkeratotic epithelium, as in hypervitaminosis A *in vivo*. In the presence of 10^{-7} M retinoic acid,

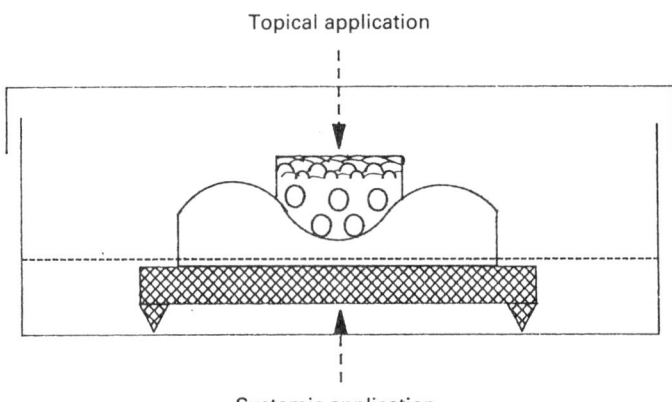

Fig. 4. Air-exposed keratinocyte cultures can be used to test preparations for both topical and systemic application.

parakeratotic epidermis formed, as in hypervitaminosis A *in vivo* (Régnier *et al.*, 1990). Retinoic acid also decreased collagenase production by keratinocytes (Régnier *et al.*, 1990).

1,25-Dihydroxyvitamin D_3 (OH_2D_3) (10^{-8}–10^{-6} M) also had dramatic effects on the organization of differentiating cultures: disappearance of the suprabasal intermediate cell compartment and thickening of the stratum corneum, a decrease in K1 and K10 synthesis and an increase of the incorporation of ^{35}S-labelled proteins into the cornified envelope (Régnier *et al.*, 1990). Mak *et al.* (1991) found a marked increase in barrier function after treatment with 10^{-6} M OH_2D_3 to the medium. They found a decrease in the number of basal and spinous layers, and a significant increase in SC thickness.

Rat reconstructed epidermis was found to respond similarly to *in vivo* skin to a vesicant (bis(β-chloroethyl) sulphide) and irritants (benzoic acid and salicyclic acid; Scavarelli-Karantsavelos *et al.*, 1990).

Addition of sodium butyrate (an inducer of morphological and biochemical cell differentiation) and 25-hyroxycholesterol (reduces the formation of cornified envelopes) resulted in accelerated differentiation and omission of a granular layer (Boyce *et al.*, 1990).

GENERAL REMARKS AND CONCLUSIONS

Although the various types of reconstructed skin described morphologically show much resemblance to normal epidermis, some deviations are still observed. The keratinocytes, although differentiating, are hyperproliferative, lipid composition of the SC is not normal and barrier function is impaired. All these features are shared with a number of skin disorders. Since dermatological research concentrates on diseased skin, this may not necessarily be a disadvantage.

Furthermore, it should be noted that in the reconstructed epidermis appendages are absent, and also Langerhans cells, Merkel cells, T cells, monocytes, neutrophils etc. are lacking. No vascularization or innervation is present, and the supply of nutrients and oxygen might be deficient. On the other hand, this model enables us to determine the effects of substances directly on a single cell type, the keratinocyte, and also makes it possible to study the metabolism of substances by keratinocytes (Régnier *et al.*, 1990), and offers the opportunity to elucidate the molecular mechanisms of drug action and transport.

The use of reconstructed epidermis offers some advantages above animal studies: greater numbers of tests can be performed simultaneously using cells from the same donor, under better controlled conditions, probably resulting in increased reproducibility. Since cultured human keratinocytes are used, extrapolation to the *in vivo* human situation might be easier. However, *in vitro* assays cannot completely replace animal experiments, since not only the skin but also other organs are very important for toxicology assessment and for the pharmacology of a great variety of drugs.

The use of reconstructed epidermis for drug testing has only just started, but the results are promising.

The problem of the availability of human dermis might be circumvented in the future by using animal dermis as a substrate.

REFERENCES
Asselineau, D., Bernhard, B., Bailly, C. and Darmon, M. (1985) Epidermal morphogenesis and induction of the 67 kD keratin polypeptide by culture of human keratinocytes at the air/liquid interface. *Exp. Cell Res.* **159** 536–539.
Barker, J. N. W. N., Mitra, R. S., Griffith, C. E. M., Dixit, V. M. and Nickoloff, B. J. (1991) Keratinocytes as initiators of inflammation. *Lancet* **337** 211–214.
Bell, E., Sher, S., Hull, B. *et al.* (1983) The reconstruction of living skin. *J. Invest. Dermatol.* **81** 2s–10s.
Bernstein, L. I. Vaughan, F. L. and Berstein, I. A. (1986) Keratinocytes grown at the air/liquid interface. *In Vitro* **22** 695–705.
Boddé, H. E., Holman, B., Spies, F., Weerheim, A., Kempenaar, J., Mommaas, M. and Ponec, M. (1990) Freeze fracture electron microscopy of *in vitro* reconstructed human epidermis. *J. Invest. Dermatol.* **95** 108–116.
Boukamp, P., Breitkreutz, D., Stark, H.-J. and Fusenig, N. E. (1990) Mesenchyme-mediated and endogeneous regulation of growth and differentiation of human skin keratinocytes derived from different body sites. *Differentiation* **44** 150–161.
Bowden, P. E., Stark, H. J., Breitkreutz, D. and Fusenig, N. E. (1987) Expression and modification of keratins during terminal differentiation of mammalian epidermis. *Curr. Top. Dev. Biol.* **22** 35–68.
Bowser, P. A., White, R. J. and Nugteren, D. H. (1986) Location and nature of the epidermal permeability barrier. *Int. J. Cosmet. Sci.* **8** 125–134.
Boyce, S., Michel, S., Reichert, U., Shroot, B. and Schmidt, R. (1990) Reconstructed skin from cultured human keratinocytes and fibroblasts on a collagen–glycosaminoglycan biopolymer substrate. *Skin Pharmacol.* **3** 136–143.
Burton, J. L. (1969) Dietary fatty acids and inflammatory skin diseases. *Lancet* **i** 27–31.
Coulomb, B., Saiag, P., Bell, E. *et al.* (1986) A new method for studying epidermalization. *Br. J. Dermatol.* **114** 91–101.
Dober, R. and Watt, F. M. (1987) Measurement of the rate of epidermal terminal differentiation: expression of involucrin by S-phase keratinocytes in culture and in psoriatic plaques. *J. Invest. Dermatol.* **89** 349–352.
Dubertret, L. (1990) Reconstruction of the human skin equivalent *in vitro*: a new tool for skin biology. *Skin Pharmacol.* **3** 144–148.
Elias, P. M. (1983) Epidermal lipids, barrier function, and desquamation. *J. Invest. Dermatol.* **80** 44–49.
Franz, T. J. (1978) The finite dose technique as valid *in vitro* model for the study of percutaneous absorption in man. *Curr. Probl. Dermatol.* **7** 58–68.
Fuchs, E. and Green, H. (1981) Regulation of terminal differentiation of cultured human keratinocytes by vitamin A. *Cell* **25** 617–625.

Goldberg, A M. and Frazier, J. M. (1989) Alternatives to animals in toxicity testing. *Sci. Am.* **261**(2) 24–30.

Hashimoto, K., Matsumoto, K., Higashiyama, M., Nishida, Y. and Yoshikawa, K. (1990) Growth-inhibitory effects of 1,25-dihydroxyvitamin D3 on normal and psoriatic keratinocytes. *Br. J. Dermatol.* **123** 93–98.

Hennings, H., Michael, D., Cheng, C., Steinert, P., Holbrook, K. and Yuspa, S. H. (1980) Calcium regulation of growth and differentiation of mouse epidermal cells in culture. *Cell* **19** 245–254.

Holbrook, K. A. and Steinert, P. M. (1978) Assembly of stratum corneum basic protein and keratin filaments in macrofibrils. *Nature (London)* **276** 729–731.

Hunziker, T., Boillat, C., Gerber, H. A., Wiesmann, U. and Wintroub, B. U. (1989) In vitro pemphigus vulgaris model using organotypic cultures of human epidermal keratinocytes. *J. Invest. Dermatol.* **93** 263–267.

Igel, H. J., Freeman, A. E., Boeckman, C. R. and Kleinfeld, K. F. (1974) A new method for covering large surface area wounds with autografts. *Arch. Surg.* **108** 724–729.

Köck, A., den Brok, J. and Wauben-Penris, P. J. J. (1991) Effects of various corticosteroids on cytokine production in human keratinocytes. In: *Pharmacology and the Skin,* Vol. 4, *Immunological and Pharmacological Aspects of Atopic and Contact Eczema.* 32–38.

Kopan, R., Trasa, G. and Fuchs, E. (1987) Retinoids as important regulators of terminal differentiation: examining keratin expression in individual epidermal cells at various stages of keratinization. *J. Cell Biol.* **105** 427–440.

Lénoir, M. C., Bernard, B. A., Pautrat, G. et al. (1988) Outer root sheath cells of human hair follicle are able to regenerate a fully differentiated epidermis In vitro. *Dev. Biol.* **130** 610–620.

Luger, T. A. and Schwarz, T. (1990) Epidermal cell derived cytokines. In: Bos, J. D. (ed.) *Skin Immune System (SIS).* CRC Press, Boca Raton, FL, pp. 257–291.

Madison, K. C., Wertz, P. W., Strauss, J. S. and Downing, D. T. (1988) Lamellar granule extrusion and stratum corneum intercellular lamellae in murine keratinocyte cultures. *J. Invest. Dermatol.* **90** 110–116.

Mak, V. H. W., Cumpstone, M. B., Kennedy, A. H., Harmon, C. S., Guy, R. H. and Potts, R. O. (1991) Barrier function of human keratinocyte cultures grown at the air–liquid interface. *J. Invest. Dermatol.* **96** 323–327.

Moll, R., Franke, W. W., Schiller, D. L., Geiger, B. and Krepler, R. (1982) The catalog of human cytokeratins: patterns of expression in normal epithelia, tumours and cultured cells. *Cell* **31** 11–24.

Ponec, M. (1991) Human epidermis reconstructed on de-epidermized dermis: expression of differentiation-specific protein markers and lipid composition. Submitted.

Ponec, M., Weerheim, A., Kempenaar, J. and Boonstra, J. (1988a) Proliferation and differentiation of human squamous carcinoma cell lines and normal keratinocytes: effects of epidermal growth factor, retinoid, and hydrocortisone. *In Vitro Cell Dev. Biol.* **24** 764–770.

Ponec, M., Weerheim, A., Kempenaar, J., Mommaas, A.-M. and Nugteren, D. H. (1988b) Lipid composition of cultured human keratinocytes in relation to their differentiation. *J. Lipid Res.* **29** 949–961.

Ponec, M., Haverkort, M., Soei, Y. L. and Kempenaar, J. (1989) Toxicity screening of N-alkylazacycloheptan-2-one derivatives in cultured human skin cells: structure–toxicity relationships. *J. Pharm. Sci.* **78** 738–741.

Ponec, M., Wauben-Penris, P. J. J., Burger, A., Kempenaaar, J. and Boddé, H. E. (1990) Nitroglycerin and sucrose permeability as quality markers for reconstructed human epidermis. *Skin Parmacol.* **3** 126–135.

Potts, R. O. (1989) Physical characterization of the stratum corneum: the relationship of mechanical and barrier properties to lipid and protein structure. In: Hadgraft, J. and Guy, R. H. (eds) *Transdermal Drug Delivery*. Dekker, New York, pp. 23–57.

Prunieras, M., Delescluse, C., Régnier, M. and Schlotterer, M. (1979) Nouveau procédé de culture des cellules épidermiques humaines sur derme homologue ou hétérologue. Préparation de greffons recombinés. *Ann. Chir. Plast.* **24** 357–362.

Régnier, M. and Darmon, M. (1989) Human epidermis reconstructed in vitro: a model to study keratinocyte differentiation and its modulation by retinoic acid. In *Vitro Cell Dev. Biol.* **25** 1000–1008.

Régnier, M., Desbas, C., Bailly, C. and Darmon, M. (1988) Differentiation of normal and tumoral human keratinocytes cultured on dermis. Reconstruction of either normal or tumoral architecture. *In Vitro Cell Dev. Biol.* **24** 625–632.

Régnier, M., Asselineau, D. and Lénoir, M. C. (1990) Human epidermis reconstructed on dermal substrates *in vitro*: an alternative to animals in skin pharmacology. *Skin Pharmacol.* **3** 70–85.

Reichert, U. (1986) Skin toxicity and cellular metabolism: *in vitro* models. *Br. J. Dermatol.* **115** s31.

Rheinwald, J. G. and Green, H. (1975) Serial cultivation of strains of human keratinocytes: the formation of keratinizing colonies from single cells. *Cell* **6** 331–343.

Rice, R. H. and Green, H. (1979) Presence in human epidermal cells of a soluble protein precursor of the cross-linking envelope: activation of the cross-linking by calcium ions. *Cell* **18** 681–694.

Rosdy, M. and Clauss, L.-C. (1990) Terminal epidermal differentiation of human keratinocytes grown in chemically defined medium on inert filter substrates at the air–liquid interface. *J. Invest. Dermatol.* **95** 409–414.

Scavarelli-Karantsavelos, R. M., Saroya, S. Z., Vaughan, F. L. and Bernstein, I. A. (1990) Pseudoepidermis, constructed *in vitro*, for the use in toxicological and pharmacological studies. *Skin Pharmacol.* **3** 115–125.

Shahabeddin, L., Berthod, F., Damour, O. and Collombel, C. (1990) Characterization of skin reconstructed on a chitosan-cross-linked collagen–glycosaminoglycan matrix. *Skin Pharmacol.* **3** 107–114.

Vermorken, A. J. H., Verhagen, H., Vermeesch-Markslag, A. M. G., Wirtz, P., Bernard, B. A., Asselineau, D., Lénoir, M. C, Kimenai, P. M. and Shroot, B. (1985) Differentiation of keratinocytes *in vitro*: a new culture vessel mimicking the *in vivo* situation. *Mol. Biol. Res.* **109** 205–213.

Watt, F. M. and Green, H. (1981) Involucrin synthesis is correlated with cell size in human epidermal cultures. *J. Cell Biol.* **90** 738–742.

Wertz, P. W. and Downing, D. T. (1983) Ceramides of pig epidermis: structure determination. *J. Lipid Res.* **24** 759–765.

Williams, M. L., Brown, B. E., Monger, D. J., Grayson, S. and Elias, P. M. (1988) Lipid content and metabolism of human keratinocyte cultures grown at the air–medium interface. *J. Cell Physiol.* **136** 103–110.

Woodley, D. T., Saurat, J. H., Prunieras, M. *et al.* (1982) Pemphigoid pemphigus and Pr antigens in adult human keratinocytes grown on non-viable substrates. *J. Invest. Dermatol.* **79** 23–29.

Ziboh, V. A. (1989) Epidermal lipogenesis (essential fatty acids and lipid inhibitors). In: Greaves, M. W. and Shuster, S. (eds) *Pharmacology of the Skin*, Vol. 1. Springer, Berlin, pp. 59–68.

14

Trends in transdermal drug delivery systems

Wilfried Fischer

INTRODUCTION

In order to achieve an effective treatment of chronic diseases by transdermal application of drugs the cellular barrier of the skin must be passed to reach the systemic circulation. Transdermal drug delivery systems (TDDSs) are drug-containing technical devices that form an environmentally protected temporal unit with the skin. By this they offer the chance for a reproducible overcoming–passing by of the skin barrier, especially the horny layer. To reach this aim physicochemical and physiological functions of the skin have to be considered in order to find a compromise between sufficient drug absorption, skin compatibility and technological expenditure. At least all efforts should lead to a benefit at minimal risk for the patient. In addition, economic requirements have to be taken into account.

This chapter deals with technical means to overcome biological membrane barriers. The basic equation for steady state mass transport through homogeneous membranes is derived from Fick's diffusion law:

$$J = \frac{KDA}{h}(C_v - C_s) \qquad (1)$$

where J is the transmembrane flux, K the partition coefficient between membrane and vehicle, D the diffusion coefficient in the membrane, A the area, h the membrane thickness, C_v the concentration in the vehicle and C_s the concentration in the skin (sink). Based on this equation the theoretical possibilities and practically used techniques to control the transdermal flux of a drug substance will be discussed.

TECHNOLOGIES INFLUENCING THE DIFFUSIONAL BEHAVIOUR

As the flux J of a drug through a membrane is directly proportional to the diffusion coefficient D in the membrane an enhanced flux will be obtained by raising D. D depends on the properties of the drug, which cannot be changed, and its interaction with the membrane, here skin. The barrier properties of skin can be changed in two different ways: chemically or physically.

In the following, 'physical means' refers to techniques without the aid of chemical additives. Currently different physical means to change the membrane properties are under research: electricity, ultrasound, and heat.

The fascinating aspect of physical absorption control is the theoretical ability to switch on and off the drug permeation by modulation of the physical force applied. So biofeedback or circadian drug level profiles could be possible. In the case of peptide and protein drugs in particular, this could advance the therapy.

Iontophoresis

The use of an electric current to force the flux of ionized drugs through the skin is very old (Leduc 1908). This is called iontophoresis and has to be distinguished from electrophoresis or electro-osmosis. Clinically iontophoresis is used to treat hyperhydrosis or to induce sweating by iontophoretic delivery of pilocarpine for diagnosis of cystic fibrosis (Chien and Banga, 1989). The main physical principle is to overlay the natural with an external electric field.

As the isoelectric point of the stratum corneum is about pH 3 to 4 the surface of the skin bears a negative charge at natural pH (5 to 6). In this way the skin acts as a capacitor with a surface that attracts cations and repulses anions. By the aid of an external controllable electrical field cations can be driven into the skin by the anode and anions by the cathode. The resulting electrical field can be enlarged or reversed by the polarization of the external field. So, charged particles are thought to migrate within the skin along the direction of the field vectors.

The flux can be described by a modified Nernst–Planck equation:

$$J_{tot} = K_s \, dC/h_s + (Z_i D_i F/RT) C_i \, dE/h_s + k C_s I_d \tag{2}$$

where J_{tot} is total flux, K_s the partition coefficient between skin and vehicle, D_s the diffusion coefficient across the skin, C the drug concentration in the skin, h_s the skin thickness, Z_i the electric valence of ion i, D_i the diffusion coefficient of ion i in the skin, F the Faraday constant, R the gas constant, T the absolute temperature, C_i the concentration of ion i in the vehicle, E the electric potential, C_s the concentration in the skin, and I_d the current density. The total flux is the sum of passive, electrical and convective flux. The term $kC_s I_d$ describes the electrically generated convective flux.

An iontophoretic device is composed of

- an adhering element,
- a cathode,
- an anode,
- a current-controlling element,
- a drug reservoir, and
- an energy source.

The adhering element may be a ring coated with a pressure-sensitive adhesive that fixes the electrodes and drug reservoir. Metallic electrodes should not be in direct contact with skin in order to avoid burning. The contact to the skin should be made by drug–electrolyte solutions. The distance of the electrodes should avoid direct charge transfer between them without penetration into the skin. The current control element should be a re-useable microchip that can be worn in a separate device with the battery. The drug reservoir will be coupled with one of the electrodes and will also act as a contact medium.

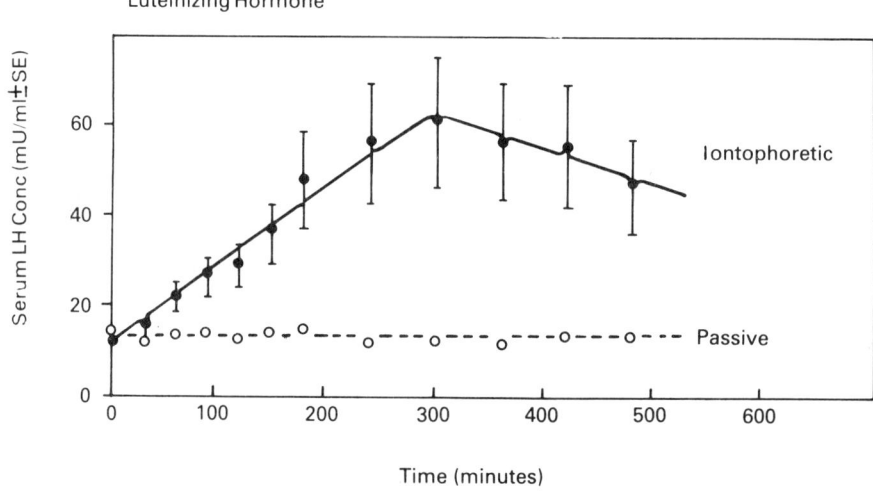

Fig. 1. Comparative serum concentration profiles of LH in 13 normal subjects following transdermal delivery of leuprolide, a synthetic LHRH analogue, by iontophoresis treatment with the direct current (0.2 mA over 70 cm^2) generated by the Powerpatch applicator (●) and by passive diffusion alone (○). (From Chien et al. (1990).)

Iontophoretically enhanced transport by constant direct current was demonstrated by Meyer et al. (1988) with LHRH (Fig. 1). Constant current leads to polarization of the skin. Polarization can result in electrolysis of the skin fluids and injury by burning and can be avoided by pulsed direct current. Pulses with different characteristics can be applied. This has an effect on the drug absorption (Fig. 2) (Chien et al., 1990). Thus, one can optimize the extent and rate of drug absorption by varying the on:off ratio, waveform and frequency of pulses.

The electric field can enlarge the apparent diffusion coefficient of — mainly charged — molecules. It has also been found that uncharged molecules could be transported indirectly by the field-induced water flow. This results from small ions such as sodium and chloride that are added to the drug solution. This electro-osmotic phenomenon is called iontohydrokinesis (Gangarosa et al., 1980).

As ions migrate in the field an electric current flows. The current is proportional to the mass flow:

$$Q = t_j it/zF \text{ or } K = t_j i/zF \qquad (3)$$

where J is the flux, Q the amount of drug, t the time, t_j the transference number parameter (fraction of current transported by the ions of interest), i the current, z the valence

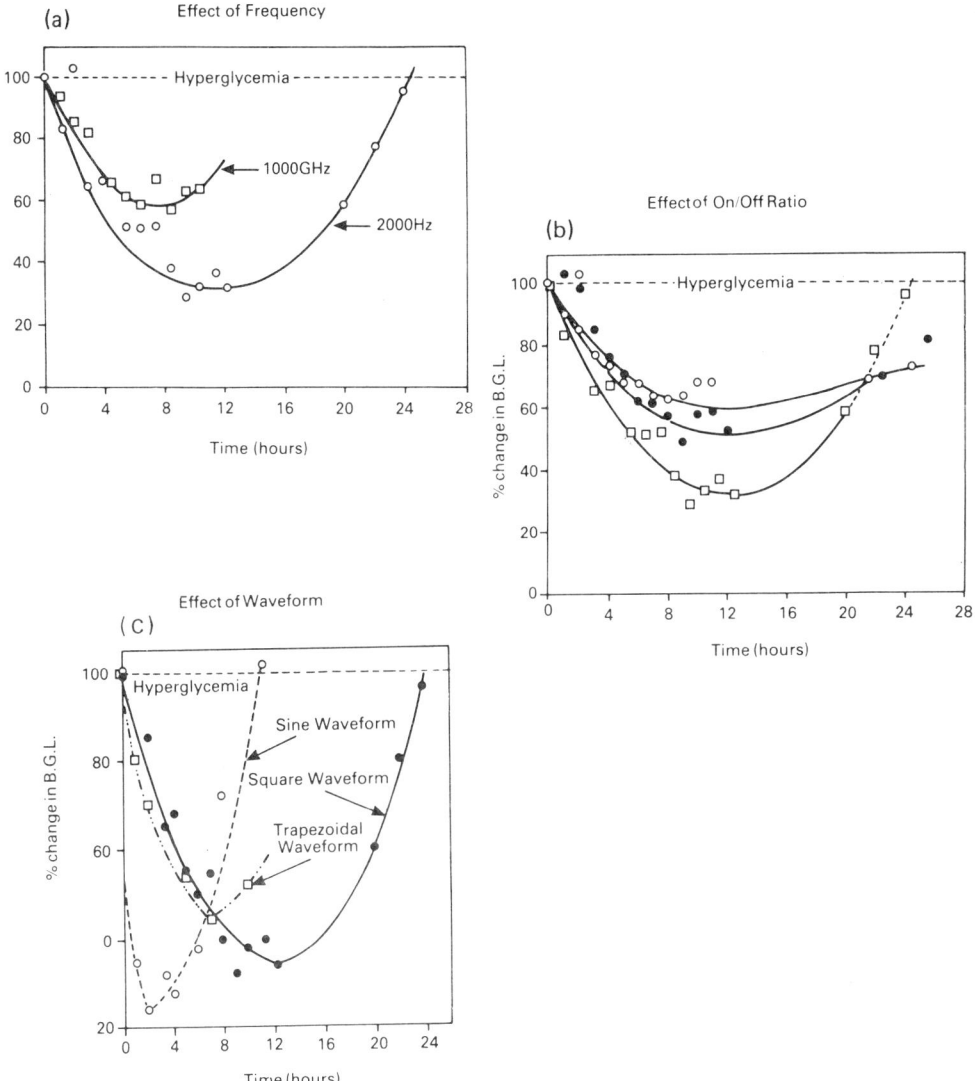

Fig. 2. (a) Effect of various waveforms of the pulse current on the oset, extent and duration of the hypoglycaemic effect (change in blood glucose levels (B.G.L.)) of insulin delivered transdermally by TPIS: transdermal pulsed iontophoretic system. (b) Effect of the frequency of pulse current on the onset, extent and duration of the hypoglycaemic effect of insulin delivered transdermally by TPIS. (c) Effect of the on:off ratio of pulse current on the onset, extent and duration of the hypoglyacemic effect of insulin delivered transdermally by TPIS. (From Chien et al. (1990).)

number, and F the Faraday constant. Consequently, a linear correlation between current density and flux has been shown (Fig. 3) (Burnette and Marero, 1986; Banga and Chien, 1990). Typical iontophoretic parameters from the literature are as follows: voltage, 1.5–7 V; current, 0.01–1 mA; frequency, 2 kHz; application time, 10–20 min.

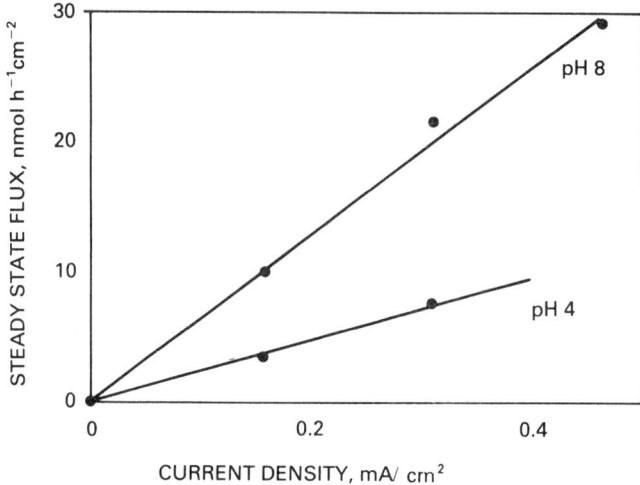

Fig. 3. A plot of skin permeation flux of thyrotropin-releasing hormone at steady state vs current density and the effect of pH (temperature $30 \pm 0.2°C$). (From Burnette and Marero (1986).)

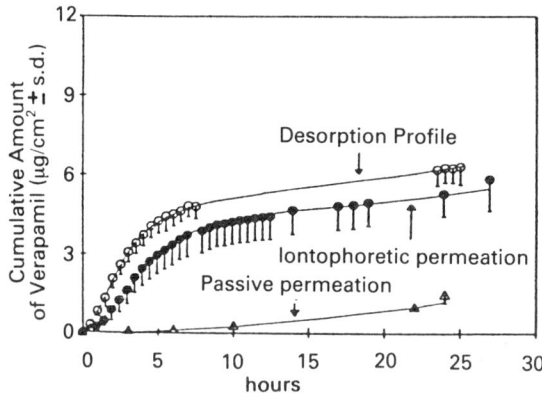

Fig. 4. Skin permeation profile of verapamil by passive diffusion (▲), and after iontophoresis treatment with pulse current at 0.1 mA for 10 min (●). The desorption profile of verapamil after the iontophoretic treatment is also shown (○). (From Wearley et al. (1989).)

Wearley et al. (1989) observed that the increased flux of the model drug verapamil hydrochloride lasted for a much longer time period than the current application. So, 10 min application of a current of 0.15 mA resulted in a 5 h enhanced absorption, compared with nontreatment (Fig. 4). From the desorption profile it can be concluded that under iontophoretic treatment the drug concentration in the skin dramatically rose. The desorption of verapamil from the skin after turning off the current may last up to 20 h, depending on the applied drug concentration (Fig. 5). This is because under iontophoresis a dispersion of charges occurs and a high drug concentration is achieved within the skin. When the current is turned off the field breaks down slowly as the charge equilibrium is approached by diffusion of the ions. That means that the capacitor 'skin' is unloaded very slowly.

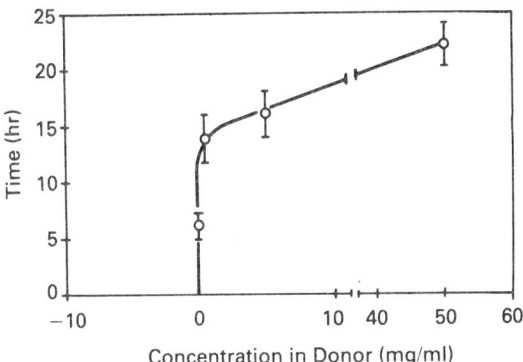

Fig. 5. Desorption time after iontophoresis treatment vs concentration of verapamil hydrochloride in the donor solution. (From Wearley et al. (1989).)

These limitations have to be taken into account if a regulating TDDS is to be developed. Techniques for an immediate stop of the drug permeation will be needed if highly active drugs such as insulin or narcotics are to be delivered by this technique.

Phonophoresis

Phonophoresis is the application of ultrasound to drug molecules dispersed in a contact agent in order to facilitate the permeation through membranes. Enhanced drug penetration can result from mechanical, thermal and chemical alterations of biological tissues under the influence of ultrasonic waves.

Upon ultrasonic irradiation, at first mechanical disturbances of the tissue occurs. The absorbed mechanical energy is transformed into heat. Secondly, ultrasound can cause cavitation in the tissue fluids and this may be the reason for an altered chemical reactivity and cleavage of macromolecules and therefore changed membrane properties. This can be controlled by the energy density and should be avoided in order to avoid irreversible damages of the tissues. Thirdly, it can cause the generation of microcurrents in membranes by heterogeneous distribution of energy in the fluids. This may lead to a reduction of the thickness of the diffusion layer and therefore enhanced diffusivity of molecules (Singh and Singh, 1990).

A phonophoretic device is composed of a power supply, an HF generator, a transducer probe, soundhead, a coupling medium, gel, and a drug reservoir.

The power supply–HF generator at the moment is a stationary apparatus with variable power output. The transducer probe is in principle a piezoelectric crystal that starts to vibrate as an alternating current is applied to it. The ultrasonic waves need a coupling medium, which can contain drugs, in order to transfer the ultrasound energy.

The clinical applications of ultrasound include diagnostics, hyperthermia, wound healing and pain treatment. In the 1960s it was observed that hydrocortisone was driven through the skin by ultrasound (Griffin et al., 1965). Since then many drugs have been applied phonophoretically, including anti-inflammatory drugs such as dexamethasone, fluocinolone acetonide, ibuprofen, indomethacin, anticancer drugs such as arabinosyl cytosine, cyclophosphamide metabolite, local anaesthetics such as lidocaine, lignocaine, carbocaine, antibiotics as streptomycin and tetracycline. The clinical results are contradictory. Whereas some researchers find enhanced permeation of drugs others find no effect (Tyle and Agrawala, 1989). The comparison of different results is difficult as the studies have been performed using different methods. Many parameters can be varied, and there is a lack of a standard method.

Clinically, ultrasonic power in the range from 0.001 to 2 W/cm^2, is applied, depending on the kind of application. Usually the ultrasonic head is moved over the application site. With this technique one can tolerate 2 W/cm^2, whereas with stationary application only 0.2 W/cm^2 for up to 2 min can be tolerated. The typical application time is 5 to 20 min.

Phonophoretic TDDS will require a stationary energy application. Instead of moving around the head, the energy can be pulsed in order to avoid local overheating. With pulsed ultrasound energy it may be possible to raise the energy without damaging the tissues (Benson et al., 1988). The high frequency is 20 kHz up to 10 MHz. The range from 0.5 to 3 MHz is used most commonly.

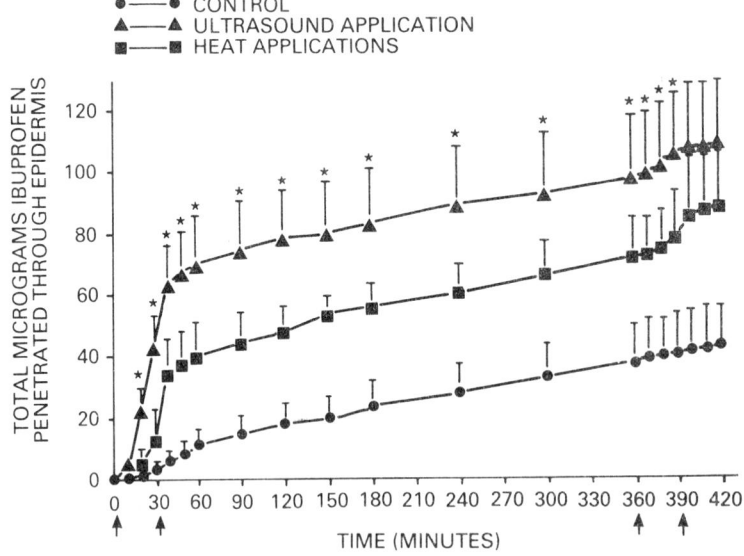

Fig. 6. Total mass (mean ± SD) of ibuprofen penetrated vs time. Ultrasound and heat applied from time 0 to 30 min and from 360 to 390 min as indicated by the arrows. Asterisks denote where ultrasound is significantly different ($p < 0.05$) from heat application and control. (From Brucks et al. (1989).)

In order to differentiate between the thermal and mechanical effects of ultrasound irradiation, Brucks et al. (1989) applied a constant ultrasound energy, 1 W/cm^2, for 30 min at 1 MHz to excised human skin *in vitro*. The ibuprofen flux under ultrasound irradiation and after heating the skin to the same temperature as under irradiation was measured (Fig. 6). The flux rose to 11.3 times the value without treatment, but obviously the temperature elevation alone enhances the absorption. The ultrasonic 'nonthermal' contribution may be an effect on the lipids of the stratum corneum: it may be increased diffusion or a reduced activation energy of diffusion.

One main difference compared with iontophoresis is the short hysteresis that makes phonophoresis better suited if short pulses of drug are needed.

There are limitations to the wide application of such systems. The energy applied in this experiment (0.5 Wn/cm^2) is much higher than the energy tolerable by patients (0.0067 W h/cm^2). A compromise between tolerability and effect has to be found which for example may be pulsed application. In my opinion the technical complexity and energy consumption may prevent the development of cheap, easy-to-use and portable phonophoretic TDDSs.

Temperature-activated systems

Temperature-activated TDDSs are a new class of systems that include an enhanced drug release by temperature elevation. The results of the temperature rise is an enhanced absorption. In principle in these systems the drug release is controlled by membranes. The membranes are thermoresponsive in such a way that the permeability sharply increases with temperature. Nozawa et al. (1991) reported a system containing a liquid-crystalline phase as a membrane. The phase transition temperature of the liquid crystal was 38°C. Below this temperature the membrane material has low permeabilities for drugs; above this temperature the permeabilities sharply rise. The material reported was monooxyethylene trimethylolpropane tristearate (MTTS).

TDDSs for nonsteroidal anti-inflammatory drugs were developed with drug release controlled by the temperature-dependent MTTS membrane. *In vivo* studies in rabbits with this system have been performed. They show that upon an externally controlled temperature rise the plasma level profiles clearly rise with temperature (Fig. 7).

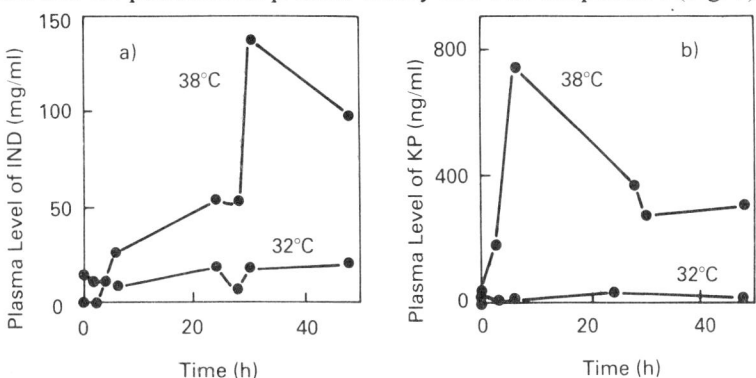

Fig. 7. Plasma levels of (a) indomethacin and (b) ketoprofen in rabbits after application to the skin with the MTTS membrane. (From Nozawa et al. (1991).)

It would be desirable to combine a thermoresponsive membrane with an integrated heating device in one TDDS. Such systems offer the option for a safe therapeutic application by external control of drug release and enhanced drug absorption resulting from increased temperature. The drug absorption can be switched on and off by temperature alteration.

TECHNOLOGIES INFLUENCING THE THERMODYNAMIC ACTIVITY OF THE DRUG

Thermodynamic activity

The motor for drug absorption from passive TDDS is the gradient of chemical potential within the absorption limiting membrane

$$J \sim d\mu/dh \tag{4}$$

$$\mu = \mu_0 + RT\ln(\tau c) \tag{5}$$

where J is the flux, μ the chemical potential, μ_0 the standard chemical potential, R the gas constant, T the absolute temperature, τ the activity coefficient, c the concentration, and τc the thermodynamic activity. So, increasing the concentration of the drug will increase the thermodynamic activity of the drug in the membrane and raise the diffusion rate.

There are several ways to increase the thermodynamic activity in the membrane:
- increase $C_{s,v}$, the solubility in the vehicle;
- increase $K_{m/v}$, the membrane–vehicle partition coefficient;
- increase $C_{s,m}$, the solubility in the membrane.

An increase of $C_{s,v}$ in the vehicle generally results in an increased C_m, under the assumption that $K_{m/v}$ does not change. The maximum flux is determined by

$$J_{max} = PAC_{s,v} \tag{6}$$

where J_{max} is the maximal flux, P the permeability coefficient, and A the absorption area. The higher $C_{s,v}$ the higher J_{max} should be. In reality this is true only in very rare cases. The increase of $C_{s,v}$ is mostly associated with the change of K. Increasing $C_{s,v}$ means that K is lowered, so that both effects tend to cancel each other. In the following equation the partition coefficient is replaced by the corresponding solubilities:

$$J_{max} = (C_{s,m}/C_{s,v})DA/hC_{s,v} \tag{7}$$

As a result, the flux of drugs from saturated solutions of different solvents is identical, unless the solvents change the skin properties.

More precisely, one has to compare the thermodynamic activities in saturated solutions. In a distribution equilibrium of saturated solutions of different solvents the chemical potential difference is zero:

$$\mu_0^m + RT\ln(C_{s,m}\tau_m) = \mu_0^v + RT\ln(C_{s,v}\tau_v) \tag{8}$$

where the indices m and v indicate the membrane and vehicle. From this the partition coefficient can be expressed as

$$K_{m/v} = \tau_v/\tau_m \tag{9}$$

and as $C_{s,v} = a/\tau_v$ one can write

$$J_{max} = (a/\tau_m)DA/h \tag{10}$$

where a is the thermodynamic activity. This means that the flux is dependent on the thermodynamic activity in the vehicle and the activity coefficient in the membrane. As the thermodynamic activities of saturated solutions are equal, equal fluxes should result from different solvents. This phenomenon, called 'thermodynamic control', has been observed for example by Flynn and Smith (1972) and Woodford and Barry (1982).

For matrix-type TDDSs this is a very important finding, because from these considerations it is not possible to enhance the absorption of drugs by the polymer itself. If the drug is dissolved in the polymer the maximum absorption can be achieved by saturated solutions independent of the polymer type assuming the most probable case of D_v being greater than D_m. The polymer acts as a reservoir and the solubility of drug is important for the duration of drug release, the skin compatibility, comfort of wearing and physical stability such control of cold flow or peel force.

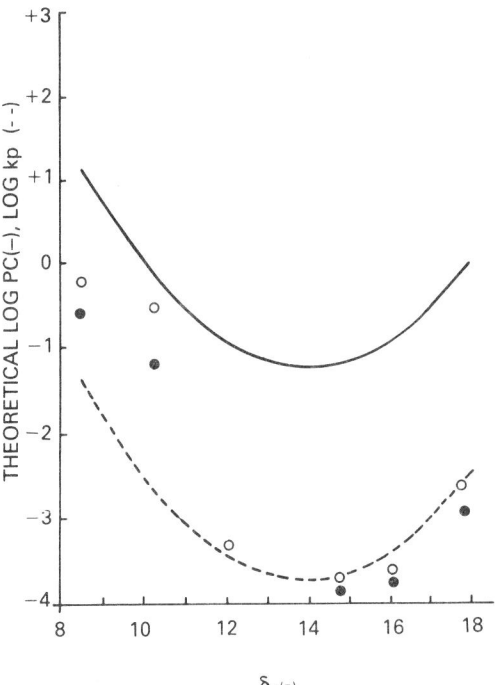

Fig. 8. A plot of theoretical log $K_{m/v}$ (———) vs $\delta_{v(n)}$ including values for steady state of the experimentally determined log k_p (- - - -). (Modified from Sloan et al. (1986).)

Based on flux measurements of theophylline from different saturated solvents, Sloan et al. (1986) found an inverse dependence of solubility and permeability coefficient. Calculating the theoretical partition coefficient from solubility parameters of theophylline and skin he found a good correlation between theoretical partition coefficients and experimentally determined permeability coefficients (Fig. 8). Thermodynamic control was not able to predict this behaviour. Although the used solvents did not change the diffusion coefficient in skin the observed fluxes depended on the solubility parameters of the solvents. Deviations from this correlation occurred with solvents having solubility parameters close to that of the skin (10 $(cal/cm^3)^{1/2}$). Here enhanced fluxes were observed.

It would be interesting to investigate the dependence of flux on solubility parameters of nonpenetrating solvents such as polymers in order to differentiate between the pure partitioning process and the possible dissolution of skin components in the solvents. So, the choice of polymers for matrix TDDS could be brought to a more rational basis.

Supersaturated systems

If an enhancement of flux is required, in some cases it can be obtained by using supersaturated polymer solutions. So, Davis (1986) could increase the amount of drug permeated by a factor of 8 with liquid solutions and gels (Fig. 9). With this method the partition coefficient is kept nearly constant, but the thermodynamic activity of the drug in the vehicle is raised, so the flux proportionally rises. The concept of supersaturation makes sense if $K_{m/v}C_{s,v}$ is less than $C_{s,m}$. The flux cannot be enhanced beyond the saturation of the membrane. Davis has determined the solubility of hydrocortisone acetate in the artificial membrane (personal communication) and concluded that a supersaturation of the membrane itself has taken place. Whether supersaturation of the skin can occur has not been shown yet. One main obstacle in this approach is that supersaturated solutions are metastable. The time for recrystallization depends on the degree of supersaturation

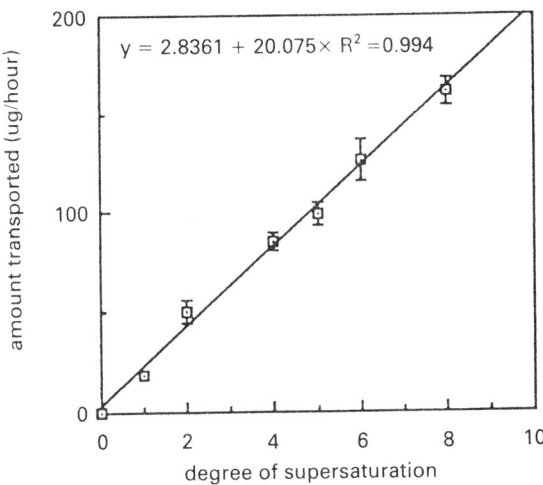

Fig. 9. Transport of hydrocortisone acetate, 0.02% w/w, from supersaturated vehicles. Demonstration of response to degree of supersaturation. Mean ± standard errors, $n = 6$. (From Davis, 1986.)

$$V_{cryst} \sim (C_v - C_{s,v})^4 \tag{11}$$

where V_{cryst} is the crystallization rate, and C_v the viscosity of the solvents. In the case of adhesive polymers this may last for several months. If the advantage of supersaturated systems could be shown *in vivo* too, this technique may be a safe method to enhance drug permeation, as no additional skin-irritating substances are necessary.

The problem of stability could be overcome by user-activated systems that were described by Ebert *et al.* (1987). During storage the drug could be in one phase at saturation. Upon activation a second phase could be admixed to form a supersaturated state. With these systems a higher, less stable degree of supersaturation could be achieved than with conventional systems.

CONCLUSION

Dermal application of drugs in order to reach the systemic circulation requires one of the most effective biological barriers, the protective stratum corneum, to be overcome. For most drugs the barrier function has to be reduced if therapeutically relevant plasma levels are to be obtained. The use of chemical absorption promoters may fulfil this aspect of transdermal drug delivery. However, in the case of a controlled drug absorption physical methods are needed. On the one hand it is possible to enhance the drug uptake by physical means such as iontophoresis, phonophoresis or supersaturation. On the other hand iontophoresis offer the chance of an active control of pharmacological effects. With these techniques future biofeedback-controlled transdermal drug delivery systems may become possible.

REFERENCES

Banga, A. K. and Chien, Y. W. (1990) Iontophoretic delivery of drugs: fundamentals, developments and biomedical applications. *J. Control. Release* **7** 1–24.

Benson, H. A. E., McElnay, J. C. and Harland, R. (1988) Phonophoresis of lignocaine and prilocaine for Emla cream. *Int. J. Pharm.* **44** 65–69.

Brucks, R., Nanavaty, M., Jung, D. and Siegel, F. (1989) The effect of ultrasound on the *in vitro* penetration of ibuprofen through human epidermis *Pharm. Res.* **6** 697–701.

Burnette, R. R. and Marero, D. (1986) Comparison between the iontophoretic and passive transport of thyrotropin releasing hormone across excised nude mouse skin. *J. Pharm. Sci.* **75** 738–743.

Chien, Y. W. and Banga, A. K. (1989) Iontophoretic (transdermal) delivery of drugs: overview of historical development. *J. Pharm. Sci.* **78** 353–354.

Chien, Y. W., Lelawongs, P., Siddiqui, O., Sun, Y. and Shi, W. M. (1990) Facilitated transdermal delivery of therapeutic peptides and proteins by iontophoretic delivery devices. *J. Control. Release* **13** 263–278.

Davis, A. F. (1986) Two-phase supersaturated topical drug release system. *GB 86-29639*, 11 December 1986.

Ebert, C. D., Heiber, W., Andriola, R. and Williams, P. (1987) Development of a novel transdermal system design. *J. Control. Release* **6** 107–111.

Flynn, G. L. and Smith, R. W. (1972) Membrane diffusion III: influence of solvent composition and permanent solubility on membrane transport. *J. Pharm. Sci.* **61** 61–66.

Gangarosa, L. P., Park, N.-H., Wiggins, C. A. and Hill, J. M. (1980) Increased penetration of nonelectrolytes into mouse skin during iontophoretic water transport (iontohydrokinesis). *J. Pharmacol. Exp. Ther.* **212** 377–381.

Griffin, J. E., Touchstone, J. C. and Liu, A. C. (1965) Ultrasonic movement of cortisol into pig tissues. II. Movement into paravertebral tissues. *Am. J. Phys. Med.* **44** 20–25.

Leduc, S. (1908) *Electric Ions and Their Uses in Medicine*. Rebman, London.

Meyer, B. R., Kreis, W., Eschbach, J., O'Mara, V., Rosen, S. and Sibalis, D. (1988) Successful transdermal administration of therapeutic doses of a polypeptide to normal human volunteers. *Clin. Pharmacol. Ther.* **44** 607.

Nozawa, I., Suzuki, Y., Sato, S., Sugibayashi, K. and Morimoto, Y. (1991) Application of a thermo-responsive membrane to the transdermal delivery of non-steroidal anti-inflammatory drugs and antipyretic drugs. *J. Control. Release* **15** 29–37.

Singh, S. and Singh, J. (1990) Transdermal delivery of drugs by phonophoresis. A review. *Drug Des. Deliv.* **5** 259–265.

Sloan, K. B., Koch, S. A. M., Siver, K. G. and Flowers, F. P. (1986) Use of solubility parameters of drug and vehicle to predict flux through skin. *J. Invest. Dermatol.* **87** 244–252.

Tyle, P. and Agrawala, P. (1989) Drug delivery by phonophoresis. *Pharm. Res.* **6** 355–361.

Wearley, L., Liu, J.-C. and Chien, Y. W. (1989) Iontophoresis-facilitated transdermal delivery of verapamil. II. Factors affecting the reversibility of skin permeability. *J. Control. Release* **9** 231–242.

Woodford, R. and Barry, B. W. (1982) Optimisation of bioavailability of topical steroids: thermodynamic control. *J. Invest. Dermatol.* **79** 388–391.

15

Interactions between liposomes and human stratum corneum *in vitro*

J. A. Bouwstra, H. E. J. Hofland, F. Spies, G. S. Gooris and H. E. Junginger

INTRODUCTION

One of the major drawbacks in transdermal drug delivery is the slow penetration rate of drugs through the skin. Several methods are being used to increase the penetration rate of substances through the skin, e.g. the use of penetration enhancers, electric forces (Hadgraft and Guy, 1989), patches and colloidal carriers, such as liposomes (Schäfer-Korting *et al.*, 1989) and other types of vesicles (Hofland *et al.*, 1991).

Concerning liposomes, several studies have been performed that rendered conflicting results. In some studies liposomes increased the flux of drugs through the skin compared with traditional creams (Weiner *et al.*, 1989; Jacobs *et al.*, 1988; Mezei and Gulasekharem, 1980; Gehring *et al.*, 1990; Michel *et al.*, 1991; Lasch and Wohlrab, 1986; Wohlrab and Lasch 1987), while in other studies no increase in drug transport was observed (Ganesan *et al.*, 1984; Knepp *et al.*, 1988, 1990; Komatsu *et al.*, 1986a,b). These differences in results might be explained by the different physicochemical properties of the liposomes, different drugs (Ganesan *et al.*, 1984) (lipophilic vs hydrophilic) and different control experiments (the type of ointment or cream used). Only in few of those studies were the liposomes varied systematically in physical or chemical properties (Ganesan *et al.*, 1984; Knepp *et al.*, 1988, 1990).

Not only were differences with respect to the influence of vesicles on the drug transport through the skin reported, but also differences in the ability of components of liposomes to penetrate into the skin were observed. Penetration of molecularly dispersed liposomal components has been supported by several groups (Weiner *et al.*, 1989; Michel *et al.*, 1991; Lasch and Wohlrab, 1986; Wohlrab and Lasch, 1987), while others reported no penetration of the phospholipids (Ganesan *et al.*, 1984; Komatsu *et al.*, 1986a,b).

One of the questions which most frequently arises is whether intact liposomes are able to penetrate into the stratum corneum or even into deeper layers of the skin. In one of the studies on this subject Mezei and Gulasekharem (1980) and Cevc and Blume (1991) found support for the penetration of liposomes into the skin. Mezei and

Gulasekharem concluded that intact liposomes not only pass the stratum corneum but even penetrate into deeper layers of the skin. However, other studies (Weiner et al., 1989; Ganesan et al., 1984; Knepp et al., 1990) showed evidence opposing these results. These studies support a mechanism in which the deposition of drugs is facilitated when they are intercalated in the bilayers of liposomes.

Because of the variability in the studies it is still not clear which factors influence the liposome–skin interactions and play an important role in determining the efficiency of drug transport through the skin.

In this study the interactions between liposomes and skin have been investigated using freeze fracture electron microscopy (FFEM) and small angle X-ray scattering (SAXS). Human stratum corneum was treated in vitro with three types of liposomes prepared from commercially available lipid compositions. The liposomes had comparable sizes and were mainly unilamellar. The main differences between the different types of liposomes were the hydrophilicity and the charge of the head groups of the lipids. This study is focussed on stratum corneum since it is thought that the main barrier for drug transport is localized in the stratum corneum.

FFEM has been used in order to visualize full skin, epidermis and epidermal junction. Holman et al. (1990) introduced a new fracture procedure, in which the fracture occurs perpendicular to the skin surface.

SAXS has been used to elucidate the structure of mouse and human stratum corneum (Bouwstra et al., 1991, 1992a,b). Using this method it is possible to obtain information on the 'bulk' structure of the stratum corneum without any pretreatments, and it is therefore an excellent complementary technique to FFEM.

CHANGES IN THE STRUCTURE OF STRATUM CORNEUM INDUCED BY LIPOSOMES

Three types of liposomes were prepared from commercially available phospholipids NAT 50, NAT 89, and NAT 106. These mixtures were a generous gift from Nattermann Phospholipids GmbH (Cologne, Germany). The compositions of the phospholipid mixtures are given in Table 1.

The aqueous phase consisted of a phosphate-buffered saline (PBS) solution: 139 mM NaCl, 2.5 mM KCl, 8 mM Na_2HPO_4; the pH was adjusted to 7.4. The NAT 106 liposomes were prepared using the film method. Both the NAT 50 and the NAT 89 liposomes were prepared according to the method of Hager et al. (1989).

The stratum corneum was soaked in a 10% w/w liposome solution at room temperature for a period of 48 h. Control samples were submerged in PBS under the same conditions.

Small angle X-ray scattering

The liposomes and human stratum corneum after treatment either with PBS or with liposomes have been studied by SAXS. The measurements were performed at Daresbury Synchrotron Radiation Source using Station 8.2, which has been built as part of a NWO/SERC agreement. A more detailed description of the apparatus and the sample holder is given elsewhere (Bouwstra et al., 1991). After treatment, the stratum corneum was rinsed in PBS in order to remove the excess liposome suspension. All measurements were performed at 20°C. The scattering intensities were plotted as a function of the scattering vector Q, which is defined as $4\pi \sin \theta/\lambda$. θ and λ are the scattering angle and wavelength (0.154 nm), respectively. According to Bragg's law, $n\lambda = 2d \sin \theta$, the scattering vector Q at the positions of the diffraction peaks is directly related to the repeat distance d by $d = 2\pi n/Q$, in which n is the order of the diffraction peak. In the case of a lamellar structure the diffraction peaks are all located at equal interpeak distances.

Table 1. Compositions of the phospholipid mixtures

Formulation	Composition	
NAT 106	PC (with LPC)	85%
	PE	10%
	PA and N-acyl PE	5%
NAT 50	PC (with LPC)	28%
	PE	2%
	PI and PA	11%
	N-acyl PE	32%
	Sterine and derivatives	12%
	Soya oil	21%
NAT 89	PC (with LPC)	10%
	PE	25%
	N-acyl PE	4%
	PI	20%
	Sterine and derivatives	n.d.

Liposomes were prepared from 10% w/w lipid in PBS. The lipid compositions of the three mixtures that were used are given in this table. Abbreviations: PA, phosphatidic acid; PC, phosphatidylcholine; PE, phosphatidylethanolamine; PI, phosphatidylinositol; LPC, lysophosphatidylcholine.

The scattering curves of the three types of liposomes are shown in Fig. 1, 2, and 3. Mainly unilamellar vesicles are present in the three different dispersions, since only very broad peaks are shown on the scattering curves (Jousma et al., 1987). The three scattering curves of the liposome suspensions all exhibit a shoulder on the left-hand side of the broad diffraction peak. Although the exact origin is not completely understood, it might be due to either the presence of two different populations of vesicles in the suspensions or a few bi- or trilamellar vesicles in the suspensions. The shoulder is most pronounced in the case of liposomes prepared from NAT 50 lipids.

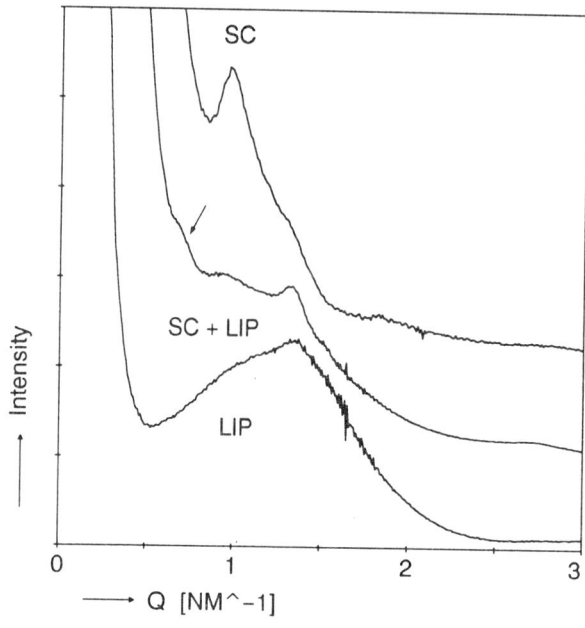

Fig. 1. Small angle X-ray scattering curves (intensity is plotted against the scattering vector Q) for NAT 89 liposomes (LIP), stratum coreum after incubation in PBS (SC) and stratum corneum after incubation in 10% w/w NAT 89 liposomes (SC+LIP). The latter curve exhibits an additional diffraction peak and shoulder (see arrow).

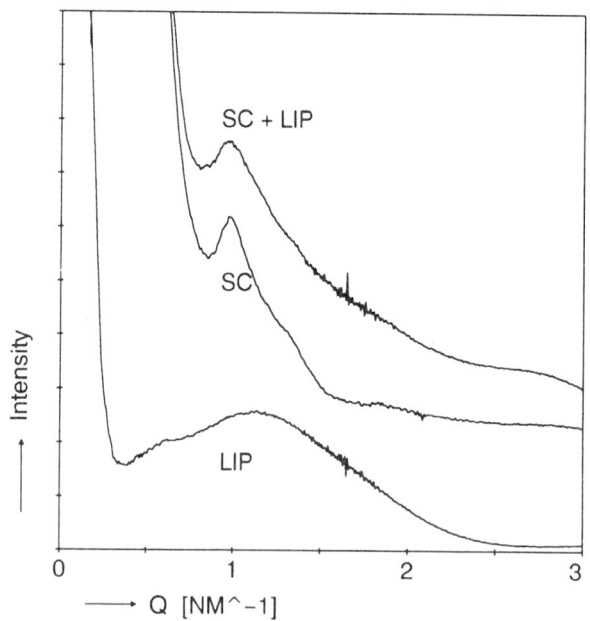

Fig. 2. Small-angle X-ray scattering curves (intensity is plotted against scattering vector Q) for NAT 106 liposomes (LIP), stratum corneum after incubation in PBS (SC) and stratum coreum after incubation in 10% w/w NAT 106 liposomes (SC + LIP). In the scattering curve of treated stratum corneum (SC + LIP) an additional diffraction peak is observed.

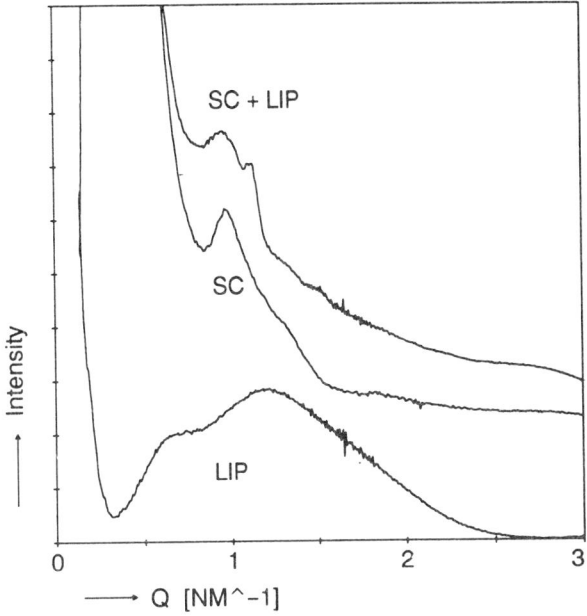

Fig. 3. Small-angle X-ray scattering curves (intensity is plotted against scattering vector Q) for NAT 50 liposomes (LIP), stratum corneum after incubation in PBS (SC) and stratum corneum after incubation in 10% w/w NAT 50 liposomes (SC + LIP).

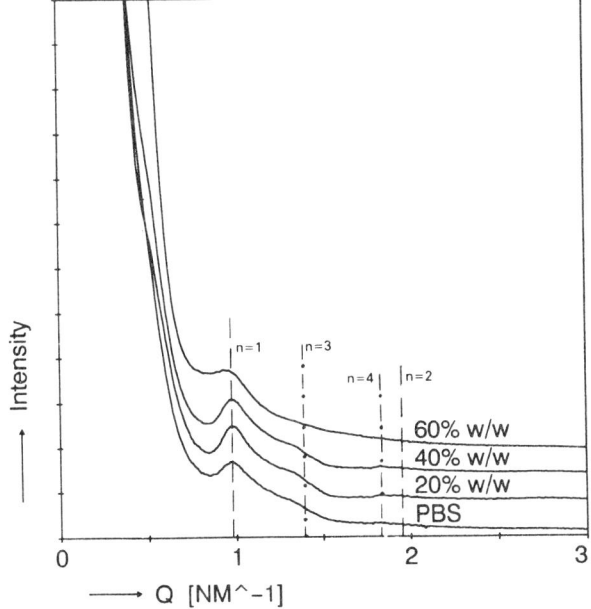

Fig. 4. Small angle X-ray scattering curves of human stratum corneum at various hydration levels and after treatment with PBS. The position of the main diffraction peak did not change. $n = 1,2$ are the first- and second-order positions of the diffraction peaks based on a repeat distance of 6.4 nm. $n = 3,4$ are the third- and fourth-order diffraction peaks based on a structure with a repeat distance of 13.4 nm.

The scattering curves of untreated stratum that was hydrated to three different water levels and stratum corneum after treatment with a PBS solution are shown in Fig. 4. The curves are characterized by a high scattering intensity at low Q values (nm^{-1}), a broad doublet peak consisting of a main position and a shoulder on the right-hand side and a weak diffraction doublet, also consisting of a main position and a shoulder on the right-hand side. Recently (Bouwstra et al., 1991) it has been shown that the scattering profile can be explained by two different lamellar structures with repeat distances of 6.4 and 13.4 nm, respectively, as is shown in Fig. 4.

Variation in hydration between 20% and 60% w/w of the stratum corneum did not influence the 6.4 nm repeat distance. No swelling of the bilayers occurred upon hydration, which is quite exceptional. Using wide angle X-ray scattering (Bouwstra et al., 1992a) it became apparent that even no lateral swelling occurred upon increasing the hydration level. Also, treatment with a PBS solution did not lead to a change in the peak position of the main diffraction peak, and therefore did not change the 6.4 nm repeat distance.

In Fig. 1 the scattering curve of stratum corneum treated with NAT 89 liposomes was shown. The treatment induced the following changes in the scattering curve.

(1) The main diffraction peak shifted slightly to a smaller Q value the repeat distance being 6.6 nm. It is not clear whether this is caused by a change in background scattering due to the presence of phospholipids in the stratum corneum or whether liposome treatment resulted in a shift in repeat distance. A shift in repeat distance should directly imply a mixing of the lipids originating from the vesicles with those originating from the stratum corneum.

(2) The liposome treatment resulted also in an additional shoulder and diffraction peak at $Q = 0.71$ and 1.34 nm^{-1} ($d = 8.8$ and 4.7 nm) respectively. The position of the additional shoulder cannot be determined with high accuracy, and therefore it is not possible to conclude whether we deal with a first- and second-order diffraction peak of one lamellar structure. An explanation for the additional peak and shoulder might be as follows. The shoulder at $Q = 0.71$ nm^{-1} is located at approximately the same position as the fully hydrated lipid bilayers ($d = 8.1 \pm 0.5$ nm) obtained from multilamellar liposomes prepared from the same lipids by the film method (scattering curve not shown). Therefore it is possible that the shoulder at 0.71 nm^{-1} is due to lamellar stacks based on the lipids originating from the NAT 89 liposomes. The scattering curve of the multilamellar liposomes did not exhibit a second-order diffraction peak. It might be that the additional peak ($Q = 1.34$ nm^{-1}) is due to a mixing of lipids originating from the stratum corneum and those from the NAT 89 liposomes. In a previous study also additional peaks were observed in the scattering curve of human stratum corneum after treatment with liposomes (Garson et al., 1990).

In Fig. 2 the scattering curve of human stratum corneum is shown after treatment with liposomes prepared from NAT 106 lipids. No swelling of the lamellar structure corresponding to repeat distance of 6.4 nm was observed. A very well-defined additional peak was observed at $Q = 1.22$ nm^{-1} ($d = 5.15$ nm). Multilamellar vesicles prepared from the same lipids by the film method resulted in a repeat distance of 8.9 ± 0.5 nm. The most likely explanation for the additional peak on the scattering curve of human stratum corneum is a mixing of lipids from liposomes and from stratum corneum, thereby forming a regular new structure which might be lamellar.

The scattering curve of human stratum corneum after treatment of liposomes prepared from NAT 50 is shown in Fig. 3. No change in the scattering curve of human stratum corneum was observed, which strongly indicates that the interactions between NAT 50 liposomes do not lead to changes in the lamellar stacking in the stratum corneum.

Freeze fracture electron microscopy
The stratum corneum was cut into small pieces approximately 3 × 15 mm in size and put into silver cylinder holder. The samples were cryofixed by quenching. The frozen samples were fractured and shadowed as described by Holman *et al.* (1990). The replicas were cleaned according to the method of Hofland *et al.* (1992).

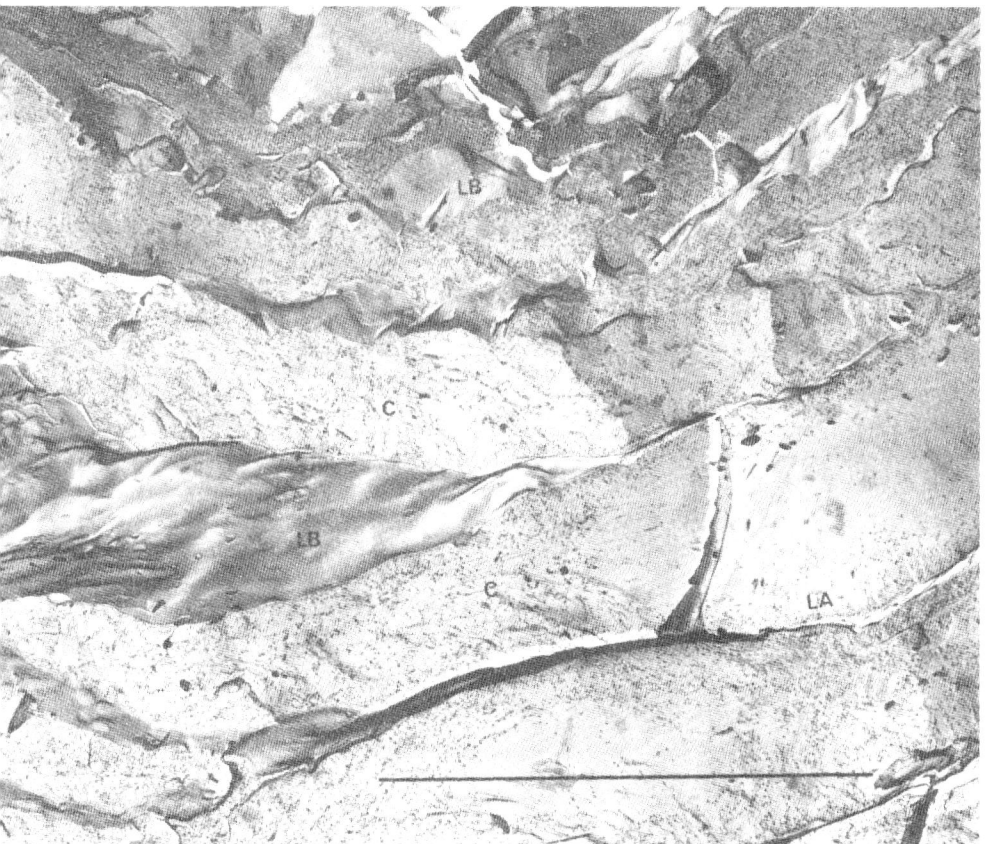

Fig. 5. PBS-treated human stratum corneum. The micrograph depicts the corneocytes (C) between which the lipid bilayers are located (LB). Keratin filaments are shown as particles that fill the interior space of the corneocytes. Close to the fracture face of the plasma membrane these keratin filaments are arranged in linear arrays (LA). The intercellular lipid regions (LB) are presented as smooth surfaces. Sharp edges appear where the fracture plane crosses the bilayers. Sometimes desmosomes are observed. The scale bar represents 1 μm.

An electron micrograph of stratum corneum treated with PBS is shown in Fig. 5. Corneocytes which are flattened hexagonal cells of approximately 30 μm in diameter and 0.5 μm in height are characterized by protein particles which are clearly depicted in the micrograph. No cell organelles are present inside the corneocytes. Close to the cell envelope inside the cells linear arrays of keratin filaments are present. Between the corneocytes smooth surfaces are located which originate from fractures through lipid regions parallel to the lamellae. Sometimes sharp edges in these surfaces are recognized which are caused by fractures perpendicular to the lamellae. In this micrograph desmosomes are shown in the intercellular spaces.

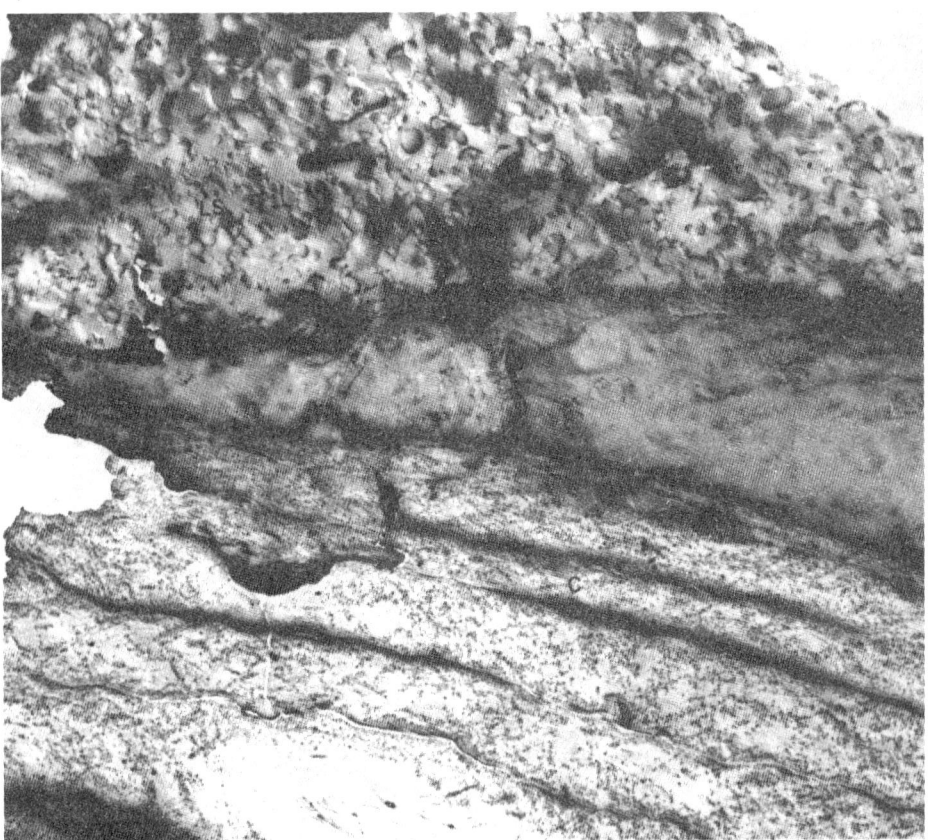

Fig. 6. Stratum corneum incubated with NAT 50 liposomes. At the upper part of the micrograph NAT 50 liposomal suspension (LS) is visualized. At the lower part of the micrograph the fracture is across the stratum corneum. In the middle part the fracture is along the interface. At this interface the liposomes fuse edge to edge, forming patches of lamellar stacks (P).

In Fig. 6 the stratum corneum is shown after incubation with liposomes prepared from NAT 50 lipids. The upper part of this micrograph depicts the liposome dispersion, while the lower part shows a fracture through the stratum corneum. Between these two regions the fracture plane is approximately along the interface between liposomes and stratum corneum. In the lipid lamellar regions in the stratum corneum no changes in the structure were observed, not even between the first and second corneocyte layer. At the interface it seems that liposomes fuse edge to edge, forming a lamellar structure. At higher magnification of the interface the fusion process is shown in Fig. 7. Using SAXS it was shown that the scattering curve after treatment with NAT 50 liposomes and PBS did not change significantly. This can be explained in three ways.

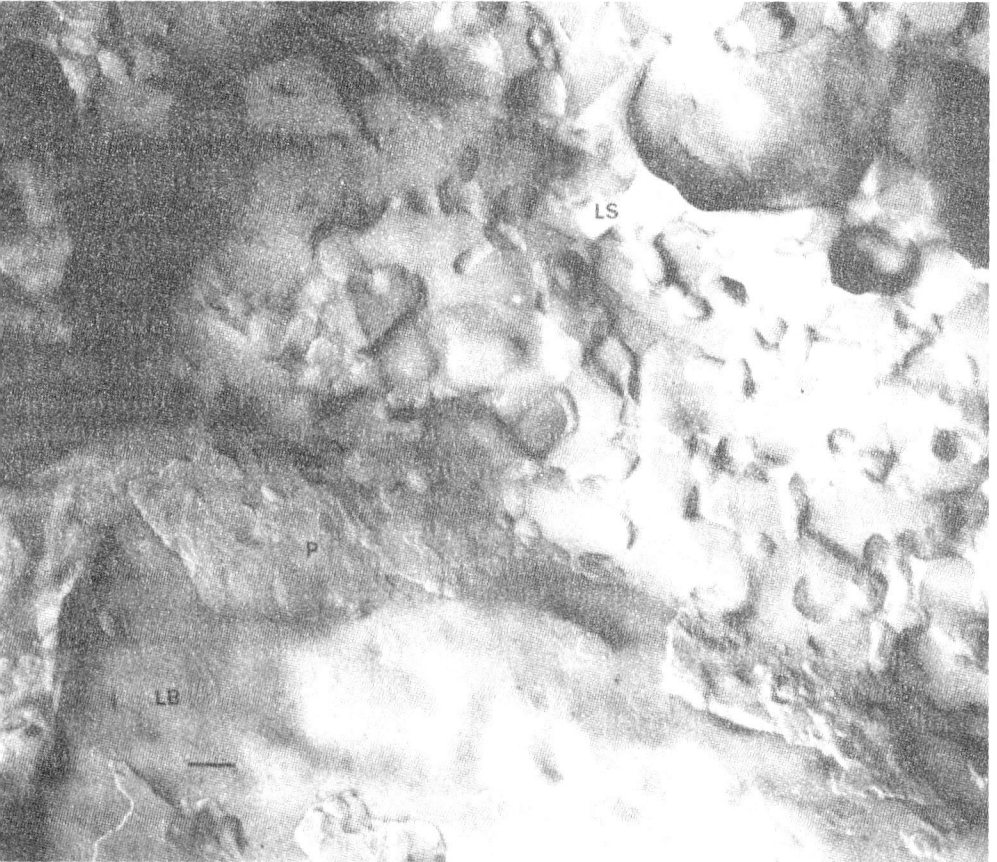

Fig. 7. A micrograph of the interface between NAT 50 liposomal suspension and stratum corneum. The fusion between the vesicles which occurs at the interface is clearly depicted (P). The scale bar represents 100 nm.

(1) The measurements were performed after rinsing the stratum corneum. It is possible that during the rinsing process the lipid bilayers formed at the interface as is shown by FFEM were "dissolved" in the excess PBS.

(2) The repeat distance between the bilayers is not very well defined. This will not result in a scattering curve with very clearly detectable diffraction peaks.

(3) Using SAXS bulk changes in the structure are detected, while using electron microscopy local changes can be detected. It is possible that the amount of material at the interface is to small to be detected using SAXS.

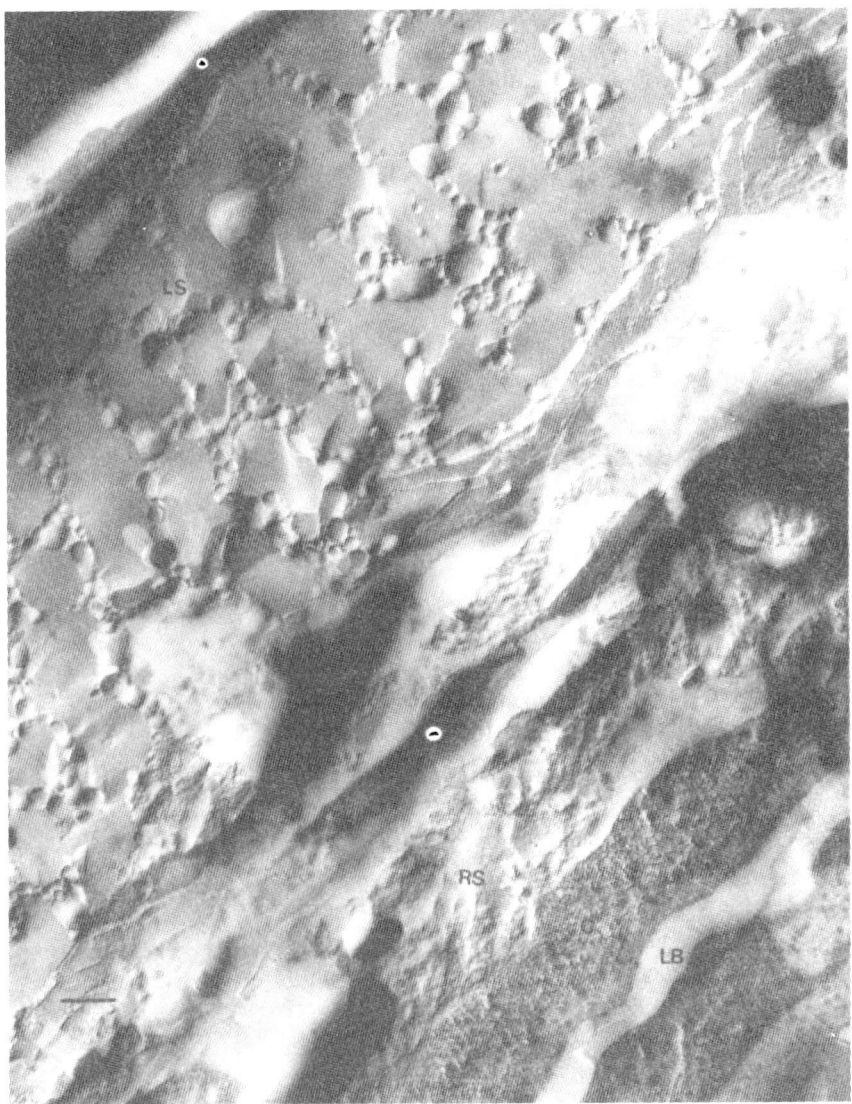

Fig. 8. Stratum corneum incubated with NAT 89 liposomes (LS). The liposomes tend to adsorb at the interface. Fusion into rough structures (RS) occurs. Lipid bilayer regions are depicted deeper in the stratum corneum. The scale bar represents 100 nm.

In Fig. 8 the influence of liposomes prepared from NAT 89 lipids on the structure of the stratum corneum is shown. In the upper left-hand corner of the micrograph the liposome suspension is visualized, while in the lower right-hand corner a cross-section

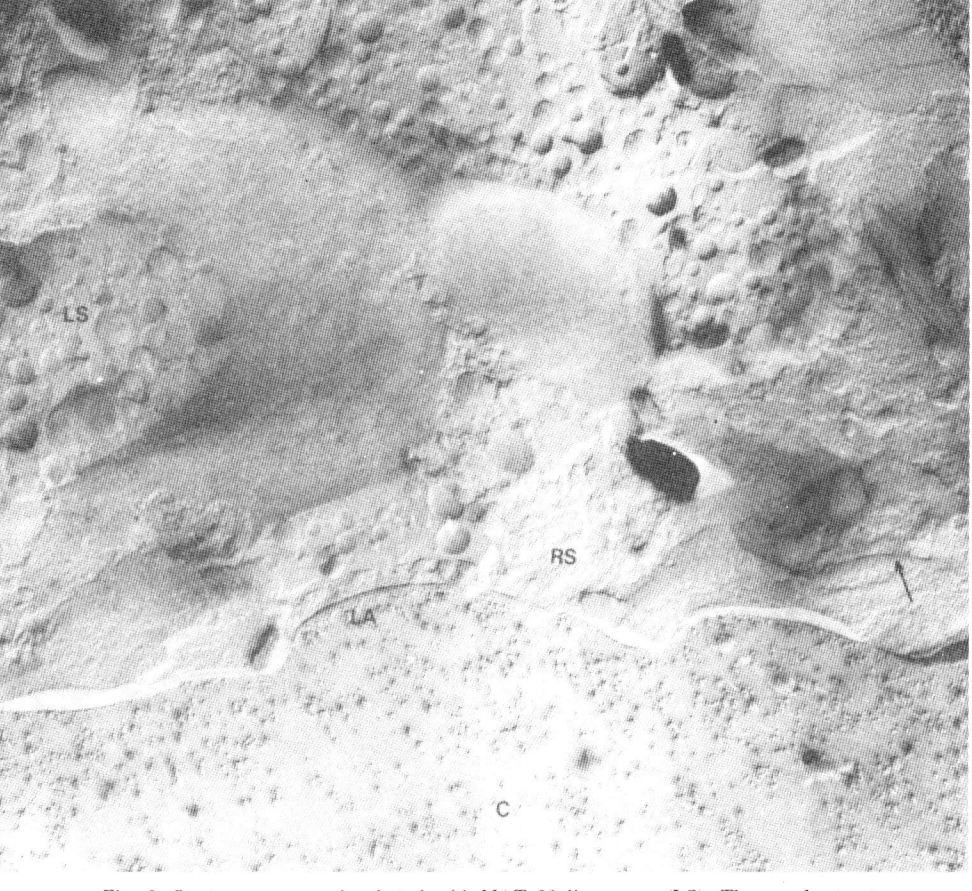

Fig. 9. Stratum corneum incubated with NAT 89 liposomes (LS). The rough structures sometimes exhibit a layered structure (see arrow). The linear arrays of keratin filaments are still present. No structural changes in the corneocytes could be found.

through the stratum corneum is shown. The NAT 89 liposomes stick at the interface between suspension and stratum corneum. It seems that vesicles fuse, resulting in rough structures. These rough structures also depict edges, but these are less sharp and less defined than in the case of the lipid lamellar structure of the stratum corneum (see arrow in Fig. 9). Rough structures are also shown in deeper layers of the stratum corneum up to the fourth cell layer (see Fig. 10), which is approximately 2 µm deep, but these are smoother than those close to the interface. The rough structures may be caused either by alteration of the lipid bilayer structure present in the stratum corneum or by a lipid structure formed by fusion of lipids mainly originating from the vesicles. Strong changes in the lipid structure of the stratum corneum has been shown also in previous studies (Bodde *et al.*, 1988). Treatment of stratum corneum with a cream in a hexagonal mesophase resulted in hexagonal structures in the intercellular region of the stratum corneum. The additional diffraction peak(s) in the scattering curve of human stratum corneum after treatment with NAT 89 liposomes may be correlated with the rough lipid structures found by FFEM. This could explain the presence of the additional diffraction peaks even after rinsing with PBS, since the rough structures are present in deeper layers of the stratum corneum. NAT 89 liposomes did not induce changes in the structure of the corneocytes. The linear arrays of keratin filaments are clearly depicted in Figs 8–10.

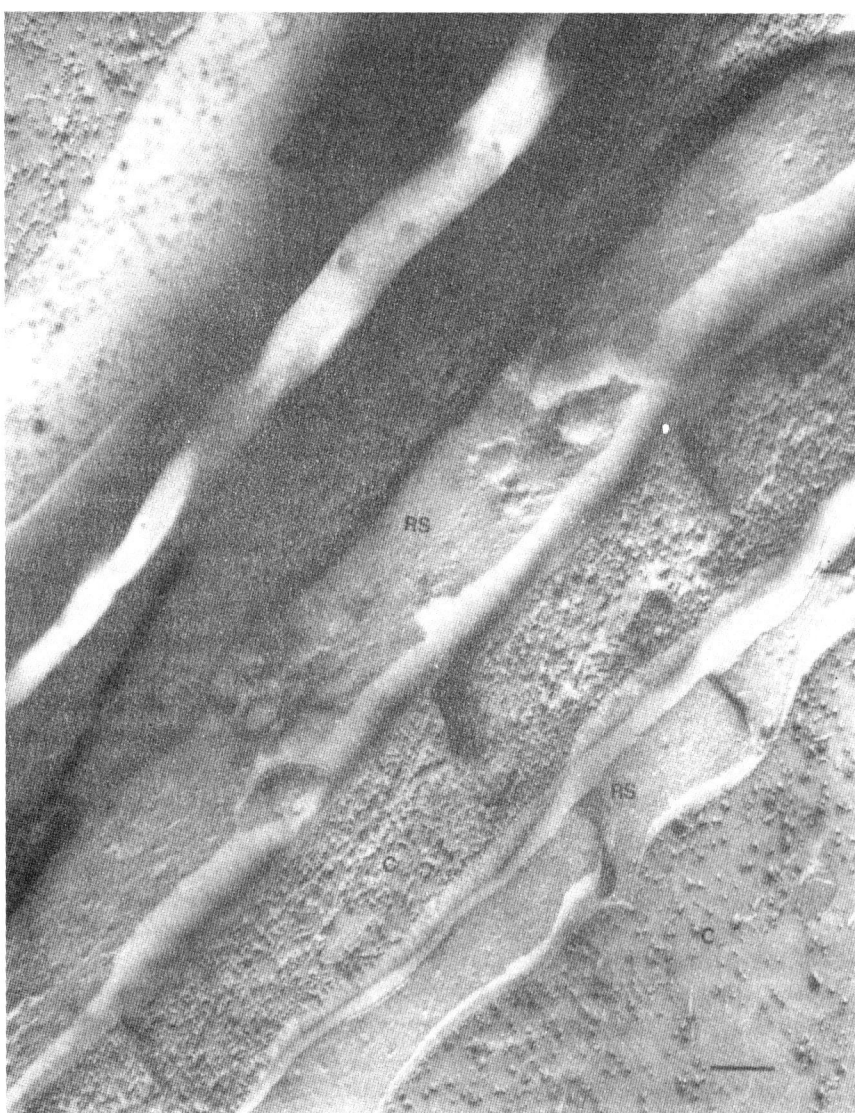

Fig. 10. Stratum corneum incubated with NAT 89 liposomes. The rough structures (RS) are also found in deeper layers of the stratum corneum.

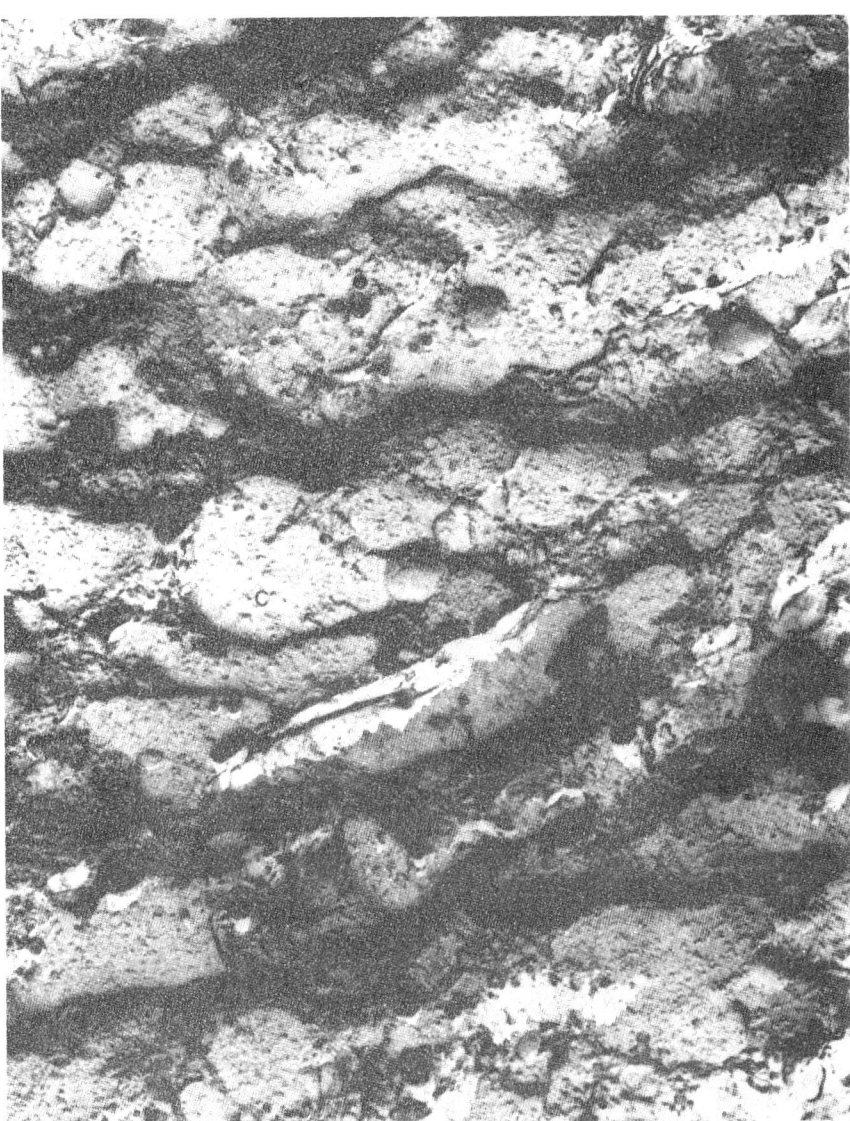

Fig. 11. (a) NAT 106 liposomes have a very strong effect on the microstructure of the stratum corneum. Te corneocytes (C) were swollen considerably and the smooth ultrastructure of the intercellular lipid bilayers showed flattened spherical structures (FS). These flattened spherical structures are not always completely circular. The linearly arranged keratin filaments along the plasma membrane completely disappeared. The scale bar represent 100 μm.

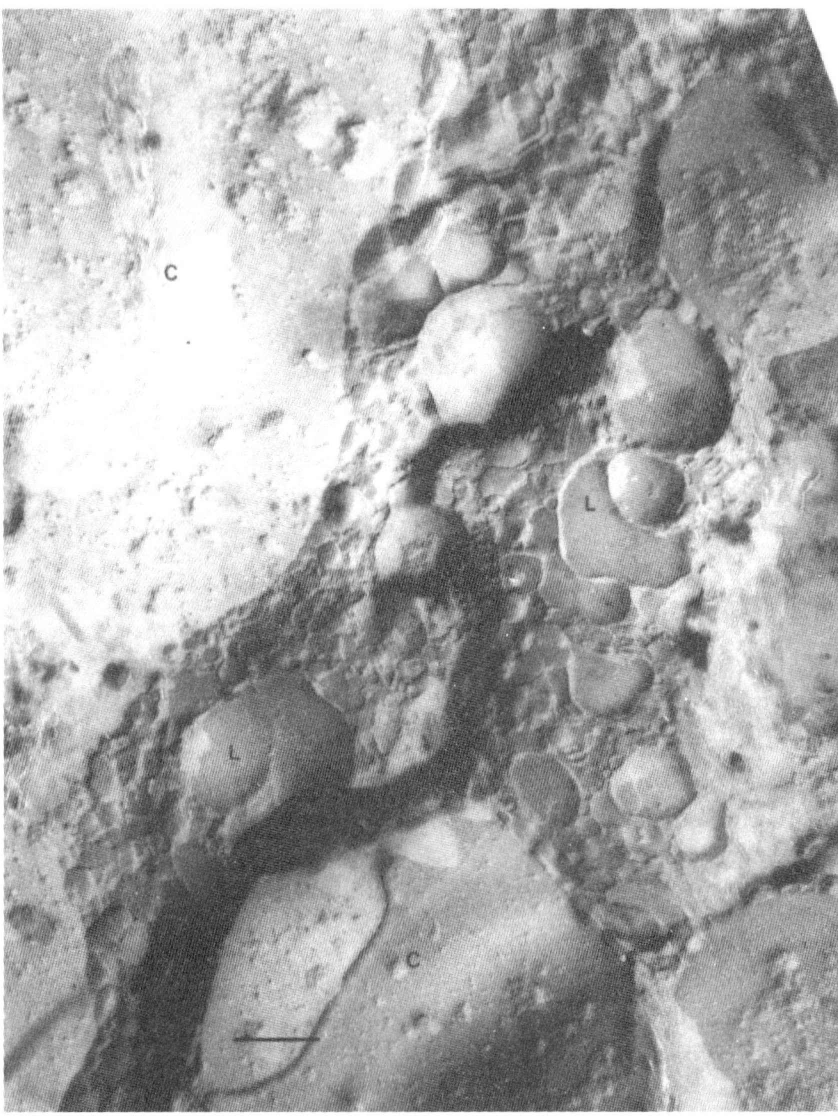

Fig. 11. (b) A higher magnification photograph of the structure of human stratum corneum after incubation with NAT 106 liposomes. Flattened spherical (L) structures are clearly depicted. The corneocytes (C) are considerably swollen. The scale bar represents 100 nm.

The NAT 106 liposomes had a very strong interaction with the stratum corneum (see Fig. 11). After 48 h of incubation the corneocytes were swollen considerably compared with the control skin. Note that the linearly arranged keratin filaments along the plasma membranes of the corneocytes are absent. The ultrastructure of the intercellular lipid bilayers showed flattened spherical structures. The diameter of the flattened structures varied between 10 and 200 nm. The small structures are not all spherical. Their fracture pattern indicates that these are multilamellar. Although the presence of these spherical structures might indicate the presence of intact liposomes in the stratum corneum, a more likely explanation involves diffusion of lipids molecularly dispersed in the lipid matrix in the stratum corneum causing a change of its structure. These changes in structure were observed in very large regions of the replica, but because the interface could not be visualized it is not known to what depth the intercellular lipid structure was modified.

CONCLUSION

There is a strong indication that the degree of interaction between vesicular dispersions and skin mainly depends on physicochemical properties of the compounds of which the liposomes are composed. The interaction is most likely to be dependent on both the size and the mean number of bilayers of the liposomes. Although the different types of liposomes had comparable sizes, lamellarity and alkyl chain length, the compositional differences between the vesicles were very complex. Therefore it is difficult to draw conclusions on the effect of each of the phospholipids on the interactions between vesicles and stratum corneum from these experiments. From the results obtained in this study it is obvious that the interactions between liposomes and skin depend to a large extent on the composition of the vesicles. The interactions can be limited to only the interface (NAT 50 liposomes), but the changes in the lipid structure can also be extended to deeper layers of the stratum corneum (NAT 89 and NAT 106 liposomes).

ACKNOWLEDGEMENTS

We thank the Nederlandse Organisatie voor Wetenschappelijk Onderzoek (NWO) and Nattermann Phospholipids GmbH (Cologne, Germany) for financial support. We thank Nattermann Phospholipids GmbH for supply of the phospholipids. The very helpful assistance of the station scientist Dr W. Bras during the SAXS measurements is acknowledged.

REFERENCES

Boddé, H. E., Holman, B. P., Brussee, J. and Spies, F. (1988) Effect of pharmaceutical preparations on human skin: an ultrastructural *in vitro* study using freeze fracture electron microscopy. *Proc. Int. Symp. Control. Release. Bioact. Mater.* **15** 276–277.

Bouwstra, J. A., Gooris, G. S., van der Spek, J. A. and Bras, W. (1991) Structural investigations of human stratum corneum by small angle X-ray scattering. *J. Invest. Dermatol.* **97** 1005–1012.

Bouwstra, J. A., Gooris, G. S., de Vries, M. A., van der Spek, J. A. and Bras, W. (1992a) The structure of human stratum corneum. A wide angle X-ray study. *Int. J. Pharm.* in press.

Bouwstra, J. A., Gooris, G. S. and Bras, W. (1992b) New aspects on the structure of the skin barrier. In: Gurny, R. (ed.) Wissenschaftliche Verlagsgesellschaft, Stuttgart, in press.

Cevc, G. and Blume, G. (1991) Lipid vesicles penetrate into intact skin owing the transdermal osmotic gradients and hydration. Submitted to *FEBS Lett.*

Ganesan, M. G., Weiner, N. D., Flynn, G. L. and Ho, N. F. H. (1984) Influence of liposomal drug entrapment on percutaneous absorption. *Int. J. Pharm.* **20** 139–154.

Garson, J. C., Doucet, J., Tsoucaris, G. and Leveque, J. L. (1990) Study of lipid and non-lipid structure in human stratum corneum by X-ray diffraction. *J. Soc. Cosmet. Chem.* **41** 347–358.

Gehring, W., Ghyczy, M., Gloor, M., Hertzler, Ch. and Rêdoing, J. (1990) Significance of empty liposomes alone and as drug carriers in dermatology. *Arzneim.-Forsch. Drug Res.* **40** 1368–1371.

Hadgraft, J. and Guy, R. H. (eds) (1989) *Transdermal Drug Delivery.* Dekker, New York.

Hager, J., Ghyczy, M., Feyen, V., Ingberge, P., Brandenburg, U. and Wilperath, P. (1989) *US Patent 4,874,552.*

Hofland, H. E. J., Bouwstra, J. A., Ponec, M., Bodde, H. E., Spies, F. and Junginger, H. E. (1991) Interactions of non-ionic surfactant vesicles with cultured keratinocytes and human skin *in vitro:* a survey of toxicological aspects and ultrastructural changes in stratum corneum, *J. Control. Release* **16** 155–168.

Hofland, H. E. J., Bouwstra, J. A., Bodde, H. E., Spies, F. and Junginger, H. E. (1992) Interactions between liposomes and human skin. Submitted to *Br. J. Dermatol.*

Holman, B. P., Spies, F. and Bodde, H. E. (1990) An optimized freeze-fracture replication procedure for human skin. *J. Invest. Dermatol.* **94** 332–335.

Jacobs, M., Martin, G. P. and Marriott, C. (1988) Effects of phosphatidylcholine on the topical bioavailability of corticosteroids assessed by human skin blanching assay. *J. Pharm. Pharmacol.* **40** 829–833.

Jousma, H., Talsma, H., Spies, F., Joosten, J. G. H., Junginger, H. E. and Crommelin, D. J. A. (1987) Characterization of liposomes. *Int. J. Pharm.* **35** 263–274.

Knepp, V. M., Hinz, R. S., Szoka, F. C. and Guy, R. H. (1988) Controlled drug release from a novel liposomal drug delivery system. I. Investigation of transdermal potential. *J. Control. Release* **10** 211–221.

Knepp, V. M., Szoka, F. C. and Guy, R. H. (1990) Controlled drug release from a novel liposomal delivery system. II. Transdermal delivery characteristics. *J. Control. Release* **12** 25–30.

Komatsu, H., Higaki, K., Okamoto, H., Miyagawa, K., Hashida, M. and Sezaki, H. (1986a) Preservative activity and *in vivo* percutaneous penetration of butyl paraben entrapped liposomes. *Chem. Pharm. Bull.* **34** 3415–3422.

Komatsu, H., Okamoto, H., Miyagawa, K., Hashida, M. and Sezaki, H. (1986b) Percutaneous absorption of butyl paraben *in vitro. Chem. Pharm. Bull.* **34** 3423–3430.

Lasch, J. and Wohlrab, W. (1986) Liposome bound cortisol. A new approach to cutaneous therapy. *Biomed. Biochem. Acta* **45** 1295–1299.

Mezei, M. and Gulasekharem, V. (1980) Liposomes — a selective drug delivery system for the topical route of administration. *Life Sci.* **26** 1473–1477.

Michel, Ch., Purmann, Th., Mentrup, E., Michel, G. and Kreuter, J. (1991) Topical application of an antiphlogistic drug in liposomes. *Proc. Int. Symp. Control. Release Bioact. Mater.* **18** 485–486.

Schäfer-Korting, M., Korting, H. C. and Braun-Falco, O. (1989) Liposome preparations: a step forward in topical drug therapy for skin disease? *J. Am. Acad. Dermatol.* **21** 1271–1275.

Weiner, N., Williams, N., Birch, G., Ramachandran, C., Shipman, C. and Flynn, G. (1989) Topical delivery of liposomally encapsulated interferon evaluated in cutaneous herpes guinea pig model, *Antimicrob. Agents Chem. Ther.* **33** 1217–1221.

Wohlrab, W. and Lasch, J. (1987) Penetration kinetics of liposomal cortison in human skin, *Dermatologica* **174** 18–22.

Part V
Nasal route

16

Nasal membranes — structure and permeability

William A. Lee and Patricia A. Baldwin

INTRODUCTION

The human nose functions as a heater and humidifier of inspired air, a filter against airborne particulates, a chemical sensor for environmental irritants, and as the principal organ of olfaction. The specialized anatomy and physiology of the naval cavity and its ready accessibility make the nasal cavity a particularly attractive delivery site for the systemic administration of drugs. Like other epithelia, the permeability of the nasal epithelium to drug molecules varies greatly depending on the chemical and physical properties of the drug. For those molecules which do not readily cross the nasal membrane, such as biopharmaceuticals, a number of strategies have been explored to increase the nasal membrane permeability. In this chapter, the structure of the nasal epithelium will be reviewed with a focus on the barrier properties of the nasal membrane. In addition, the strategies which have been designed to increase mucosal permeability will be examined and results from our laboratory describing one such approach will be detailed.

NASAL MEMBRANE STRUCTURE

The nasal cavity is located posterior to the external vestibule of the nose and is lined with three types of epithelia: (1) squamous, (2) respiratory and (3) olfactory. The squamous epithelium is found lining the nostrils and in the anterior portion of the cavity up to and partially covering the turbinates. In humans, the respiratory epithelium covers the majority of the nasal cavity. The olfactory epithelium represents approximately 5% of the epithelial tissue and is located in the dorsal portion of the cavity. The architecture and the location of the different epithelia in the human nose are shown in Fig. 1. The percentage of each epithelia type varies from species to species; largely dependant on the degree to which a species relies on olfaction (Sch∴ ∋ider, 1986).

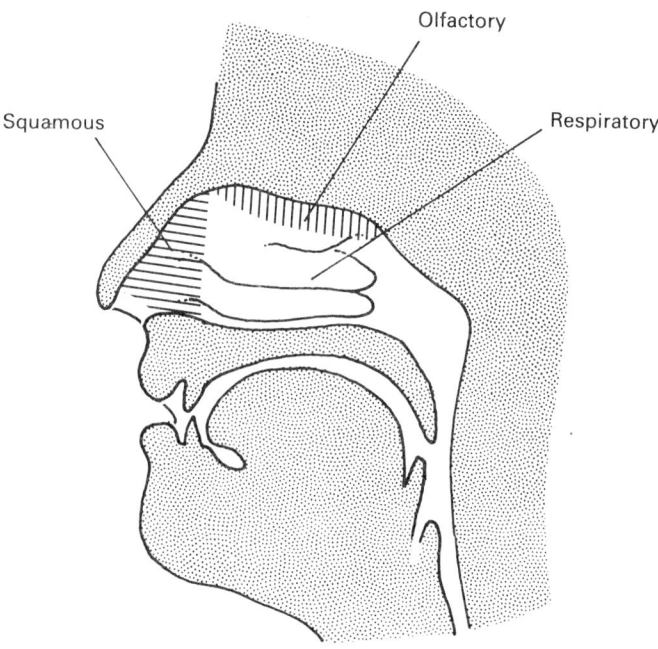

Fig. 1. Locations of the different types of epithelia in the nose.

The respiratory epithelium is a mucous membrane and as such serves as an interfacial exchange surface between the body cavity and the environment. It is also the primary site of drug deposition and absorption after intranasal administration. The respiratory mucosa has much in common with the other mucosal membranes of the body, especially with regard to cell types. Histologically the nasal mucosa is a pseudo-stratified epithelium consisting of up to 6 major cell types, (in man only 4 cell types have been identified) (Popp *et al.*, 1986). In the anterior third of the mucosa, the cell types found are mostly non-ciliated columnar and goblet cells. There is a smooth transition to a more ciliated epithelium in the middle region and in the posterior third, the entire mucosa appears to be covered by cilia. Scanning electron micrographs of the two latter sections are shown in Fig. 2. Hidden among the ciliated columnar cells in the posterior region of the turbinates are mucus-secreting goblet cells. These specialized cells along with submucosal glands are responsible for covering the epithelial surface with a blanket of mucus. The synchronized motion of the cilia results in the constant transport of this surface layer of mucus towards the posterior of the nasal cavity, removing with it any trapped particulate matter. Fig. 3 is a light micrograph of a cross-section of the rat nasal septum showing a thick clear mucous layer coating the apical cell surfaces. The cells in the epithelial layer containing this non-staining clear fluid are goblet cells filled with mucus.

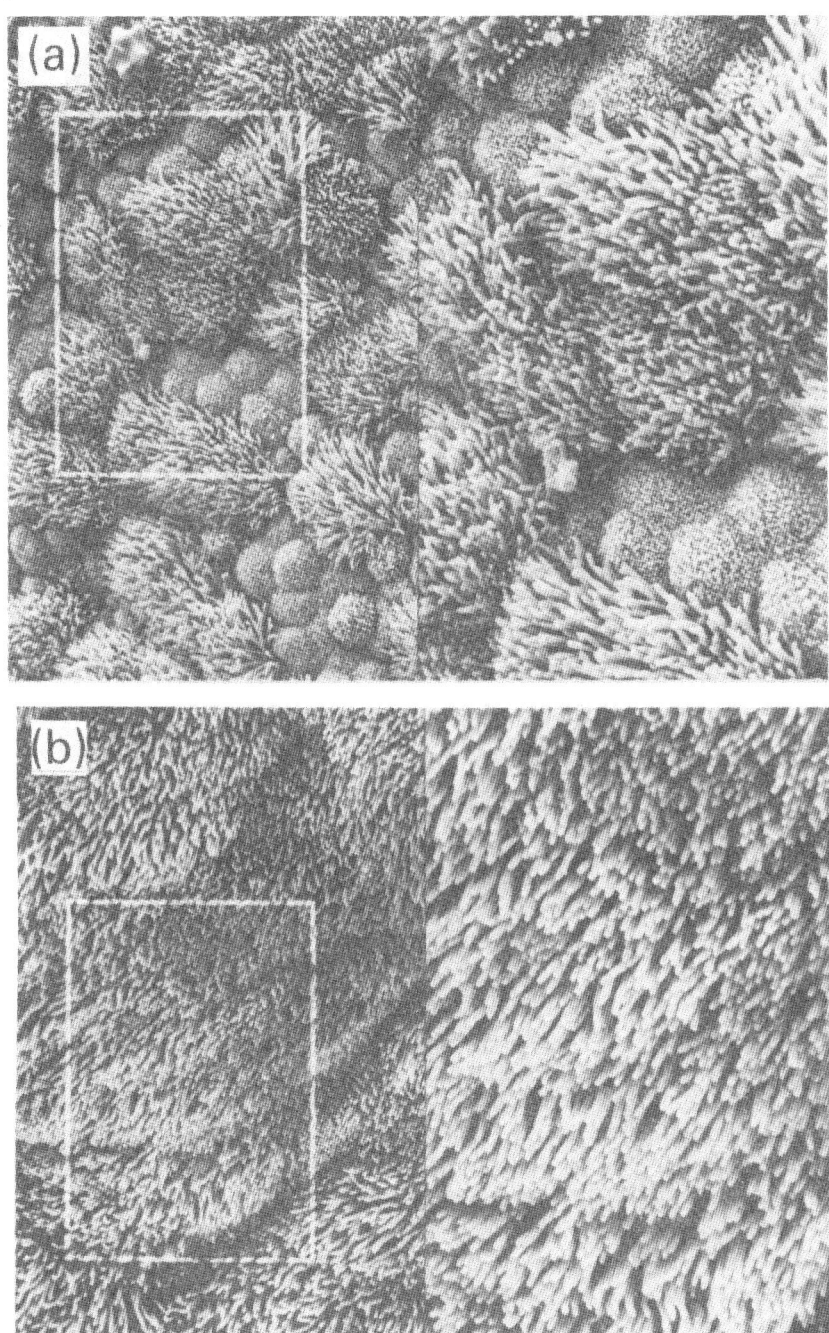

Fig. 2. Scanning electron micrographs of nasal mucosa: (a) middle turbinates; (b) posterior turbinates.

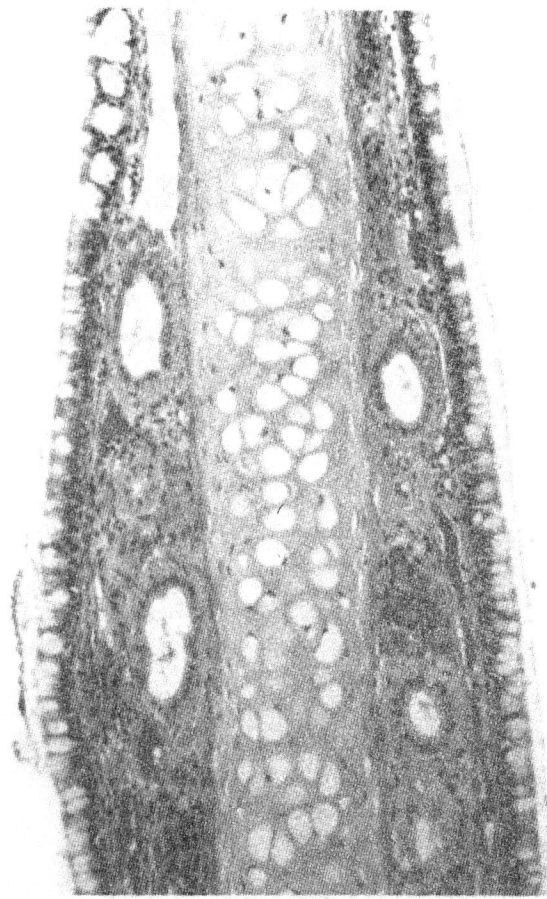

Fig. 3. Light micrograph of a cross-section of the nasal mucosa.

In order to reach the systemic circulation, there are numerous barriers a drug must cross. After administration as a nebulized spray or as large droplets, the majority of the drug is deposited in the anterior portion of the mucosa. The clearance of a spray from the site of deposition is retarded relative to an instilled liquid, resulting in a greater contact time with the mucosa.(Hardy et al., 1984). The drug first comes into contact with the mucous layer which varies between 5 and 20 µm in depth (Fig. 3). Mucus is a viscoelastic material composed of hydrated mucin glycoproteins consisting of a single polypeptide chain with multiple branched carbohydrate chains (50–80% carbohydrate). Major portions of the carbohydrate are negatively charged because of terminal sialic acid residues or sulphonated residues of the oligosaccharide chains. Individual glycoproteins are covalently bonded through disulphide linkages between the protein cores to increase further the viscosity and gelling properties of the mucus (Allen, 1978). Linear association of these glycoproteins can result in molecular weights as high as 20 000 000 Da (Marriott, 1987). The mucus layer acts both as a physical barrier to entrap inspired particulates and as a medium to maintain hydration at the epithelial surface. The coordinated ciliary movement at the epithelial surface results in the net transport of mucus from the anterior to the posterior nasal cavity and down the oesophagus, with a net turnover time for mucus in the nasal cavity between 10 and 15 min. Drugs delivered in a solution or as powders must rapidly dissolve in the mucous layer and diffuse through the mucous layer before reaching the epithelium. Although mucus acts as a physical barrier to bulk water transport, diffusion of smaller molecules through the mucus is not significantly slowed. Radomsky et al. (1990), using mid-cycle mucus, have shown that the diffusion rate of fluorescein (MW ~300 Da) is the same in mucus as in unstirred water, $D_m/D_w > 0.9$. For bovine serum albumin (MW ~68 000 Da) the ratio of D_m/D_w is 0.86; however, for IgG (MW ~146 000 Da) the ratio drops to 0.32 (Radomsky et al., 1990). The authors suggest that IgG is being impeded by the limited pore radius (10–100 nm) of the mucin lattice. The net negative charge on the glycoproteins of the mucous layer can also act as a selective ion exchange medium, thus slowing the diffusion of positively charged drug molecules. Lee and Nichols (1987) have utilized a diffusion chamber to study the diffusion of potassium ions through a neutral starch gel and negatively charged pig gastric mucus. Diffusion through the gastric mucus was significantly slower than through the starch gel (D_m/D_s = 0.58). Reducing the negative charge of the gastric mucus by treatment with N-acetylneuraminidase resulted in less diffusional retardation reactive to the untreated mucus.For larger proteins with basic isoelectric points, the combination of size and electrostatic interactions will result in significant diffusional impedance through nasal mucus. An additional barrier is presented by the apical membranes of the epithelial membrane which are covered with a layer of negatively charged membrane-bound glycoproteins and glycolipids which together constitute the glycocalyx. Electrostatic interactions between drug and glycocalyx can further retard the absorption of positively charged molecules. In addition to glycoproteins, mucus contains a number of proteins, including albumin, immunoglobulins and lysozyme (Widdicombe and Wells 1982). Albumin concentration can be as high as 10 mg/ml and the non-specific binding of a drug to albumin can prevent or inhibit penetration through the mucosa. As noted above, the mucus layer is subject to continuous clearance by the action of the cilia and thus, diffusional or other retardation (e.g. binding to albumin) will increase drug clearance from the mucosal surface and therefore lower the drug available for systemic delivery.

After the mucous layer, the lipophilic plasma membrane presents the next barrier to drug absorption. The plasma membrane functions specifically to restrict the unregulated diffusion of hydrophilic molecules in and out of the cells. Furthermore, enzymes associated with the plasma membrane surface or in the cytoplasm have been shown to significantly degrade peptide drugs (Hussain et al., 1990; Stratford and Lee, 1986). Transport across the plasma membrane, irrespective of the mechanism, results in the cytoplasmic localization of the drug. To reach the systemic circulation the drug must then survive the intracellular environment and diffuse out through the basolateral membrane to the subepithelial space. An alternative route of entry to this subepithelial region is via diffusion through the intercellular spaces. Inhibiting this diffusional pathway are contiguous interlocking proteins found at the apical cellular junctions. These belt like proteins constitute the tight junctions or zonula occludens which are responsible for the separation of the apical and basolateral plasma membrane. They also act as a barrier to diffusion in and out of the submucosa. Under normal resting conditions the tight junctions are very impermeable (150–300 Ω/cm^2); however, with chronic exposure to tobacco smoke or allergic rhinitis, the junctions can become leaky (Inagaki et al., 1985). It has recently become clear that the tight junctions are not static barriers, but instead they are dynamic and can be regulated by intracellular messengers such as cAMP (Madara, 1988). It has been shown that in the intestinal mucosa, water-facilitated diffusion of glucose through the tight junctions may account for greater than 50% of the glucose absorbed by the body (Pappenheimer and Zeiss, 1987). Once a drug reaches the subepithelial space, either by diffusion out of the epithelial cell via the basolateral membrane or by diffusion through the tight junctions, there are few if any significant barriers to cross before reaching the nasal vasculature. The submucosal space is a loose network of connective tissue that presents little diffusional resistance. Likewise, the vasculature of the nose is highly permeable. Watanabe et al. (1980) have demonstrated that, after 10 s, horseradish (HRP) injected intravenously into the tail vein of rats was found in the pericapillary spaces of the nasal mucosa. The high permeability of the nasal vasculature is due to the loose endothelial cell junctions and the highly fenestrated nature of the capillaries similar to those found in liver sinusoid. For the majority of drugs administered to the nose, it is the epithelial membrane which is the primary barrier to systemic absorption.

DRUG PERMEABILITY

Despite the interest in the nose as a delivery site for systemic administration, relatively few intranasal products on the market today are intended for this purpose. The majority of the nasal products available are intended for topical administration to the nasal cavity (e.g. antihistamines, vasoconstrictors) and little work has been published describing the systemic levels of these drugs after intranasal application. In animal and in vitro models, the permeability of the nasal mucosa to a large number of small organic drugs has been extensively studied. Much of this work has previously been reviewed (Chien and Chang, 1985).

When comparing intranasal data, the characteristics and limitations of each model must be considered. Using an in situ rat perfusion model, Gibson and Olanoff (1987), determined that the initial absorption rate constants for alkaloid acids were dependent on the ionization state of the acid moiety. The maximal absorption rate constant was at the pH equivalent to the pK_a value of the acids (~4.8), dropping off at higher and lower pH. Also interesting was the finding that the acyl chain length did not significantly affect the permeability, suggesting that simple oil–water partitioning behaviour does not explain the penetration of fatty acids through the nasal mucosa. In the same study, the rate of absorption for hydrocortisone and progesterone was also evaluated. The rate constant for absorption was shown to be a linear function of the logarithm of the partition coefficient (PC), indicating that for these steroids a simple partition mechanism does account for the absorption process. However, using an in vivo rabbit model, Corbo et al. (1989) showed that the bioavailability for progesterone and its hydroxy derivatives did not correlate with the log PC. The bioavailability, however, did correlate with the nasal mucosa partition coefficients by incubating the steroid solutions with 20 mg sections of rabbit nasal mucosa. This led the authors to conclude that nasal absorption of small molecules was not a simple partition phenomena and that multiple *in vivo* factors influence the rate and extent of nasal absorption. McMartin and coworkers have attempted the noble task of correlating the intranasal bioavailability with molecular weight, charge, hydrophobicity, and susceptibility to amino peptidase for 25 small organic, peptide and protein drugs (McMartin *et al.*, 1987). As can be expected, the data show a high degree of scatter; however, there does appear to be a correlation with molecular weight, and perhaps a weaker correlation with charge and polarity.

Because of their hydrophilic nature, high charge density and large molecular weights, peptides and proteins would not be expected to have good permeability across the nasal membrane. Lee and Longenecker (1988) have summarized the bioavailabilities of a series of peptide and protein molecules and with few exceptions the data show a clear drop in bioavailability with increasing molecular weight. Above 10 amino acids the bioavailability is generally less than 1%. Despite the low bioavailability of peptide drugs, there are a number of intranasal peptide products on the market intended for systemic delivery (Table 1). The lack of alternatives to parenteral administration, the high therapeutic indices, and the low costs of goods make the intranasal route an acceptable alternative for these peptides. In the case of protein therapeutics which generally have even lower bioavailability, this is not the case.

Table 1. Intranasal peptide products for systemic administration on the world market

Product	Drug	Number of amino acids
Syntocinon	Oxytocin	9
DDAVP	Desmopressin	9
Diapid	Lypressin	9
Suprefact	Buserelin	9
Synarel	Nafrelin	10
Miacalcic	Salmon calcitonin	32
Turbocalcin	Elcatonin	32

PERMEATION ENHANCEMENT

Three principal strategies have evolved to overcome the low permeability of macromolecules across the nasal mucosa: (1) increase residence time of the drug in the nasal mucosa, (2) increase blood flow to the nasal mucosa, and (3) modify drug-membrane characteristics with surfactants. Each of these strategies relies on the inclusion of an agent(s) in the drug formulation to effect net drug transport across the mucosa.

Many investigators have studied the possibility of increasing net drug transport across the nasal mucosa by increasing the residence time of the drug on the mucosa. This strategy is valid if the clearance rate of the mucus from the cavity is rate determining. Morimoto *et al.* (1985) used polyacrylic acid to increase the viscosity of an intranasal calcitonin formulation and reported an increase in bioavailability in rats relative to a simple aqueous formulation. Using solid mixtures of insulin and crystalline cellulose, hydroxypropyl cellulose, or carbopol 934, Nagai *et al.* (1984) showed enhanced absorption in dogs and they attributed this to both the improved dispersion of insulin and the gelling of the solids in the nasal cavity. Using a similar strategy, Vickery *et al.* (1989) showed that larger molecular weight dextrans can similarly increase nafrelin bioavailability in monkeys. The most well-characterized system, introduced by Illum, uses degradable starch microspheres coated with drug (Illum *et al.*, 1987). These microspheres are known to swell in contact with the mucosa, are bioadhesive, and remain in the cavity for up to 3 hours, thus increasing the probability of drug transport during this time. Bjørk and Edman (1988) have used starch microspheres in combination with insulin and reported a bioavailability of ~30% in rats. The insulin peak concentration in serum was reached after 8 min and glucose was reduced maximally between 30 and 40 min. The increase in bioavailability using the starch microspheres is impressive; however, the rationale based on an increase in drug residence time on the mucosa is seemingly flawed. Alternatively, the rapid T_{max} and clearance observed suggest that the microspheres are inducing a permeability effect that involves active chemical interaction with the mucosa and is independent of residence time of the microsphere.

Olanoff and coworkers have employed 'physiological modifiers' in intranasal formulations to increase mucosal blood flow. In principal, increased blood flow could increase the concentration gradient across the mucosa and thus result in higher bioavailabilities for those drugs which can already cross the epithelial barrier. Using histamine as a physiologic modifier, Olanoff *et al.* (1987) examined both nasal blood flow and urine osmolarity after intranasal administration of desmopressin in healthy volunteers. Nasal blood flow did show a histamine dose dependence, but the effect on urine osmolarity after desmopressin administration was slight. This suggests that increased blood flow alone is not sufficient to increase mucosal permeability dramatically for peptide drugs which are poorly transported across the epithelial barrier.

The most widely employed strategy for enhancing mucosal permeability is the co-administration of surfactants to modify the drug and/or membrane properties. Hirai *et al.* (1981) pioneered this strategy by examining the effects of the non-ionic ether and ester, anionic, and amphoteric surfactants on the intranasal absorption of insulin. They found that many types of surfactants of differing structural types enhance absorption; however, in many cases the degree of enhancement was roughly correlated to damage to the mucosa. A notable exception was the bile salts which showed good enhancing properties with little correlation to membrane erosion or red blood cells lysis. In the 1980s clinical studies were published using bile salts as permeation enhancers (Frauman *et al.*, 1987; Pontiroli *et al.*, 1985, 1989). Gordon (1985) examined the ability of eight different bile salts to increase insulin absorption in forty normal subjects. The greatest enhancement was observed for those bile salts whose nucleus contained two hydroxyl substitutions. Conjugation of a taurine or glycine group to the free acid of deoxycholate appeared to decrease irritation caused by the bile salt without decreasing bioavailability. Those results suggest that irritation and/or mucosal damage can be separated from permeation enhancement. This has led to the exploration of a variety of other surfactant molecules as potential permeation enhancers.

In our laboratory we have extensively examined the molecule sodium tauro-24,25-dihydrofusidate (STDHF) as a potential permeation enhancer for intranasal administration of protein and peptide drugs (Longenecker et al., 1987; Baldwin et al., 1990; Lee et al., 1991). STDHF is a steroidal surfactant and is structurally related to bile salts. Like the bile salts, STDHF aggregates above a certain concentration (CMC) to form micelles. STDHF was selected as a permeation enhancer based on efficacy, wide protein compatibility, and preliminary safety data.

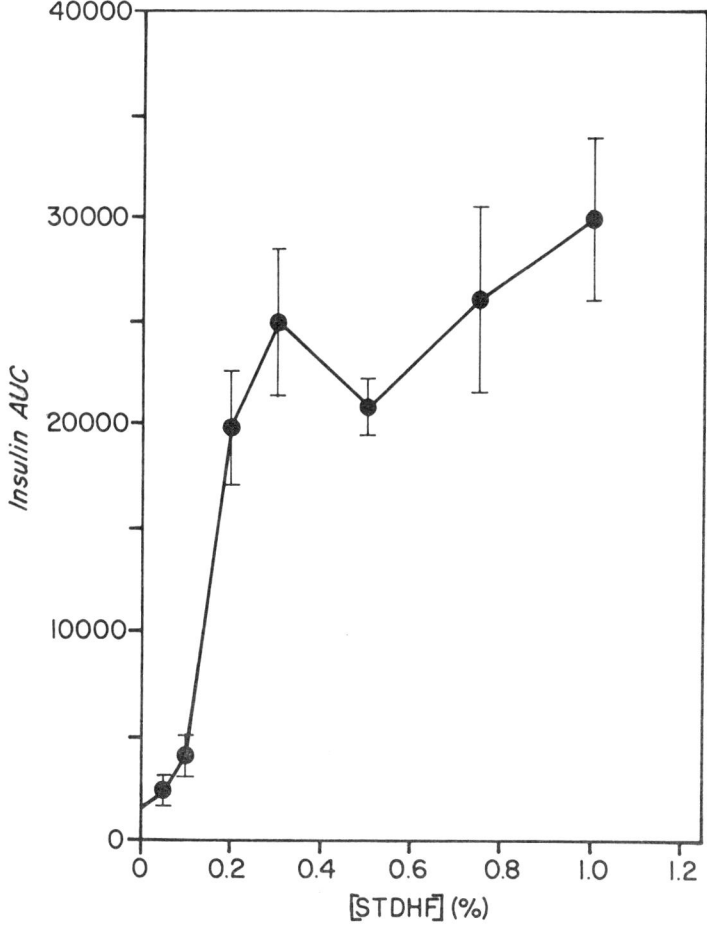

Fig. 4. Area under the plasma insulin concentration vs time curve (AUC) as a function of STDHF concentration.

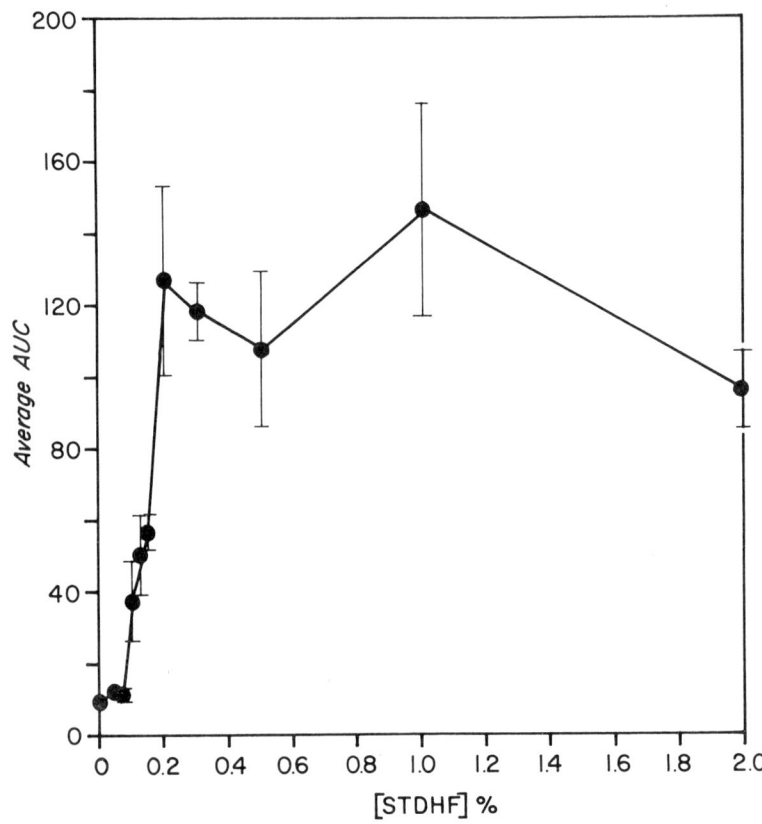

Fig. 5. Area under the plasma FITC-dextran concentration vs time curve (AUC) as a function of STDHF concentration.

Table 2. The effect of FITC-dextran molecular weight on bioavailability in the rat

Molecular weight (daltons)	Bioavailability (%)	
	Without STDHF	With STDHF
4000	2	72
10000	3	47
20000	1	18
40000	<1	4
70000	<1	1

The absorption of macromolecules including FITC-labelled dextrans shows a marked dependence on STDHF concentration. In Figs 4 and 5, the areas under the serum concentration vs time curves are plotted against STDHF concentration for human insulin and a 20 000 Da FITC- labelled dextran. In both cases, the data show a steep rise in AUC values starting at concentrations slightly below the CMC of STDHF (~0.16%) to concentrations above the CMC. Above 0.3% STDHF the AUC values do not increase significantly. Since the monomer concentration is constant above the CMC value and only the number of micelles increases, we conclude the concentration of monomer species is an important variable in the enhancement mechanism. Micelles may play a secondary role in helping to solubilize drug or as a reservoir for monomers.

The effect of molecular size on the permeability of the mucosa in the presence of STDHF has been studied using FITC- labelled dextrans. Table 2 lists the percent bioavailability of FITC- dextrans after intranasal administration with and without 1% STDHF in the rat model. For the 4000 Da dextran, bioavailability is greater than 70% in the presence of STDHF. Above 40 000 Da, the bioavailability is less than 5% even in the presence of STDHF. Because of its expanded structure, a 40 000 Da dextran occupies a volume far larger than a protein of the same molecular weight and thus the size exclusion limit for proteins is expected to exceed 40 000 Da.

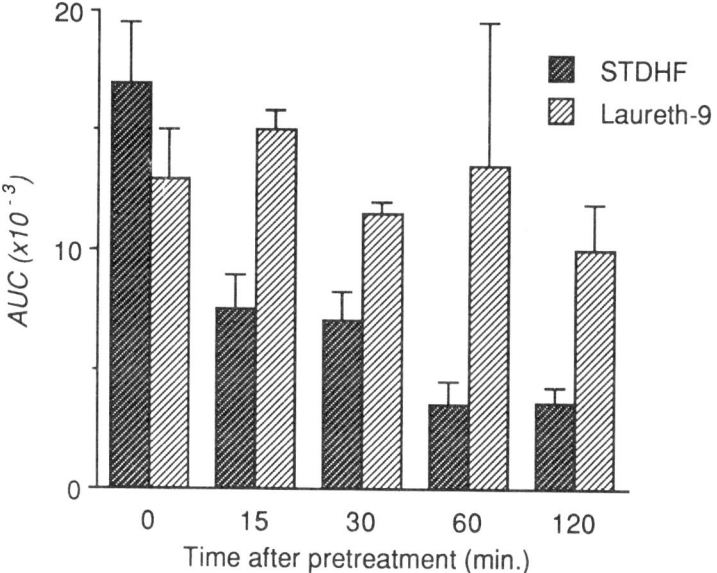

Fig. 6. Area under the plasma human growth hormone concentration vs time curve (AUC) as a function of the time between surfactant administration and hormone administration.

The duration of the permeability effect in the presence of STDHF and another non-ionic surfactant, Laureth-9, has been studied. Human growth hormone (hGH) was administered at fixed time intervals after administration of STDHF or Laureth-9. With STDHF, the AUC has decreased by seven-fold after 60 min, whereas with Laureth-9 the AUC remains constant (Fig. 6). This suggests a transient permeability effect resulting from STDHF. This is advantageous for a delivery technology since an extended permeability could expose the systemic circulation to a variety of foreign substances.

We have attempted to localize the absorption pathway created by STDHF by looking at the distribution of insulin in the rat nasal mucosa after intranasal administration. Using a double antibody technique, insulin can be localized in the mucosa using a colloidal gold–silver stain. In Fig. 7, the staining results are shown from a sample fixed 5 min after administration of a 1% insulin, 0.5% STDHF solution. After co-administration with STDHF, insulin can be visualized both inside the cells of the mucosa and in the intercellular spaces. Without STDHF, no insulin penetrates the mucosa. Unfortunately, we cannot determine the relative flux between the two pathways or whether the intracellular insulin actually escapes the cell. It is clear that the gross cellular damage is not required in order to enhance absorption.

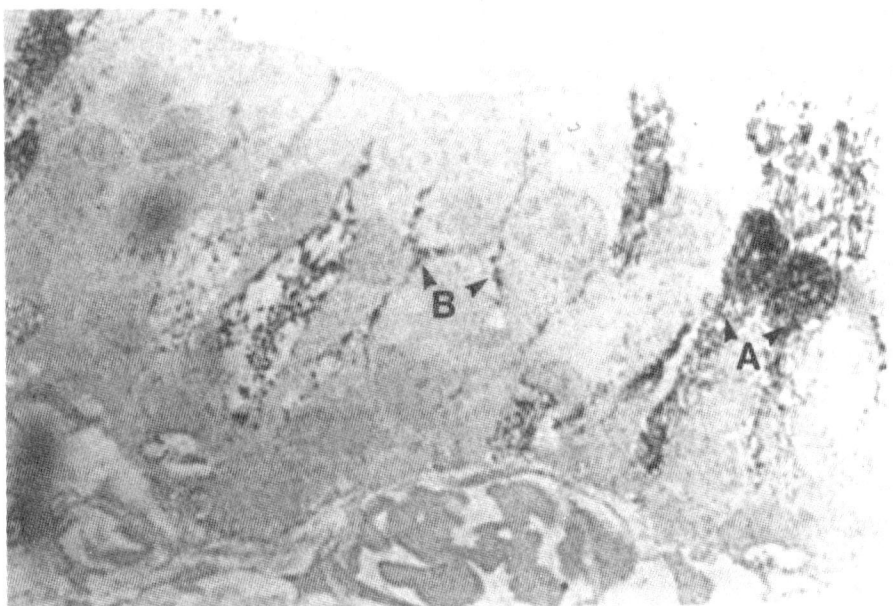

Fig. 7. Localization of insulin in the nasal mucosa after fixation 5 min after delivery of a solution containing 1% insulin, 0.5% STDHF. Insulin is seen in both intracellular (A) and intercellular (B) locations.

Various mechanisms have been proposed for surfactant-based permeation enhancement. These include (1) the formation of transient membrane pores, (2) endocytosis, (3) ion pairing, (4) protease inhibition, (5) cellular erosion and (6) the loosening of tight junctions. From our mechanistic and immunohistochemical studies we can eliminate several of these proposals. We believe ion pairing and protease inhibition are relatively minor components, histological evidence suggests that cellular erosion does not occur, and the time course for appearance of drug in the systemic circulation is too rapid to support an endocytotic mechanism (Ennis *et al.*, 1990). This leaves either a transcellular or a paracellular mechanism. Our data does not allow us to differentiate between the two. The ability of STDHF, however, to enhance the delivery of the hydrophilic dextran molecules leads us to suggest that the primary mechanism of transport involves a paracellular pathway. It is highly unlikely that a 20 000 Da dextran molecule could pass through two bilayers without at the same time disrupting the ionic gradients which exist between the intra- and the intercellular environments and, in the process, killing the cell.

SUMMARY

The nasal cavity is an attractive site for the systemic administration of drugs. For small molecules with the appropriate physical properties, the various mucous and epithelial barriers can be readily overcome. In the case of macromolecules, absorption across the nasal mucosa is severely limited. Three strategies have evolved to circumvent this limitation and encouraging results have been observed in animals and in the clinic. Each of these strategies involves the addition of a substance to increase mucosal permeability. The viability of each of these enhanced strategies will be dependent on establishment of a long term safety profile for both the adjuvant and the final drug formulation.

ACKNOWLEDGMENTS

The authors would like to acknowledge the contributions of John Barackman, Theresa Benkert, Maria Botet, Lucy Cesar and Richard Ennis to the work presented here.

REFERENCES

Allen, A. (1978) *Br. Med. Bull.* 34 28–33.
Baldwin, P. A., Klingbeil, C. K., Grimm, C. J. and Longenecker, J. P. (1990) *Pharm. Res.* 7 547–552.
Bjørk, E. and Edman, P. (1988) *Int. J. Pharm.* 47 233–238.
Chien, Y. W. and Chang, S. F. (1985) In: Chien, Y. W. (ed.) *Transnasal Systemic Medications.* Elsevier, Amsterdam, pp. 1–99.
Corbo, D. C., Huang, Y. C. and Chien, Y. W. (1989) *Int. J. Pharm.* 50 253–260.
Ennis, R. D., Borden, L. A. and Lee, W. A. (1990) *Pharm. Res.* 7 468–475.
Frauman, A., Gerum, G. and Luis, W. J. (1987) *Diabetes Res. Clin. Pract.* 3 197–202.
Gibson, R. E. and Olanoff, L. S. (1987) *J. Control. Release* 6 361–366.
Gordon, G. S. (1985) *Proc. Natl. Acad. Sci. USA* 82 7419–7423.
Hardy, J. G., Lee, S. W. and Wilson, C G. (1984) *J. Pharm. Pharmacol.* 37 294–297.
Hirai, S., Yashiki, T. and Mima, H. (1981) *Int. J. Pharm.* 9 165–172.
Hussain, A. A., Iseki, K., Kagoshima, M. and Dittert, L. W. (1990) *J. Pharm. Sci.* 79 947–948.
Illum, L., Jorgensen, H., Bisgaard, H., Krogsgaard, O. and Rossing, N. (1987) *Int. J. Pharm.* 39 189–199.
Inagaki, M., Sakakura, Y., Itoh, H., Ukai, K. and Miyoshi, M. (1985) *Rhinology* 23 213–221.
Lee, S. P. and Nichols, J. F. (1987) *Rheology* 24 565–569.

Lee, W. A. and Longenecker, J. P. (1988) *Biopharm. Manuf.* **1** 30–37.
Lee, W. A., Narog, B. A., Patapoff, T. W. and Wang, Y. J. (1991) *J. Pharm. Sci.* **80** 1–5.
Longenecker, J. P., Moses, A. L., Flier, J.S., Silver, R. D., Carey, M. C. and Dubovi, E. J. (1987) *J. Pharm. Sci.* **76** 351–355.
Madara, J. L. (1988) *Cell* **53** 497–498.
Marriott, C. (1987) In: Ganderton, D. and Jones, T. (eds) *Drug Delivery to the Respiratory Tract.* Ellis Horwood, Chichester, pp. 68–74.
McMartin, C., Hutchinson, L. E. F., Hyde, R. and Peters, G. E. (1987) *J. Pharm. Sci.* **76** 535–540.
Morimoto, K., Morisaka, K. and Kamada, A. (1985) *J. Pharm. Pharmacol.* **37** 134–136.
Nagai, T., Nishimoto, Y., Nambu, N., Suzuki, Y. and Sekine, K. (1984) *J. Control. Release* **1** 15–22.
Olanoff, L. S., Titus, C. R., Shea, M. S., Gibson, R. E. and Brooks, C. D. (1987) *J. Clin. Invest.* **80** 890–000.
Pappenheimer, J. R. and Reiss, K. Z. (1987) *J. Membr. Biol.* **100** 123–136.
Pontiroli, A. E., Alberetto, M. and Pozza, G. (1985) *Br. Med. J.* **290** 1390–1391.
Pontiroli, A. E., Calderara, A., Pajetta, E. and Alberetto, M. (1989) *Diabetes Care* **12** 604–608.
Popp, J. A., Monteiro-Riviere, D. A. and Martin, J. T. (1986) In: Barrow, C. S. (ed.) *Toxicology of the Nasal Passages* Hemisphere Publishing, Washington, DC, pp. 37–49.
Radomsky, M. L., Whaley, K. J., Cone, R. A. and Saltzman, W. M. (1990) *Biomaterials* **11** 619–624.
Schreider, J. P. (1986) In: Barrow, C. S. (ed.) *Toxicology of the Nasal Passages.* Hemisphere Publishing, Washington, DC, pp. 1–25.
Stratford, R. E. and Lee, V. H. L. (1986) *Int. J. Pharm.* **30** 73–82.
Vickery, B. H., Fu, C.-C., Benjamin, E. J. and Sanders, L. M. (1989) *Europ. Pat. Appl. No. 0312052.*
Watanabe, K., Saito, Y., Watanabe, I. and Mizuhira, V. (1980) *Ann. Otol.* **89** 377–382.
Widdicombe, J. G. and Wells, U. M. (1982) In: Proctor, D. F. and Anderson, I. (eds) *The Nose.* Elsevier Biomedical Press, Amsterdam, pp. 215–244.

17

Present and future trends in pharmaceutical dosage forms for nasal application

F.W.H.M. Merkus, W.A.J.J. Hermens, N.G.M. Schipper, S.G. Romeijn and J.C. Verhoef

INTRODUCTION

Until recently nasal preparations, such as antibiotics, anti-inflammatory steroids and decongestants, were administered nasally only for the treatment of local diseases. However the nasal mucosa is also a potential site for drug absorption, as the surface of the mucosa is large and well provided with blood vessels. The nasal route is also very attractive for drug administration, since no injection is required and first pass elimination is circumvented. Nevertheless, for many drugs, particularly peptides and proteins, the nasal epithelial mucosa is a strong physical and metabolic barrier for drug absorption. The mucociliary clearance system in the nose is a key defense mechanism in the human upper airways, protecting the body against noxious materials inhaled. Impairment of mucociliary clearance predisposes to chronic infections of the respiratory system.

Nasal mucociliary clearance depends upon the interaction of the ciliary beating of the epithelial cells and the physical properties of the mucus. Ciliostasis prevents the defensive barrier from functioning properly. Cilia are microscopic, fingerlike protrusions of the epithelial cell. Each cell has about 200 cilia on its surface, all beating with a frequency of about 20 beats/s in a coordinated way, probably regulated by an intracellular pacemaker system. The factors influencing ciliary beat frequency and coordination have not yet been fully identified. Pharmacological experiments have indicated an influence of the sympathic and parasympathic nervous system on mucociliary activity.

An individual cilium is approximately 5 μm in length and 0.2 μm in diameter. The fine structure of a cilium consists of nine microtubular doublets in a ring around two central microtubules. The nine microtubular doublets have so-called dynein arms, extending from one side towards the neighbouring doublet. The motion of cilia, which is an energy-consuming process, is dependent upon the microtubules sliding past one another with the dynein providing the needed ATPase activity.

In general, nasal mucociliary clearance carries the mucus, with entrapped dust, allergens and bacteria, backward to the nasopharynx. The mucus is dispatched by a wiping action of the palate to the stomach periodically through swallowing. As ciliary beating is the most important parameter in nasal mucociliary clearance in normal circumstances, it should not be decreased by nasal medication.

To study the actions of drugs and pharmaceutical dosage forms on nasal mucociliary clearance, both measurements of the mucus transport time (MTT) and the ciliary beat frequency (CBF) are used. CBF studies allow for relative comparison of the ciliostatic potential of various excipients and for measurements of concentration-dependent effects (Hermens and Merkus, 1987; Schipper et al., 1991). Commonly, the *in vivo* effects on the nasal mucociliary clearance may be less severe than those *in vitro* because of the dilution of the formulation by the mucus and the fast elimination from the nasal epithelium by the mucociliary clearance. In Table 1 some potential ciliotoxic compounds are listed.

Table 1. Examples of ciliostatic–ciliotoxic drugs or additives[a]

Lidocaine
Cocaine
Bupivacaine
Propranolol
Diphenhydramine
Tripelennamine
Deoxycholate
Laureth-9
STDHF
Mercury-containing preservatives
L-α-Lysophosphatidylcholine

[a]Drugs and additives were tested in the general used or advised concentration.

ABSORPTION ENHANCERS

In hundreds of papers the possible utility of the nasal administration of a great number of compounds has been demonstrated (Chien et al., 1989). Nevertheless, only a few peptide drugs for intranasal systemic absorption are presently used and their therapeutic effect is undisputed. Table 2 summarizes some of these drugs.

Obviously, nasal absorption may be useful for the administration of peptide hormones. Hormone substitution therapies require repeated injections for up to long periods. The high potency of most peptides makes these substances very suitable for intranasal administration as the amount per dose is mostly small. On the other hand, the frequently large molecular size and hydrophilic properties at physiologic pH hamper absorption through the hydrophobic membranes. The absorption efficiency of intranasally administered peptides can be improved with the aid of absorption promoters such as bile salts. However, these compounds are ciliotoxic (Duchateau et al., 1986). Ciliotoxicity appeared to increase with an increase of hydrophobicity. Dihydroxy bile salts are more ciliotoxic than trihydroxy bile salts (Figs 1 and 2). Unfortunately, dihydroxy bile salts appeared to be more potent in the absorption promoting effect of insulin (Moses et al., 1984).

Table 2. Drugs used intranasally for their therapeutic systemic effects

| Calcitonin |
| Vasopressin |
| Desmopressin |
| Glucagon |
| Oxytocin |
| LHRH |
| Buserelin |
| Nafarelin |
| GHRH |

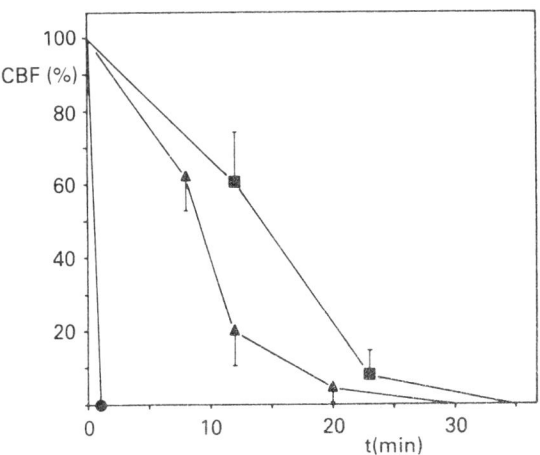

Fig. 1. Time vs frequency plot of dihydroxy BSs at a concentration of 5 mmol/l. SEM is indicated ($n = 6$). ●, DC; ▲, GDC; ■, TDC.

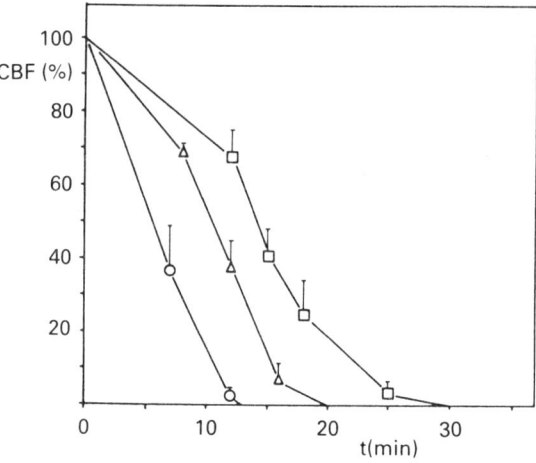

Fig. 2. Time vs frequency plot of trihydroxy BSs at a concentration of 30 mmol/l. SEM is indicated ($n = 6$). o, c: △, GC; □, TC.

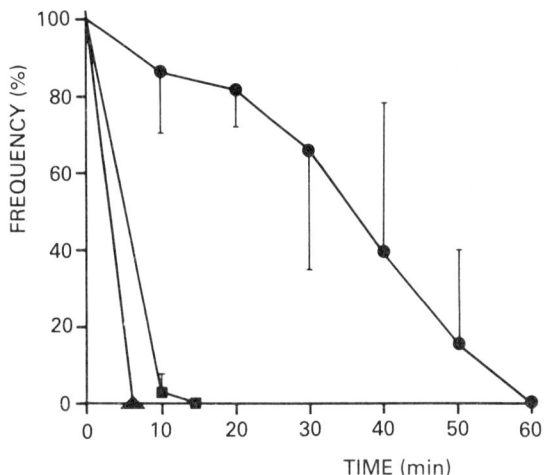

Fig. 3. Time vs frequency plot (mean ± SD) of cilia in solutions of 0.3% STDHF (●), 0.3% laureth-9 (▲) and 0.3% deoxycholate (■).

Sodium taurodihydrofusidate (STDHF) could be a promising enhancer for nasal delivery of peptide drugs. This compound greatly enhanced the nasal absorption of insulin (Longenecker et al., 1987; Deurloo et al., 1989), and of growth hormone (Baldwin et al., 1990). We studied the in vitro effect on ciliary beat frequency of STDHF in relation to bile salt and the surfactant laureth-9. STDHF was found to induce ciliostasis with concentrations of 0.3% (w/v) and higher (Fig 3). The ciliostasis is irreversible, being a serious drawback for its use in chronic nasal insulin therapy. Using similar concentrations, STDHF appears to be less ciliostatic than the well-known nasal absorption promoters deoxycholate and laureth-9, which both cause a very rapid irreversible ciliostasis (Table 3). The absorption enhancers glycocholate and taurocholate exhibit a very mild ciliostatic activity. Human insulin in a concentration of 1% (w/v) does not have any effect on the nasal ciliary beat frequency (Hermens et al., 1990a).

Table 3. Effects of various absorption enhancers and insulin on human nasal ciliary beat frequency (CBF)

	% (w/v)	Time (min)[a]						n
		10	20	30	40	50	60	
STDHF	0.1	93 ± 4	98 ± 5	94 ± 4	92 ± 6	90 ± 9	90 ± 9	4
STDHF	0.2	90 ± 2	92 ± 6	92 ± 9	88 ± 11	82 ± 11	82 ± 13	4
STDHF	0.3	86 ± 14	82 ± 8	64 ± 31	39 ± 39	16 ± 25	0	8
STDHF	0.5	0	0	0	0	0	0	4
STDHF	1.0	0	0	0	0	0	0	4
Laureth-9	0.3	0	0	0	0	0	0	8
Deoxycholate	0.3	2 ± 4	0	0	0	0	0	8
Taurocholate	0.3	96 ± 7	93 ± 6	90 ± 7	90 ± 10	90 ± 8	90 ± 8	8
Glycocholate	0.3	89 ± 7	87 ± 10	88 ± 8	87 ± 9	87 ± 10	85 ± 11	8
Human insulin	1.0	99 ± 3	99 ± 3	99 ± 4	99 ± 6	97 ± 10	93 ± 7	4
Human insulin with STDHF	1:1	17 ± 32	10 ± 28	3 ± 8	0	0	0	8

[a]All values are presented as percentages of the initial frequencies (t_0 = 100%) and are the mean ± SD for the number of experiments given (n).

The absorption promoting effect of medium chain fatty acid salts such as sodium caprylate, sodium caprate and sodium laurate on rat nasal insulin absorption has been studied. Among these fatty acids sodium caprylate in a concentration of 1%, exhibited the strongest insulin absorption promoting effect. This effect appeared to be partly associated with the chelating ability for calcium ions and with the inhibitory action on leucine aminopeptidase activity. The fatty acid salts showed higher haemolytic activity than glycocholate (Mishima et al., 1987).

Also the absorption enhancing effect of carbenoxolone, and glycyrrhizinic acid salt on the nasal insulin absorption was investigated in rats (Mishima et al., 1989). These compounds have structures comparable with triterpenes, and show a promoting action similar to that of bile acids or saponins. Carbenoxolone turned out to be the most effective agent. Nasal absorption of 10 IU/kg insulin in the presence of 1% carbenoxolone was 26.5% of that in the case of a 5 U/kg intravenous dose. Nasal leucine aminopeptidase activity was more strongly inhibited by carbenoxolone than by glycocholate. Intranasal insulin solutions in combination with 0.5% of L-α-lysophosphatidylcholine produced in rats a reduction in blood glucose levels similar to laureth-9. The two main constituents of L-α-lysophosphatidylcholine, being the palmitoyl component (72%) and the stearoyl component (24%), produced similar effects to that of L-α-lysophosphatidylcholine, thus indicating that both of these lysophospholipids are equally potent absorption enhancers (Illum et al., 1989). Using the enhancer didecanoyl-L-α-phosphatidylcholine in human volunteers insulin bioavailability was 8.3% and 11.5% when compared with i.v. and s.c. administered insulins, respectively (Drejer et al., 1990).

In order to reduce nasal clearance and thereby to increase nasal drug absorption, a new concept has been introduced using albumin, starch, and DEAE–Sephadex microspheres with a diameter of 40–50 μm as nasal dosage forms (Illum et al., 1987). These microsphere preparations appeared to have clearance half-life values of 3 h or more, as compared with 15 min for solutions and powder formulations. These remarkably reduced clearance times are probably caused by swelling of the microspheres, thereby forming a mucoadhesive intranasal delivery system. Starch microspheres increased the bioavailability of nasally administered insulin in rats and sheep considerably (Bjørk and Edman, 1990; Farraj et al., 1990). Other mucoadhesive delivery systems have also been used for intranasal drug administration. A polyacrylic acid gel base improved the absorption of insulin and calcitonin in rats (Morimoto et al., 1985), while cellulose derivatives and neutralized polyacrylic acid (Carbopol 934) increased the nasal absorption of insulin in dogs (Nagai et al., 1984).

CYCLODEXTRINS AS ABSORPTION ENHANCERS

In recent years we have concentrated our research on the effect of a relatively new class of compounds, cyclodextrins (CDs), on nasal drug absorption. CDs are cyclic oligosaccharides of 6, 7, or 8 glucose units: α-CD, β-CD, and γ-CD respectively.

On the one hand, CDs are able to form inclusion complexes with lipophilic drugs, thereby increasing their water-solubility. Nasal formulations of oestradiol and progesterone containing dimethyl-β-cyclodextrin (DMβCD) as solubilizer and enhancer appeared to increase substantially the bioavailability of these steroid hormones in rabbits, rats and men (Hermens et al., 1990b; Schipper et al., 1990; Hermens et al., 1991). Nasal formulations of oestradiol and progesterone with DMβCD resulted in rat experiments in bioavailabilities of 60% and 70%, respectively, as compared with only 20% for control suspension preparations (Hermens et al., 1990b; Schipper et al., 1990) (see Figs 4 and 5). These DMβCD–hormone formulations exert only minor effects on the ciliary beat frequency of human adenoid tissue, indicating that they have potential for the nasal therapy of oestradiol and progesterone (Fig 6). After nasal delivery of 0.34 mg oestradiol in three patients, concentration–time curves of oestradiol in serum and its metabolite oestrone in plasma were established. High initial oestradiol serum levels were found in the order of 5 nmol/l (Fig 7). Oestrone:oestradiol ratios were below unity, whereas, in contrast, oestrone:oestradiol ratios after oral administration of oestradiol are known to exceed unity. Biological activity, as reflected by suppression of FSH and LH, was manifest. In nine patients symptoms of oestrogen deficiency were addressed by a questionnaire. After 3 and 6 months of nasal treatment, a clinically and statistically significant decrease of the total score according to this questionnaire was found compared with the beginning of the study (Hermens et al., 1991).

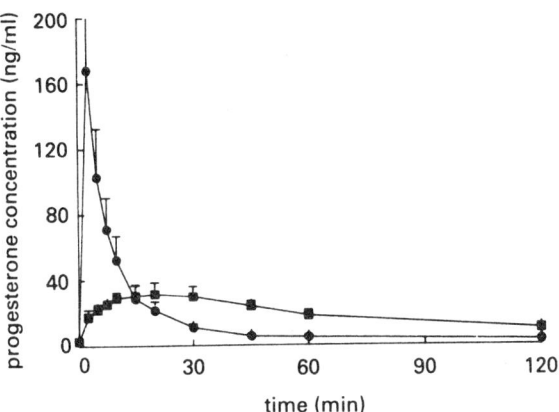

Fig. 4. Mean serum concentrations of progesterone following administration of a progesterone–oestradiol–DMβCD preparation: ●, intravenous administration of 100 µg progesterone and 5 µg oestradiol with DMβCD; ■, nasal administration of 200 µg progesterone and 10 µg oestradiol with DMβCD.

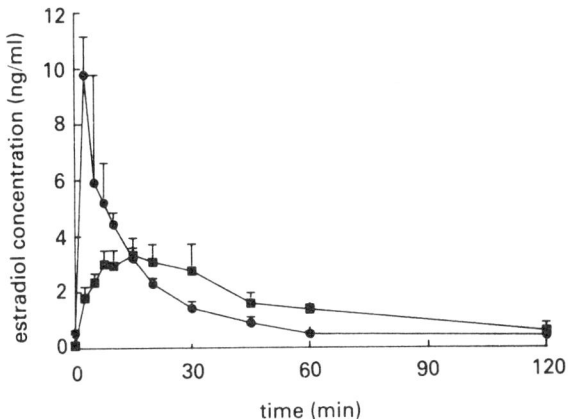

Fig. 5. Mean serum concentrations of oestradiol following administration of a progesterone–oestradiol–DMβCD preparation: ●, intravenous administration of 100 µg progesterone and 5 µg oestradiol with DMβCD; ■, nasal administration of 200 µg progesterone and 10 µg oestradiol with DMβCD.

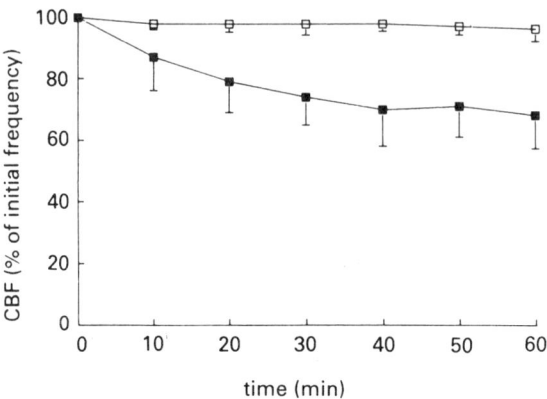

Fig. 6 Time vs CBF plot of human adenoid tissue in progesterone–oestradiol–DMβCD solutions (■) and blank Locke-Ringer solutions (□).

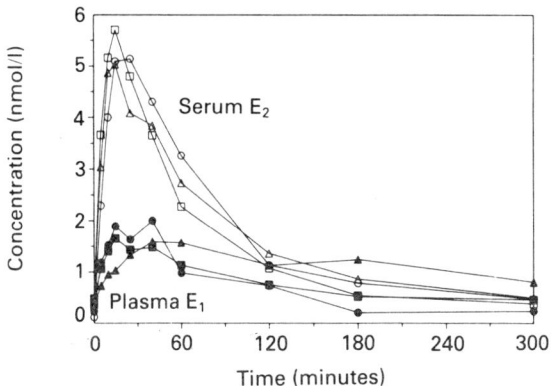

Fig. 7. Serum oestradiol (△, ○, □) and plasma oestrone (▲, ●, ■) levels after nasal administration of 0.34 mg oestradiol in three patients (△, ▲, patient 1; ○, ●, patient 2; □, ■, patient 3).

On the other hand, CDs may also have direct effects on epithelial membranes, thereby facilitating transport of hydrophilic drugs such as peptides and proteins. Studies in rats with a variety of CDs showed that some of these compounds are potent promoters of nasal insulin absorption, leading to almost complete insulin bioavailability (Merkus et al., 1991). Coadministration of 5% (w/v) DMβCD to the insulin solution resulted in a high bioavailability, $108.9 \pm 36.4\%$ (mean ± SD, $n = 6$), compared with i.v. administration, and a strong decrease in blood glucose levels, to 25% of their initial values. Coadministration of 5% α-CD gave rise to an insulin bioavailability of $27.7 \pm 11.5\%$ (mean ± SD, $n = 6$) and a decrease in blood glucose to 50% of its initial value. The rate of insulin absorption and the concomitant hypoglycaemic response were delayed for the α-CD-containing solution as compared with the DMβCD preparation. The other CDs investigated, HPβCD (5%), β-CD (1.8%), and γ-CD (5%), did not have significant effects on nasal insulin absorption.

In contrast, ongoing experiments in rabbits and human volunteers showed for insulin no absorption enhancing effect of cyclodextrins. This proves that for nasal administration the influence of CDs on insulin absorption differs substantially between animal species.

REFERENCES

Baldwin, P. A., Klingbeil, C. K., Grimm, C. J. and Longenecker, J. P. (1990). The effect of sodium taurodihydrofusidate on the nasal absorption of human growth hormone in three animal models. *Pharm.Res.* **7** 547–552.

Bjørk, E. and Edman, P. (1990) Characterization of degradable starch microspheres as a nasal delivery system for drugs. *Int J. Pharm.* **62** 187–192.

Chien, Y. W., Su, K. S. E. and Chang, S. F. (1989) *Nasal Systemic Drug Delivery.* Dekker, New York.

Deurloo, M. J. M., Hermens, W. A. J. J., Romeyn, S. G., Verhoef, J. C. and Merkus, F. W. H. M. (1989) Absorption enhancement of intranasally administered insulin by sodium taurodihydrofusidate in rabbits and rats. *Pharm. Res.* **6** 853–856.

Drejer, K., Vaag, A., Bech, K., Hansen, P. E., Sorensen, K. R. and Mygind, N. (1990) Pharmacokinetics of intranasally administered insulin with phospholipid as absorption enhancer. *26th Annual Meeting European Assoc. for the Study of Diabetes.* Abstract, 198, p. A61.

Duchateau, G. S. M. J. E., Zuidema, J. and Merkus, F. W. H. M. (1986) Bile salts and intranasal drug delivery . *Int. J. Pharm.* **31** 193–199.

Farraj, N. F., Johansen, B. R., Davis, S. S. and Illum, L. (1990) Nasal administration of insulin using bioadhesive microspheres as a delivery system . *J. Control. Release.* **13** 253–261.

Hermens, W. A. J. J. and Merkus, F. W. H. M. (1987) The influence of drugs on nasal ciliary movement. *Pharm. Res.* **4** 445–449.

Hermens, W. A. J. J., Hooymans, P. M., Verhoef, J. C. and Merkus, F. W. H. M. (1990a) Effects of absorption enhancers on human nasal tissue ciliary movement *in vitro* . *Pharm. Res.* **7** 144–146.

Hermens, W. A. J. J., Deurloo, M. J. M., Romeyn, S. G., Verhoef, J. C. and Merkus, F. W. H. M. (1990b) Nasal absorption enhancement of 17β-estradiol by dimethyl-β-cyclodextrin in rabbits and rats. *Pharm. Res.* **7** 500–503.

Hermens, W. A. J. J., Belder, C. W. J., Merkus, J. M. W. M., Hooymans, P. M., Verhoef, J. and Merkus, F. W. H. M. (1991) Intranasal estradiol administration to oophorectomized women. *Eur. J. Obstet. Gynecol. Reprod. Biol.* **40** 35–41.

Illum, L., Jörgensen, H., Bisgaard, H., Krogsgaard, O. and Rossing, N. (1987) Bioadhesive microspheres as a potential nasal drug delivery system . *Int. J. Pharm.* **39** 189–199.

Illum, L., Farraj, N. F., Critchley, H., Johansen, B. R. and Davis, S. S. (1989) Enhanced nasal absorption of insulin in rats using lysophosphatidylcholine . *Int. J. Pharm.* **57** 49–54.

Longenecker, J. P., Moses, A. C., Flier, J. S., Silver, R. D., Carey, M. C. and Dubovi, E. J. (1987) Effects of sodium taurodihydrofusidate on nasal absorption of insulin in sheep. *J. Pharm. Sci.* **76** 351–355.

Merkus, F. W. H. M., Verhoef, J., Romeyn, S. G. and Schipper, N. G. M. (1991) Absorption enhancing effect of cyclodextrins on intranasally administered insulin in rats. *Pharm. Res.* **8** 588–592.

Mishima, M., Wakita, Y., Nakano, M. (1978) Studies on the promoting effects of medium chain fatty acid salts on the nasal absorption of insulin in rats. *J. Pharmacobio-Dyn.* **10** 624–631.

Mishima, M., Okada, S., Wakita, Y. and Nakano, M. (1989) Promotion of nasal absorption of insulin by glycyrrhetinic acid derivatives. *J. Pharmacobio-Dyn.* **12** 31–36.

Morimoto, K., Morisaka, K. and Kamada, A. (1985) Enhancement of nasal absoroption of insulin and calcitonin using polyacrylic acid gel. *J. Pharm. Pharmacol.* **37** 134–136.

Moses, A. C., Flier, J. S., Gordon, G. S., Silver, R. D. and Carey, M. C. (1984) Transnasal insulin delivery: structure–function studies of absorption enhancing adjuvants. *Clin. Res.* **32** 245A.

Nagai, T., Nishimoto, J., Nambu, N., Suzuki, Y. and Sekine, K. (1984) Powder dosage form of insulin for nasal administration. *J. Control. Release.* **1** 15–22.

Schipper, N. G. M., Hermens, W. A. J. J., Romeyn, S. G., Verhoef, J. and Merkus, F. W. H. M. (1990) Nasal absorption of 17β-estradiol and progesterone from a dimethyl-β-cyclodextrin inclusion formulation in rats. *Int. J. Pharm.* **64** 61–66.

Schipper, N. G. M., Verhoef, J. C. and Merkus, F. W. H. M. (1991) The nasal mucociliary clearance : Relevance to nasal drug delivery. *Pharm. Res.* **8** 807–814.

Index

absorption
   intestinal peptide, 93
   particulate, 114
absorption of particles, gastrointestinal mucosa, unwanted, 122
absorption enhancers
   nasal, 238
   transdermal, 169
acebutolol, 68
acebutololhydrochloride, 64
acid
   arachidonic, 183
   free fatty, 170
   linoleic, 183
   oleic, 170, 172, 174
acid deficiency, fatty, 183
activation, endothelial, 7
adhesion, 58, 92
   platelet, 7
   specific, 98
adsorption, 58
adsorption–interpenetration theory, 57
agents, cytotoxic, 23
albumin, 5, 10
amphipathic polyethyleneglycol derivatives, 27
amphiphiles, 29
amphoteric surfactants, 230
anchors, hydrophobic, 22
angiotensin II, 72
anionic surfactants, 230
anti-inflammatory drugs, 196
antibiotics, 71
antibodies, monoclonal, 13
antibody–antigen system, 33
antigens, 53, 73
antiparasitic drugs, 24
antiviral drugs, 24
apolipoproteins, 14, 21, 24
1-β-D-arabinofuranosylcytosine, 72

arabinoside, cytosine, 22
arachidonic acid, 183
asialofetuin, 18, 21
astrocytes, 9
azone, 170, 175

bacterial transport, gastrointestinal mucosa, 114
barrier
   blood–brain, 9
   buccal transmucosal transport, 57, 62
   epithelial, 47
   function, 8, 45
   functions of the gastrointestinal tracts, 46
   hypothesis, steric, 29
   microvascular, 9
   skin cell cultures, 182
basal lamina, buccal, 63, 68, 69
basic physiology, pulmonary sufactant, 129
bilayers
   phospholipids, 26
   rigidity, 27, 30
   stratum corneum, 208
bile salts, 78
binding, target, 34
bioadhesion, 57, 58
   gastrointestinal transit of drug delivery systems, 94
   intestinal, 92
   microspheres, 120
   polymer fluidity, 60
   oral peptide delivery, 95
   pharmaceutical–technological aspects, 93
biochemical composition, pulmonary surfactant, 130
biodegradable lactide–glycolide microparticles, 119
biphasic emulsions, 71
bodies, lamellar, 155
Bragg's law, 205

buccal
  basal lamina, 68, 69
  drug delivery, 57
  electrical resistance, 66
  morphology, 66
  mucoadhesion, 57
  mucosa, 51, 62
  mucosa, porcine, 68
  transmucosal transport barriers, 57, 62
bupivacaine, 238
bupranolol, 68
bupranololhydrochloride, 64
buserelin, 229, 239

calcitonin, 229, 239
capillaries, 1, 2, 7, 10
  brain, 3
  continuous, 2
  permeability, 6, 8
carriers, colloidal, 203
CBF, nasal ciliary beat frequency, 242
cell cultures, skin, 178
cell layers, superficial, 50
cells
  damage, 46
  endothelial, 13, 24
  fat-storing, 13
  glandular, 46
  Kupffer, 13, 19, 24, 27, 32
  M, 53, 81, 83, 114, 122
  parenchymal, 13
  parenchymal liver, 24
  target, 38
  tumour, 23
ceramides, 50, 170
charge, surface, 27
chemical modification of lipoproteins, 21–22
cholesterol, 22, 27, 170
cholesteryl sulphate, 170
chronically isolated intestinal loop model, 94
chylomicron remnants, 24
chylomicrons, 3, 14, 24
cilia nasal epithelium, 224, 237
ciliary beat frequency (CBF), nasal, 242
ciliated columnar cells, nasal epithelium, 224
ciliostasis, 237
ciliostatic–ciliotoxic drugs, 238
ciliotoxicity, 239
circulation, prolonged, of liposomes, 34
clearance of liposomes, 27
coating granules, membrane, 50
cocaine, 238
coefficient
  combined spreading, 59
  permeability, 198
collagen, 181

colloidal
  carriers, 203
  carrier uptake, 113
  drug delivery systems, 71
colon absorption of drugs, multiple unit dose systems, 111
combined spreading coefficient, 59
composition, lipid, 27, 30
constants, permeability, 45
content of oral mucosa, lipid, 50
content of skin, lipid, 50
corneocytes, 169, 210
cornified envelope, 180
cultures
  keratinocyte, 178
  skin cell, 178
cyclodextrines, 243
cysteamine, 73
cytosine arabinoside, 22
cytotoxic
  agents, 23
  drugs, 33

d-tubocurarine, 72
damage, cellular, 46
dead epidermized dermis (DED), 181, 184
DED, dead epidermized dermis, 181, 184
deficiency, fatty acid, 183
degradable starch microspheres, 230
delivery
  buccal drug, 57
  LDL-mediated, 23
  liposomes oral, 74
  vaccine, 123
delivery systems
  colloidal drug, 71
  drug, 92
deoxycholate, 238, 242
dermatological drugs, 180
9-desglycinamide-8-arginine vasopressin (DGAVP), 94
desmopressin, 229, 239
desmosome, 50
detergent-dialysis method, 33
dextrans, 51
DGAVP, 9-desglycinamide-8-arginine vasopressin, 94
diaphragms, open, 5
differential scanning calorimetry (DSC), 171, 172
differentiation
  of keratinocyte cultures, 180
  skin cell cultures, 180
diffusion resistance, mucosa, 65
diffsion experiments, mucosa, 64
diffusional behaviour, skin membrane, 190
digestion of liposomes, 77

dioxide, titanium, 122
dipalmitoyl phosphatidylcholine (DPPC), 72, 130, 171, 175
dipeptide, muramyl, 24
diphenhydramine, 238
diphenylhydantoin, 22
distearoylphosphatidylcholine (DSPC), 30
dolichol, 73, 75
dosage forms, multi-unit, 101
drug, thermodynamic activity, 198
drug delivery, buccal, 57
drug delivery systems, 92
    colloidal, 71
    transdermal (TDDS), 190
drug testing, reconstructed skin, 184–185
drugs
    antiviral, 23
    cytotoxic, 33
    dermatological, 178
    liposome entrapped, 72
    nanocapsules, 74
drugs for gastrointestinal application, nanospheres, 73
DSC, differential scanning calorimetry, 172

elcatonin, 229
electrical resistance, mucosa, 66, 68
electron spin resonance (ESR), 171, 173
emulsions
    biphasic, 71
    triphasic, 71
endocytosis, 6
    of liposomes, 77
    of particles, 80–81
    receptor-mediated, 6, 38
endothelia
    continuous, 5
    fenestrated, 3
endothelial, 1, 8
    activation, 7
    cells, 13, 24
    microvascular, 4
    permeability, 6, 9
endothelial model, pulmonary, 33
energy
    Griffith fracture, 58, 59
    interfacial, 57
    surface, 58
enhancers, 170
    nasal absorption, 238
    penetration, 92, 203
    skin penetration, 169
    enterocytes, 53, 81, 82
    enterocyte radio binding assay (ERBA), 98
entrapped drugs, liposome, 71
envelope, cornified, 180

environment, luminal, 46
enzymes, lysosomal, 22
epidermis on DED, reconstructed, 181
epidermis skin, 49
epithelium
    barrier, 47
    gastro-intestinal, 47, 51
    keratinized oral, 50
    microvascular, 2
    nasal, 223
    oesophageal, 50
    oral, 50
    stratified squamous, 47, 50
    turnover times of, 49
ERBA, enterocyte radio binding assay, 98
ESR, electron spin resonance, 173
exchange of fluid, 5
excipients, pellets, 104
experiments, mucosa diffusion, 64
extravasation, 6, 8
extrusion, pellets, 103

factor VIII, 72
factor IX, 73
factors, growth, 178
Faraday constant, 194
fat-storing cells, 13
fatty acids
    free, 170
    deficiency, 183
    profile, 183
fenestrae, 5, 6
ferritin, 6
FFEM, freeze fracture electron microscopy, 204, 209
fibroblasts, 181
floor of mouth, 51
fluorescence spectroscopy, 171
follicles, hair, 181
Fourier transform infrared, 171, 172
fracture energy, Griffith, 58, 59
free fatty acids, 170
freeze fracture electron microscopy (FFEM), 204, 209
function, barrier, 45
functions of the gastrointestinal tracts, barrier, 46

galactose receptors, 19
gangliosides, 30
gaps, intercellular, 8
gastrointestinal mucosa, 45
    bacterial transport, 114
    latex uptake, 121
    macromolecular uptake and particulate uptake, 114
    micro- and nanoparticulate uptake, 116

transit time, 110
unwanted absorption of particles, 122
gastrointestinal application, 71
nanospheres, drugs for, 73
gastrointestinal epithelium, 51
gastrointestinal tract, 47
barrier functions of the, 46
gastrointestinal transit of drug delivery systems, bioadhesion, 94
gentamycin, 72
GHRH, 239
gingiva, 47
glandular cells, 46
glucagon, 239
glucose oxidase, 72
glycocalyx, 227
glycocholate, 242
glycoproteins, 227
glycosylceramides, 51
goblet cells, nasal epithelium, 224
gold-labelled, proteins, 6
granulation, pellets, built-up, 101
granulation liquid, pellets, 105
granules, membrane coating, 50
Griffith fracture energy, 58, 59
growth factors, 178
gut-associated lymphoid tissue, 84

hair follicles, 181
hard palate, 47
HDL, 17, 21
hemidesmosomes, 182
heparin, 73
hepatic processing, 21
high density lipoproteins (HDL), 17
histamine, 7
HIV human immunodeficiency virus, 24
horseradish peroxidase (HRPO), 52, 62, 68
hot stage microscopy, 171
HRPO, horseradish peroxidase, 52, 62, 68
human immunodeficiency virus (HIV), 24
human stratum corneum, 203
hydrogels, 93
hydrogenated phosphatidylinositol, 27
hydrolases, lysosomal, 22
hydrophobic 'anchors', 22
hypothesis, steric barrier, 29

immunization, oral route for, 123
immunoliposomes, 26, 33, 34
targeting, 38
target-sensitive, 39
temperature-sensitive, 39
immunomodulators, 24
in situ rat perfusion model, nasal drug permeability, 228

in vitro models, nasal drug permeability, 228
in vivo studies, pellets, 110
indomethacin, 73, 74, 122
insulin, 72, 73, 74, 75, 76, 79, 84, 230, 233, 234, 240, 242
interaction, ligand–receptor, 26
intercellular
gaps, 8
junctions, 5, 10
lipid bilayers, 182
interfacial energy, 57
internalization, 38
interpenetration, 60
intestinal
bioadhesives, 92
loop model, chronically isolated, 94
peptide absorption, 93
transit, 94
intestine
small, 49
larger, 49
intracellular processing, 19
iontohydrokinesis, 192
iontophoresis, 191
device, 191
parameters, 192
uncharged molecules, 192
isoelectric point, stratum corneum, 191

junctions
intercellular, 5, 10
tight, 50, 51

keratin filaments, 210
keratinized oral epithelium, 50
keratinocyte cultures, 177
differentiation, 180
lesional, 184
Kupffer cells, 13, 19, 24, 27, 32

lamellar bodies, 155
lamina, buccal basal, 63, 68, 69
Langmuir–Blodgett films, 171
latex uptake, 121
laureth-9, 238, 242
layers, superficial cell, 50
LDL, 17, 19, 21, 23
LDL receptors, 23
LDL-mediated delivery, 23
leakage, 7, 8
vascular, 7, 8
lectin, tomato, 98
lectins, 98
lesional keratinocyte cultures, 184
LHRH, 192, 239
lidocaine, 238

ligand–receptor interaction, 26
light scattering, 171
linoleic acid, 183
lipid
  composition, 27
  opsonin, 36
lipid content
  of oral mucosa, 50
  of skin, 50
Lipiodol, 74, 83
lipoproteins, 13, 22
  low density (LDL), 3, 17
  chemical modification of, 21
  high density (HDL), 17
  very low density (VLDL), 14
liposomes, 13, 18, 26, 29, 32, 71, 72, 76, 116, 175, 203, 204
  clearance of, 27
  composition, 31
  digestion of, 77
  endocytosis of, 77
  entrapped drugs following oral administration, 76
  entrapped drugs, 72
  internalization, 38
  long-circulating, 32
  multilamellar vesicles, 208
  oral delivery, 74
  phospholipid mixtures, 205
  size, 27, 31
  specific uptake of, 27
  stability, 30
  targeting, 26, 33
liver, 13, 32
long-circulating liposomes, 32
loop model, chronically isolated intestinal, 94
low density lipoproteins (LDL), 17
luminal environment, 46
lung surfactant, 155
  available surfactant, 158
  as carrier, 161
  phospholipid composition, 156
  phospholipids, 161
  physicochemistry, 157
  recombinant surfactant, 160
  SP-A, 161
  SP-B, 162
  SP-C, 163
  surfactant by design, 160
lung surfactant proteins, 161
  formation and structures, 155
  functional description, 155
  molecular aspects, 155
  use as pulmonal carriers, 155
lymphoid tissue, gut-associated, 84
lypressin, 229
L-α-lysophosphatidylcholine, 238

lysosomal, 22
  enzymes, 22
  hydrolases, 22
  membrane, 22
  route, 21
lysosomes, 22

M cells, 53, 81, 83, 114, 122
macromolecular uptake and particulate uptake, gastrointestinal mucosa, 114
macromolecules, 5, 6, 8, 10, 52
mechanical stabilization, 130
mechanism, triggered release, 39
mechanisms
  of skin penetration, 169
  of nasal permeation enhancement, 234
membrane
  basal, 5
  cell, 38
  coating granules, 50
  lysosomal, 22
  nasal plasma, 227
  nasal, 223
  plasma, 2, 5, 217
  rigidity, 31
mercury-containing preservatives, 238
method, detergent-dialyis, 33
methotrexate, 22
methylmethacrylate microspheres, 80
micelles, 113
micro- and nanoparticle uptake, gastrointestinal mucosa, 116
microemulsions, 13
microparticles
  biodegradable lactide–glycolide, 119
  oral uptake across the gastrointestinal mucosa, 113
microspheres, 94, 113
  bioadhesive, 120
  degradable starch, 230
  methylmethacrylate, 80
  polystyrene, 80, 98
microvascular
  barrier function, 9
  epithelium, 2
  permeability, 1
microviscosity, 31
mixing process, pellets, 105
model, pulmonary endothelial, 33
monoclonal antibodies, 13
monosialoganglioside, 27
morphological studies, 66
morphology, mucosa, 66
mouth, floor of, 51
mucin, 45, 46
mucoadhesion, 57, 94, 98

buccal, 57
intestinal, 94, 98
specific, 99
mucoadhesive coating, 95
mucociliary clearance, nasal, 237
mucosa
  buccal, 51, 62
  diffusion experiments, 64
  diffusion resistance, 65
  electrical resistance, 66, 68
  gastrointestinal, 45
  lipid content of oral, 50
  morphology, 66
  oral, 45
  palatal, 49
  permeability, 68
  permeability constants, 47
  porcine buccal, 68
  water permeability of oral, 50
mucus, 46, 60, 61, 226
multi-unit dosage forms, 101
multilamellar vesicles, liposomes, 208
multiple unit dose systems, 111
  colon absorption of drugs, 111
  transit times, 111
muramyl dipeptide, 24

N-acetylgalactosamine, 19
N-methyl pyrrolidone (NMP), 170
nafarelin, 229, 239
nanocapsules, 71, 74
  drugs, 74
  entrapped drugs following oral administration, 83–84
  oral delivery by, 82
nanoparticles, 13
nanospheres, 71, 73
  drugs for gastrointestinal application, 73
  entrapped drugs following oral administration, 79–80
  oral delivery by, 79
  polyacrylate, 122
  polystyrene, 80
  possible mechanisms of translocation, 80–81
  rate of translocation, 81–82
  translocation of particles, 80
nasal
  absorption enhancers, 238
  ciliated columnar cells, 224
  goblet cells, 224
  membranes, 223
  membrane structure, 223
  non-ciliated cells, 224
  olfactory, 223
  plasma membrane, 227
  respiratory, 223

  squamous, 223
nasal application of
  bupivacaine, 238
  cocaine, 238
  deoxycholate, 238
  diphenhydramine, 238
  laureth-9, 238
  lidocaine, 238
  L-α-lysophosphatidylcholine, 238
  mercury-containing preservatives, 238
  oestradiol, 243
  progesterone, 243
  propranolol, 238
  STDHF, 238
  tripelennamine, 238
nasal ciliary beat frequency (CBF), 242
nasal drug permeability, 228
  systemic administration, 228
  in situ rat perfusion model, 228
  in vitro models, 228
nasal epithelium, 223, 238
  ciliostatic–ciliotoxic drugs, 238
  permeation enhancement, 229
nasal mucociliary clearance, 237
nasal mucus, physical barrier, 227
nasal penetration (absorption) enhancers
  amphoteric surfactants, 230
  anionic surfactants, 230
  bile salts, 230
  cyclodextrines, 243
  deoxycholate, 242
  glycocholate, 242
  laureth-9, 238, 242
  non-ionic ester, 230
  non-ionic ether, 230
  sodium tauro-24,25-dihydrofusidate (STDHF), 231, 233, 238, 240, 242
  STDHF, 231, 233, 238, 240, 242
  taurocholate, 242
nasal penetration enhancers, sodium taurohydrofusidate (STDHF), 240
nasal peptide products, 229, 239
  buserelin, 229, 239
  calcitonin, 229, 239
  desmopressin, 229, 239
  elcatonin, 229
  GHRH, 239
  glucagon, 239
  LHRH, 239
  lypressin, 229
  nafarelin, 229, 239
  oxytocin, 229, 239
  salmon calcitonin, 229
  vasopressin, 239
nasal permeation enhancement, mechanisms of, 234
neutron scattering, 171

Index 253

niosomes, 71, 73
  oral delivery by, 78
nitric oxide, 7
NMP, *N*-methyl pyrrolidone, 180
NMR, nuclear magnetic resonance, 173
non-ciliated cells, nasal epithelium, 224
non-ionic ether, 230
non-ionic ester, 230
nuclear magnetic resonance (NMR), 171, 173

oesophageal epithelium, 50
oestradiol, 22, 243
oleic acid, 170
olfactory, nasal, 223
opsonin lipid, 36
oral delivery
  by liposomes, 74
  by nanocapsules, 82
  by nanospheres, 79
  by niosomes, 78
oral epithelium, 50
  keratinized, 50
oral uptake across the gastrointestinal mucosa, microparticles, 113
oral peptide delivery
  bioadhesion, 95
  vaccination, 53
oral mucosa, 45
  lipid content of, 50
  water permeability of, 50
oral route, 71, 123
  for immunization, 123
ovalbumin, 51
oxidase, glucose, 72
oxide, nitric, 7
oxytocin, 229, 239

palate, hard, 47
paracellular pathway, 50, 51
paramaters, iontophoresis, 194
parenchymal cells, 13
parenchymal liver cells, 23
particle uptake, 52, 114
particulates, 80
patches, Peyer's, 53, 78, 81, 82, 84, 114, 120, 122
pathway, paracellular, 51
PCP, polycarbophil, 97
PEG-PE, 29
pellets, 101
  built-up granulation, 101
  excipients, 104
  extrusion, 103
  granulation liquid, 105
  in vivo studies, 110
  mixing process, 105
  plasticity of mass before extrusion, 107

spheronization, 103, 108
penetration enhancers, 92, 203
  nasal, 230, 231, 242, 243
  physicochemical techniques, 171
  skin, 169
penetration enhancing effects, poly(acrylic acid), 98
penetration of proteins, 52
penetration rates, reconstructed epidermis, 183
peptide absorption, intestinal, 93
peptides, 71, 179
pericytes, 9
permeability, 6
  barrier, stratum corneum, 180
  capillary, 6, 8
  coefficients, 198
  constants, 45, 46
  endothelial, 6, 9
  microvascular, 1
  mucosa, 68
  of oral mucosa, water, 50
  of skin, water, 50
permeation enhancement
  mechanisms of nasal, 234
  nasal epithelium, 229
peroxidase (HRPO), horseradish, 52, 62, 68
persorption, 53, 81, 113
Peyer's patches, 53, 78, 81, 82, 84, 114, 120, 122
phagocytosis, 81
pharmaceutical–technological aspects, bioadhesion, 93
PHEMA poly(2-hydroxyethyl methacrylate), 94
phonophoresis, 195
  anti-inflammatory drugs, 196
  device, 195
phosphatidylcholine (PC), 28
phosphatidylinositol (PL), hydrogenated, 27
phosphatidylserine (PS), 36
phospholipids, 22, 27
  bilayers, 26
  composition, lung surfactant, 156
  mixtures, liposomes, 204
physical barrier, nasal mucus, 227
physicochemical techniques, penetration enhancers, 171
physicochemistry of lung surfactant, 157
pinocytosis, 51, 52
plasma membrane, 217
  nasal, 227
plasticity of mass before extrusion, pellets, 107
platelet adhesion, 7
polyacrylate nanospheres, 122
poly(acrylic acid), penetration enhancing effects, 98
poly(alkylcyanoacrylate), 73, 79, 82, 83
polycarbophil (PCP), 97
polyethyleneglycol, amphipathic, 27
poly(2-hydroxyethyl methacrylate) (PHEMA), 94

poly(isobutylcyanoacrylate), 82
poly(*d,l*-lactide), 73, 82, 83
poly(lactide-coglycolide), 73
polymers, bioadhesion of, 60
polystyrene
  latex, 120
  latex particles, 114
  microspheres, 80
  nanospheres, 80
porcine buccal mucosa, 68
postcapillary venules, 1, 2, 3, 7, 8, 10
primaquine, 24
processing
  hepatic, 21
  intracellular, 19
prodrugs, 22
profile, fatty acid, 183
progesterone, 243
prolonged circulation, 34
propranolol, 238
prostacyclin, 7
proteins, 6
  gold-labelled, 6
  penetration of, 52
pulmonary surfactant
  airways stabilization, 132
  average surface tension, 131
  basic physiology, 129
  biochemical composition, 130
  disturbed surfactant system, 133
  endothelial model, 33
  function of the surfactant system, 130
  local defense mechanisms, 131
  replacement therapy, 129
  surfactant as anti-oedema factor, 130

RDS, respiratory distress syndrome, 129
receptor/carrier-mediated, vesicular exchange, 10
receptors
  galactose, 19
  LDL, 23
  remnant, 24
  scavenger, 22
reconstructed epidermis
  on DED, 181
  penetration rates, 183
reconstructed skin, 178
  drug testing, 184
release mechanism, triggered, 39
remnant receptor, 24
remnants
  chylomicron, 24
  VLDL, 15
replacement therapy, pulmonary surfactant, 129
RES, reticuloendothelial system, 26, 29, 32, 34
reserpine, 22

resistance
  diffusion, 65
  electrical, 66
  mucosa diffusion, 65
  mucosa electrical, 66, 68
respiratory distress syndrome (RDS), 129
respiratory, nasal, 223
reticuloendothelial system (RES), 26, 27
rigidity
  bilayer, 27, 30
  membrane, 31

SAXS, small angle X-ray scattering, 204, 206, 207, 212
scavenger receptor, 22
sinusoidal endothelial cells, 3
size, liposome, 27, 31
skin, 47
  lipid composition, 170
  lipid content, 50
  reconstructed, 178
  water permeability, 50
skin cell cultures, 178
  barrier function, 182
  differentiation, 180
skin membrane, diffusional behaviour, 190
skin penetration
  enhancers, 169
  mechanisms, 169
small angle X-ray scattering (SAXS), 204, 206, 207, 212
sodium tauro-24,25-dihydrofusidate (STDHF), 231, 233, 238, 240, 242
specific adhesion, 98
specific targeting, 13
specific uptake of liposomes, 13
spheronization, pellets, 103, 108
sphingomyelin, 30
spreading coefficient, combined, 59
squamous epithelium
  nasal, 47, 50
  stratified, 223
SRT, surfactant replacement therapy, 134
  artificial surfactant, 134
  modified natural surfactant, 134
  natural surfactant, 134
  synthetic natural surfactant, 149
stabilization, mechanical, 130
STDHF, sodium tauro-24,25-hydrofusidate, 231, 233, 238, 240, 242
steric barrier hypothesis, 29
stratified squamous epithelium, 50
stratum corneum, 169, 170, 204, 208, 213
  bilayers, 181, 208
  human, 203
  isoelectric point, 191

Index

permeability barrier, 180
structure changes, 204
streptavidin, 29
structure, nasal membrane, 223
structure changes, stratum corneum, 204
superficial cell layers, 50
supersaturated systems, 200
surface
 charge, 27
 energy, 58
surfactant replacement therapy (SRT), 134
surfactants
 amphoteric, 230
 anionic, 230
systemic administration, nasal drug permeability, 228
systems
 antibody–antigen, 33
 colloidal drug delivery, 71
 drug delivery, 92
 reticuloendothelial, 27
 supersaturated, 200
 targeting, 26

target binding, 34
target cell, 38
target-sensitive immunoliposomes, 39
targeting
 immunoliposome, 38
 liposome, 26, 33
 specific, 13
 system, 26
taurocholate, 242
TDDS transdermal drug delivery systems, 190
 temperature-activated systems, 197
temperature-sensitive immunoliposomes, 39
theory, adsorption–interpenetration, 57
thermodynamic activity, 200
thrombocytopenia, 9
tight junctions, 50, 51
times of epithelium, turnover, 49
tissue, gut-associated lymphoid, 84
titanium dioxide, 122
tomato lectin, 98
tongue, 47
tract, barrier functions of the gastrointestinal, 46
transcutol, 170, 175
transcytosis, 5, 6, 38

receptor-mediated, 5
transdermal drug delivery systems (TDDS), 190
transit times, 110
 large intestine, 111
 multiple unit dose systems, 111
 small intestine, 111
 stomach, 111
translocation
 nanospheres, possible mechanisms of, 80
 nanospheres, rate of, 81
 of particles, nanospheres, 80
 of particles, quantification, 81
transmucosal transport barriers, buccal, 57, 62
transport barriers, buccal transmucosal, 57, 62
transport vehicles, 13
triggered release mechanism, 39
triphasic emulsions, 71
tris-gal-chol, 18, 19, 21, 23
tumour cells, 23
tumour vasculature, 38
turnover times of epithelium, 49

ultrasonic power, 196
ultrasound, 195
uncharged molecules, iontophoresis, 192
uptake, particle, 52
urokinase, 7

vaccination, 53
vaccine delivery, 123
vascular leakage, 7, 8
vasculature, tumour, 38
vasopressin, 239
vehicles, transport, 13
venules, postcapillary, 1, 2, 3, 7, 8, 10
very low density lipoproteins (VLDL), 14
vesicular exchange, receptor/carrier-mediated, 10
vincamine, 73
viruses, 53
vitamin K, 73
VLDL, 14
VLDL remants, 15

water permeability
 of oral mucosa, 50
 of skin, 50

X-ray diffraction, 171